PAIN
IN CHILDREN
AND ADULTS WITH
DEVELOPMENTAL
DISABILITIES

PAIN
IN CHILDREN
AND ADULTS WITH
DEVELOPMENTAL
DISABILITIES

---

edited by

TIM F. OBERLANDER, M.D., FRCPC

Department of Pediatrics
Centre for Community Child Health Research
University of British Columbia, Vancouver

and

FRANK J. SYMONS, PH.D.

Department of Educational Psychology
College of Education and Human Development
University of Minnesota
Minneapolis

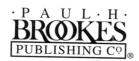

·P·A·U·L·H·
BROOKES
PUBLISHING CO.®

Baltimore • London • Sydney

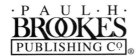

Paul H. Brookes Publishing Co.
Post Office Box 10624
Baltimore, Maryland 21285-0624

www.brookespublishing.com

Typeset by Integrated Publishing Solutions, Grand Rapids, Michigan.
Manufactured in the United States of America by Sheridan Books, Inc.,
Chelsea, Michigan.

The information provided in this book is in no way meant to substitute
for a medical practitioner's advice or expert opinion. Readers should
consult a health professional if they are interested in more information.
This book is sold without warranties of any kind, express or implied,
and the publisher and authors disclaim any liability, loss, or damage
caused by the contents of this book.

The case studies in this book are fictionalized accounts based on the
authors' clinical and research experience that do not represent the
lives of specific individuals, and no implications should be inferred.

Library of Congress Cataloging-in-Publication Data

Pain in children and adults with developmental disabilities / edited by
  Tim F. Oberlander and Frank J. Symons.
     p.;   cm.
  Includes bibliographical references and index.
  ISBN-13: 978-1-55766-869-1 (pbk.)
  ISBN-10: 1-55766-869-8 (pbk.)
  1. Developmentally disabled children.   2. Pain—Treatment.   3. Develop-
mental disabilities—Complications.   I. Oberlander, Tim F.   II. Symons, Frank
James, 1967–   .
  [DNLM: 1. Pain—diagnosis.   2. Developmental Disabilities—complications.
3. Pain—therapy.   4. Pain Measurement—methods.
WL 704 P14565 2006]
RJ135.P35 2006
618.92'0472—dc22   2006010531

British Library Cataloguing in Publication data are available
from the British Library.

CONTENTS

I
FOUNDATIONAL ISSUES

II
EPIDEMIOLOGICAL,
DEVELOPMENTAL, AND FUNCTIONAL ISSUES

III
ASSESSMENT AND TREATMENT ISSUES

IV
EPILOGUE

ABOUT THE EDITORS

Tim F. Oberlander, M.D., FRCPC, is a developmental pediatrician at British Columbia Children's Hospital (BCCH) in Vancouver. He is Associate Professor in the Department of Pediatrics, University of British Columbia (UBC), and the inaugural recipient of the R. Howard Webster Professorship in Child Development. He is supported by a Senior Scholar Award from the Human Early Learning Partnership (HELP) at UBC and is a faculty member of the Centre for Community Child Health Research.

Dr. Oberlander completed medical school training at Queen's University in Kingston and a residency in pediatrics at Montreal Children's Hospital/McGill University. Fellowship training included developmental pediatrics in Montreal and pediatric pain management in Boston at Children's Hospital. He joined the UBC Department of Pediatrics in 1993 and is a clinician with the Child Development and Rehabilitation Program as well as an attending physician with the Complex Pain Service at BCCH. As a clinician he works with children with complex pain and developmental disabilities as well as infants and children with prenatal alcohol and drug exposure.

Dr. Oberlander's research focuses on two areas: The first is directed at understanding the influence of early biological and environmental factors on childhood development. This work seeks to understand how prenatal exposure to psychotropic medications and drugs (e.g., antidepressants, alcohol) and depressed maternal mood alter the developing brain and contribute to development and behavior during infancy and childhood. A second area of research focuses on understanding pain in children with developmental disabilities. With colleagues he is studying pain reactivity in infants and children following neonatal intensive care and pain in children with cognitive and social impairments.

Dr. Oberlander's work has been supported by funding from the Canadian Institutes of Health Research, Michael Smith Foundation for Medical Research, HELP, and the March of Dimes Foundation.

Frank J. Symons, Ph.D., is Associate Professor in the Department of Educational Psychology and Coordinator of Special Education Programs at the University of Minnesota. Prior to this, Dr. Symons was Research Scientist at the FPG Child Development Institute and held faculty appointments in both the school of education and the department of psychiatry at the University of North Carolina at Chapel

Hill. Dr. Symons was formerly Research Associate at the John F. Kennedy Center for Research on Human Development at Peabody College, Vanderbilt University, as well as a postdoctoral fellow in the Institute for Developmental Neuroscience at Vanderbilt University. Dr. Symons has taught undergraduate preservice general and special education courses as well as graduate courses in the areas of applied behavior analysis, emotional and behavioral disorders, and intervention issues in developmental disabilities. Dr. Symons' research focuses on understanding the severe behavior problems of children and adults with special needs, primarily those with developmental disabilities and emotional or behavioral disorders. Dr. Symons' professional activities and publications are in the areas of behavioral assessment and severe behavior problems of individuals with disabilities. Dissemination activities include classroom-based and schoolwide in-service delivery; case consultation; and local, state, national, and international conference presentations. Dr. Symons has been supported primarily by grants funded by the National Institute of Child Health and Human Development of the National Institutes of Health investigating the early development and assessment and treatment of self-injurious behavior.

CONTRIBUTORS

James W. Bodfish, Ph.D.
Professor
Department of Psychiatry
University of North Carolina at Chapel Hill
Human Development Research and
    Training Institute at the J. Iverson Riddle
    Developmental Center
300 Enola Road
Morganton, North Carolina 28655

Shauna Bottos, B.A.
470 Laurier Avenue West
Suite 1707
Ottawa, Ontario K1R 7W9

Lynn M. Breau, Ph.D.
Registered Psychologist, Complex Pain
    Team
CIHR Strategic Training Program
    Postdoctoral
Pediatric Pain Research
IWK Health Centre
5850 University Avenue
Halifax, Nova Scotia B3K 6R8

**Christine T. Chambers, Ph.D.,
R. Psych.**
Assistant Professor of Pediatrics and
    Psychology
Dalhousie University and IWK Health
    Centre
5850/5980 University Avenue
Post Office Box 9700
Halifax, Nova Scotia B3K 6R8

Kenneth D. Craig, Ph.D.
Professor of Psychology
University of British Columbia
2136 West Mall
Vancouver, British Columbia V6T 1Z4

Jennifer M. Deacon, M.A.
Licensed Psychological Associate
University of North Carolina at Chapel Hill
Human Development Research and
    Training Institute at the J. Iverson Riddle
    Developmental Center
300 Enola Road
Morganton, North Carolina 28655

Joseph R. Deacon, Ph.D.
Associate Director
University of North Carolina at Chapel Hill
Human Development Research and
    Training Institute at the J. Iverson Riddle
    Developmental Center
300 Enola Road
Morganton, North Carolina 28655

Joyce M. Engel, Ph.D., OT
Professor
Department of Rehabilitation Medicine
University of Washington School of
    Medicine Box 356490
Seattle, Washington 98195

Gary Goldetsky, Psy.D., LP
Senior Psychologist
University of Minnesota School
    of Dentistry
Department of Diagnostic and Biological
    Sciences
Division of TMD and Orofacial Pain
Minnesota Head and Neck Pain Clinic
6-320 Moos Health Science Tower
515 Delaware Street S.E.
Minneapolis, Minnesota 55455

Ruth Eckstein Grunau, Ph.D.
Associate Professor of Pediatrics
University of British Columbia
Center for Community Child Health
    Research
SHY, F605B
4480 Oak Street
Vancouver, British Columbia V6H 3V4

Vicki N. Harper, M.A.
Licensed Psychological Associate
University of North Carolina at Chapel Hill
Human Development Research and
    Training Institute at the J. Iverson Riddle
    Developmental Center
300 Enola Road
Morganton, North Carolina 28655

Deborah Kartin, Ph.D., PT
Associate Professor
Department of Rehabilitation Medicine
University of Washington
1959 NE Pacific Street
Box 356490
Seattle, WA 98195

Lois J. Kehl, D.D.S., Ph.D.
Assistant Professor
Department of Anesthesiology
University of Minnesota Twin Cities
B 524 Mayo Building
420 Delaware Street SE
Minneapolis, Minnesota 55455

Craig H. Kennedy, Ph.D.
Professor, Special Education and
    Pediatrics
Director, Vanderbilt Kennedy Center
    Behavior Analysis Clinic
Vanderbilt University
Peabody #328
Nashville, Tennessee 37203

**Patrick J. McGrath, OC, Ph.D.,
    FRSC, FCAHS**
Professor of Psychology
Pediatrics and Psychiatry/CIHR
Distinguished Scientist/Canada Research
    Chair/ Psychologist
Dalhousie University & IWK Health
    Centre
5850/5980 University Avenue
Room K8533
Halifax, Nova Scotia B3K 6R8

Maureen E. O'Donnell, M.Sc., M.D.
Assistant Professor Developmental
    Pediatrics
University of British Columbia
Sunny Hill Health Centre
F110B
3644 Slocan Street
Vancouver, British Columbia V5M 3E8

Mark F. O'Reilly, Ph.D.
Associate Professor
Department of Special Education
University of Texas at Austin
George I. Sanchez Building 306
Austin, Texas 78712

Neil L. Schechter, M.D.
Director, Pain Relief Program
Connecticut Children's Medical Center
Hartford, CT
Professor of Pediatrics
University of Connecticut School of
    Medicine
Farmington, CT
282 Washington Street
Hartford, Connecticut 06108

Dick Sobsey, Ed.D.
Professor and Coordinator
Special Education
JP Das Developmental Disabilities Centre
Department of Educational Psychology
University of Alberta
6-102 Education North Edmonton, Alberta
    T6G 2G5

**Bonnie Stevens, Ph.D., M.Sc.N.,
    B.Sc.N.**
Signy Hildur Eaton Chair in Paediatric
    Nursing Research
Hospital for Sick Children
University of Toronto, Faculty of Nursing
50 St. George Street
Room 220
Toronto, Ontario M5S 3H4

**Anna Taddio, Ph.D., B.Sc.Phm.,
    M.Sc.**
Scientist
Department of Pharmacy and Population
    Health Sciences
The Hospital for Sick Children
555 University Avenue
Toronto, Ontario M5G 1X8

Marc Zabalia, Ph.D., MRSH
Maître de Conférences en psychologie
Université de Caen Basse-Normandie
Esplanade de la Paix
Caen, France 14400

FOREWORD

Well, it is about time there was a volume like this! Editors Tim F. Oberlander and Frank J. Symons have assembled a superb collection of dedicated researchers and clinicians with expertise in various aspects of pain and pain management to address—more accurately, begin to address—the critical issues of pain experiences in individuals with developmental disabilities. And, as the volume attests, there really are multiple issues. Despite the fact that pain is a universal behavioral experience, it remains a challenge to define, measure, understand its functional consequences, treat, and investigate. All of these challenges are inherent even at the best of times and the least complicated circumstances. As the editors point out in the preface—and it is echoed many times throughout the volume—addressing these challenges with individuals with developmental disabilities is even more challenging, especially if their experiences are different because of the underlying condition and/or their expression of the pain. Communicating differently does not mean that one is unable to communicate. In these cases, it is contingent on professionals to understand and interpret the communication.

And why shouldn't we be able to make some progress in doing so? Many, if not all, of us can remember the excitement that accompanied the early reconceptualization of pain experience and mechanisms that Melzack and Wall (1970) proposed. We can still remember how that opened our eyes and our minds to understanding and investigating pain in fundamentally different ways. The pain experience, and our investigations of it, became much more nuanced and multidimensional. Even more of us can probably remember the dramatic effect of early studies on premature infants undergoing patent ductus arteriosus closure operations by Anand and colleagues, which changed almost everyone's beliefs about whether human infants, especially preterm infants, experienced pain (Anand et al., 1985; Anand, Carr, & Hickey, 1987; Anand, Sippell, & Aynsley-Green, 1987). The increased understanding of infant and preterm pain since these studies—thanks in part to the contributions of many who contribute to this volume—has been truly remarkable. It is time for that same kind of attention, energy, thought, and conviction to be applied to the challenges of addressing pain in individuals with developmental disabilities.

But, despite all of these impressive advances, our understanding of the pain experience still has a sense of being somehow an approximation. Why is that? Infants with colic illustrate three key challenges that are faced when we try to understand pain in individuals with developmental delays and serious neurological impairment: "How do we know whether, and if so when, an infant with colic is in pain?" The answers are telling and arguably relate to these challenges. First, because infants with colic are preverbal, our ability to understand whether they are in pain can only be inferential, limited to indirect behavioral and physiological measures. In some cases, infants and children with disabilities are preverbal or verbal in different or atypical ways. Similar inferential arguments will be required. Second, such inferences might be possible if there were specific ("pathognomic") relationships between behavioral and physiological responses and known stimuli. Although there is plenty of evidence that there are characteristic responses to known pain stimuli, these responses are also seen in nonpain stress situations and therefore are not specific to pain experience (Barr, 1998; White, Gunnar, Larson, Donzella, & Barr, 2000). Third, most of our understanding of pain behavior in infants derives from responses to procedures in which the pain is acute and the timing and nature of the noxious stimuli are known. By contrast, the crying bouts and associated behavior typical of colic occurs recurrently and paroxysmally (unexpectedly and seemingly unrelated to anything in the environment), and the nature of the stimulus (or stimuli) is unknown. Consequently, even evidence for a specific behavioral and physiological response to acute pain stimuli (a pain signature) would not necessarily generalize to the phenomenology of colic. This, too, is likely to be analogous in individuals with disabilities; although some of the pain they experience will be directly related to known stimuli, much of it will be chronic and recurring.

As an illustration of the challenge, it has long been believed that there was a specific pain cry in infants, based on the early recognition studies in normal newborns. However, with more methodologically sound studies, the weight of evidence now seems to support the concept that infant crying is a graded stimulus rather than a typological distress behavior (i.e., a specific cry type for a specific cause) (Gustafson, Wood, & Green, 2000). The characteristic features of pain cries following a pain stimulus, such as higher fundamental frequencies, hyperphonemic breaks, bifurcations on acoustic analysis, and increased pitch and dysphonation when listening, are more likely a function of the increased energy being delivered to the "speaker system" because of the intensity of the pain stimulus, rather than a specific manifestation of the pain experience itself. Furthermore, even though these features may be seen in the first or second expiratory cry, the ongoing crying soon resolves to a more basic cry pattern (Green, Gustafson, & McGhie, 1998; Wolff, 1969). Unless individuals with developmental disabilities show us differently (and they may), the lack of a specific behavioral signature is likely to be a challenge in deciphering their pain as well.

A second illustration of the challenge that infants with colic help to demonstrate is the more widely recognized principle that behavioral measures (overt) manifestations of pain and stress are only weakly, sometimes not at all, associated with physiological (covert) manifestations of pain and stress. When infants with and without colic were subjected to a nonpainful physical examination, all infants showed responses in both behavioral (crying) measures and physiological (heart rate, vagal tone, and salivary cortisol) measures, but only the behavioral measures were different between the groups (White et al., 2000). Similarly, newborn infants undergoing heel stick procedures were differentially responsive to sucrose, holding, or sucrose and holding interventions depending on whether behavioral (facial activity) and physiological (heart rate and vagal tone) responses were considered (Gormally et al., 2001). This principle is used, appropriately enough, to argue for multimodal measures of pain. However, that does not relieve us of the obligation to understand what is evidence of pain in any one patient at any one time. If we use only crying as an indicator of pain, then we may change the behavior but not the physiology; if we use only changes in physiological measures, then we may underestimate the pain experience and undertreat it (Barr, 1998). Even worse, a strong, lusty cry is actually a sign of vigor (an honest signal of health and robustness) rather than of illness and pain (Barr, 1998). If more crying is associated with more treatment, then we may actually provide more treatment to those who need it less and less to those who need it more. This biobehavioral discordance is equally true in individuals with severe neurological impairment and can have potentially serious adverse consequences both for clinical and research approaches to them and their pain experiences.

So it is little wonder that we still cannot quite understand the pain experience of infants with colic or of infants in general, despite all the progress that has been made. The challenge in trying to understand the pain experience for preverbal newborns and infants with colic is likely to be similar to that for children and adults with developmental disabilities. On the one hand, the fact that their underlying conditions may result in behavioral and physiological manifestations of pain that are largely or even completely different than those of infants and individuals without disabilities may result in additional challenges. On the other hand, the initiatives taken by the editors and the authors in this volume to describe, document, measure, assess and intervene, and grapple with the underlying biology and physiology in these individuals may reveal some principles about pain experience that we have not been able to discover in otherwise typical infants. As with many systems, whether mechanical or biological, it is often difficult to really understand how they work until one encounters an example that does not work or works differently from the rest.

The increasing focus on and intensive study of the pain experience in individuals with developmental disabilities may be just what is needed to help address the puzzle of pain (Melzack, 1973) in traditional ways and in new ways. These editors and their authors deserve great credit for putting this important volume together. It is likely, indeed virtually certain, that there are still considerable challenges ahead. But this is a great start, and it is about time.

Ronald G. Barr, MDCM, FRCPC
Canada Research Chair in Community Child Health Research
Professor of Pediatrics, University of British Columbia Faculty of Medicine
Director, Centre for Community Child Health Research
Child & Family Research Centre, British Columbia Children's Hospital

REFERENCES

Anand, K.J.S., Brown, R.C., Causon, R., Christofides, S.R., Bloom, S.R., & Aynsley-Green, A. (1985). Can the human neonate mount an endocrine and metabolic response to surgery? *Journal of Pediatric Surgery, 20,* 41–48.

Anand, K.J.S., Carr, D.B., & Hickey, P.R. (1987). Randomized trial of high-dose anesthesia in neonates undergoing cardiac surgery: hormonal and hemodynamic stress responses. *Anesthesiology, 67,* A501.

Anand, K.J.S., Sippell, W.G., & Aynsley-Green, A. (1987). A randomized trial of fentanyl anesthesia undergoing surgery: Effect on the stress response. *Lancet, 1,* 243–248.

Barr, R.G. (1998). Reflections on measuring pain in infants: dissociation in responsive systems and "honest signalling." *Archives of Disease in Childhood Fetal Neonatal Edition, 79,* F152–F156.

Gormally, S.M., Barr, R.G., Wertheim, L., Alkawaf, R., Calinoiu, N., & Young, S.N. (2001). Contact and nutrient caregiving effects on newborn infant pain responses. *Developmental Medicine and Child Neurology, 43,* 28–38.

Green, J.A., Gustafson, G.E., & McGhie, A.C. (1998). Changes in infants' cries as a function of time in a cry bout. *Child Development, 69,* 271–279.

Gustafson, G.E., Wood, R.M., & Green, J.A. (2000). Can we hear the causes of infants' crying? In R.G. Barr, B. Hopkins, & J.A. Green (Eds.), *Crying as a sign, a symptom, and a signal: clinical, emotional and developmental aspects of infant and toddler crying* (pp. 8–22). London: MacKeith Press.

Melzack, R. (1973). *The puzzle of pain.* New York: Basic Books.

Melzack, R., & Wall, P.D. (1970). Psychophysiology of pain. *Internal Anesthesiology Clinics, 8,* 3–34.

White, B.P., Gunnar, M.R., Larson, M.C., Donzella, B., & Barr, R.G. (2000). Behavioral and physiological responsivity, sleep and patterns of daily cortisol production in infants with and without colic. *Child Development, 71,* 862–877.

Wolff, P.H. (1969). The natural history of crying and other vocalizations in early infancy. In B.M. Foss (Ed.), *Determinants of infant behavior* (pp. 81–108). London: Methuen.

PREFACE

This volume is the outcome of a commitment to improve our understanding of the field of pain in developmental disabilities and is a direct outcome of a January 2000 workshop funded by the Mayday Fund (New York) and organized by Tim F. Oberlander and Kenneth D. Craig. This gathering brought together a stimulating, expert, and varied group of basic and clinical scientists to examine what was known about pain in individuals who, as a consequence of cognitive, motor, or language impairments, have altered or reduced capacities to communicate distress. As demonstrated by disagreement concerning the definition of pain among individuals with developmental disabilities, it became clear that there were substantial gaps in basic and clinical knowledge of pain. It was agreed that a definition of pain was needed that would reflect both the common features of pain among all people and unique features of pain among those with disabilities.

Individuals with developmental disabilities are likely to experience increased daily pain relative to people without disabilities; for many, it is poorly recognized and incompletely managed, leading to increased distress and suffering. Failure to directly address unique features in both the expression and experience of pain in individuals with developmental disabilities contributes to this. With the recognition that the health and well-being of individuals with developmental disabilities was most likely compromised by inadequate understanding of the basic and clinical nature of pain, we realized that we lacked the knowledge from systematic and sustained attention to this group that had led to substantially improved outcomes in other vulnerable populations (e.g., preterm infants, the elderly). It was clear that systematic attention was urgently needed to improve our understanding of pain and health among individuals with developmental disabilities.

At the outset, three questions were asked: "How can our understanding of the basic neurobiology of pain help our clinical practice in this population?," "What do we know about assessment?," and "What are the unique requirements for optimal management of pain?" Workshop participants, who represented a range of scientific disciplines, were able to comment on both human and animal issues and to provide commentary encompassing basic molecular through social issues in both laboratory and clinical practice and community care settings. The importance of interdisciplinary collaboration in the study of pain became particularly evident during the workshop. In particular, we recognized that a narrow biomedical perspective was inadequate because it does not encompass the broad range of psychological, social, community, and cultural issues involved in the understanding of disability and pain.

We were all acutely aware of the difficulties we faced in starting a conversation about pain in a setting in which signals of distress are frequently ambiguous and nonspecific, particularly with a diverse group of professionals who were unlikely to have met before or talked with each other. To begin a systematic process of understanding pain in this setting, we deliberately included in this group individuals with expertise in studying pain in verbal and nonverbal infants, children, adults, and the elderly, as well as in nonhuman populations.

We soon recognized that the likelihood for substantial and undertreated pain and suffering among individuals with a range of developmental disabilities was considerable. It was clear that individuals with limited motor, communication, and/ or cognitive abilities were vulnerable not only to all of the sources of pain afflicting people without impairments but also to pain and discomfort arising from the medical conditions leading to brain impairment and the resulting increased requirements for medical intervention. Thus, pain among individuals with developmental disabilities was likely to be even more prevalent than in populations without impairments. Given that the capacity for expression is often limited, confusing, contradictory, and confounded by concurrent disease or illness associated with developmental disability, caregivers can find providing care a frustrating task, and it is not unusual for unfortunate attitudes to emerge.

The critical issues presented within the workshop context led to many of the contributions presented in this volume. We have limited knowledge about pain among individuals with developmental disabilities despite recognition of the broad scope of the problem. There is also limited knowledge of the extent of the problem, given evidence that pain is often unrecognized, not assessed using systematic measures, and underestimated. In addition, there is a fundamental limited understanding of the nature of pain in individuals with communication, motor, and cognitive limitations or impairments. Perhaps not surprising, the differing definitions and terms associated with various disabilities create unique difficulties related to characterizing and classifying pain-related problems. It was recognized that the definition of pain itself had historically failed to include the possibility that pain could be effectively expressed by an individual with an impairment. When the expression of pain is ambiguous, decision making becomes highly subjective, and both the assessment and management of pain present tremendous challenges.

Several trends make this book timely. Since the mid-1990s, there has been tremendous growth in research activity in the field, spanning from interests in the unique challenges of preterm infants to children with cognitive and communication impairments to adults with cerebral palsy to frail older adults with dementias. Since the 2000 workshop, the definition of pain was revised to recognize that "the inability to communicate verbally does not negate the possibility that an individual is experiencing pain and is in need of appropriate pain-relieving treatment" (http://www.iasp-pain.org/terms-p.html). This evidence-based and eminently sensible revision dramatically highlights the plight of those with communication limitations and effectively recognizes the useful transfer of research advances to applications satisfying the needs of often neglected people. A number of scales and checklists specific to assessing pain among individuals with developmental disabilities have been published. They usually provide descriptions of the expression of pain in certain disabilities and often satisfy psychometric standards, including face validity, reliability, some empirical validity, and perhaps clinical utility. It is to be hoped that there will not be a proliferation of poorly developed scales and that existing scales will continue to be studied and improved.

Studies of novel treatment strategies uniquely adapted to the needs of individuals with developmental disabilities are still lacking. Although the number of publications in the field remains small, the recent growth parallels similar trends in pain-related pediatric research presented at national and international professional and research meetings (e.g., Pediatric Academic Societies, Canadian Pain Society, American Pain Society, IASP World Congresses on Pain). Finally, current standards of practice, care guidelines, and accreditation standards mandate continual monitoring of pain. The Joint Commission on Accreditation of Healthcare Organizations in the United States has issued standards requiring explicit pain assessment in hospitals, ambulatory care facilities, health care networks, home care, and related long-term care organizations. We look forward to learning that these standards are being applied to and adapted for people with disabilities.

Pain in the context of developmental disability and related neurological impairment has emerged in recent years as an area requiring increased scientific attention. There is evidence of unnecessary pain and suffering, and the pain experience among individuals with developmental disabilities often is complex and confusing, frequently raising questions about the nature of pain itself. The editors and contributors to this volume believe the work described in the following chapters represents a "topography" of the field and contributes another step toward sharpening the focus on what we are beginning to know about pain in people with developmental disabilities, and where we might proceed in the coming years in the expectation that improved understanding of pain will lead to better health outcomes and improved quality of life for individuals with developmental disabilities.

We are very grateful to the Mayday Foundation for their original funding, without which this volume would not have been possible. We are equally grateful for the support provided by the Peter Wall Institute for Advanced Studies (PWIAS) at the University of British Columbia, which made it possible for the initial and continuing collaborations leading to this volume.

ACKNOWLEDGMENTS

My contribution to this volume would not have been possible without the convergence of five key factors. The first is the inspiration from the children and their families with whom I work at Sunny Hill Health Centre of Children and British Columbia Children's Hospital. Second is the wonderfully creative greenhouse in which I work at the Centre for Community Child Health Research, Early Human Learning Partnership (University of British Columbia) and my department of pediatrics. Third are my mentors Ron Barr, Chuck Berde, and Neil Schechter, who guided me into child development and childhood pain and taught me how to combine these two worlds. Fourth is the patience and wisdom of Frank Symons for bearing with me on producing this volume. Finally, none of this work would have been possible without the love and support of my wife Julie and my children Ariel, Talia, and Malka, whose encouragement continuously sustains me and reminds me of the priorities of life.

Tim F. Oberlander

My role in this book would not exist if Patrick McGrath had decided not to answer a naive telephone call inquiring about the nature of his work; if Ken Craig and Tim Oberlander had not invited me to participate in the Millcroft Symposia convened in the woods north of Toronto; if the Peter Wall Institute for Advanced Studies at the University of British Columbia did not have a visiting junior scholar program; if Jim Bodfish was unwilling to translate ideas into real-world effort for the benefit of behavioral science research and individuals with developmental disabilities; if Heather Shrestha from Paul H. Brookes Publishing Co. had not been so responsive to my e-mail; if Tim had disagreed with me that he was the right person and this was the right time; and if Raymond Tervo at Gillette Children's Specialty Healthcare had not introduced me to Patrick Rivard. To you all I am grateful; you are the moving force behind much of this work and the limited role I have played in it. I am indebted to the contributors to this book who have, without exception, prepared exceptionally competent, outstanding chapters and accepted our editorial suggestions graciously. I am grateful for all of the parents and their children for whom the work in this volume represents. I am thankful for the support provided, in part, by the National Institute of Child Health and Human Development of the National Institutes of Health for my work and for the McKnight Land-Grant Professorship from the University of Minnesota. And, finally, I am thankful for the unwavering support of my spouse Stacy Coleman Symons, whose patient understanding, along with that of Stewart and Elisabeth, was immeasurably helpful over the course of this project. Special thanks to Alicia Vegell for persistence and dedication above and beyond the call of duty in the editing of this volume.

Frank J. Symons

1

AN INTRODUCTION TO THE PROBLEM OF PAIN IN DEVELOPMENTAL DISABILITY

Tim F. Oberlander and Frank J. Symons

Until recently, pain in people with developmental disabilities received very little scientific attention. Individuals with developmental disabilities have been systematically excluded as study participants from research studies on pain, and little was known about the pain in daily life, the expression of pain in the absence of words, or the challenges of pain management in the context of a substantial neurological injury. Expression of pain by individuals with developmental disabilities can be ambiguous, and its recognition by caregivers and health care providers can be highly subjective. Even when pain-specific behaviors are present, such behaviors may be regarded as altered or blunted, may be confused with other sources of generalized stress or arousal, or, in the extreme, may be misinterpreted as a behavior disorder of psychiatric origin. This presents a tremendous challenge to the individual, caregiver, clinician, and researcher alike.

Pain is a universal biological experience that is essential to promoting health (it alerts us to danger), but it is also associated with tremendous suffering that compromises the quality of life when underrecognized or poorly treated. There is no reason to believe that pain is any less frequent in the lives of those with developmental or acquired disabilities that alter the way they communicate or that such individuals would be insensitive or indifferent to pain. Regardless of the degree of the disability and the underlying neurological condition, functional limitations frequently confound the presentation of pain that is often a part of daily life for individuals with developmental disabilities. How can pain be assessed and managed when typical means of verbal or nonverbal communication or cognition are altered or absent? In the absence of easily recognized verbal or motor-dependent forms of communication, it remains uncertain if the pain experience itself is different or only the expressive manifestations are altered. Indeed, without easily recognizable means of communication or motor skills, pain may not be recognized or treated. In spite of the potential for altered nociception and pain expression, there is no evidence that individuals with cognitive or motor impairments are spared any of the miseries of a noxious experience. In this book, we review progress and a number of key challenges facing this field. These include aspects of the definition of pain as it relates to the unique challenges faced by individuals with developmental disabilities, the epidemiology and functional impact of pain in people with disabilities, issues in the management of pain, pain in individuals with self-injurious and severe behavior disorders, and the difficulties of assessing pain in children with severe intellectual and communicative disabilities. Many fundamental questions about how the pain system functions when its underlying neural substrate is altered remain unanswered, limiting our understanding of how to assess and manage pain in individuals with developmental disabilities.

There is a growing recognition that the study of pain in individuals with developmental disabilities is an opportunity to reexamine our understanding of what constitutes the universal but highly personal human experience of pain. This book was designed, in part, to capitalize on this opportunity by providing a forum for critical discussion of pain in the context of a developmental disability. We worked with a broad definition of developmental disability that included any disability that is manifested before the person reaches 22 years of age, that constitutes a substantial disability to the affected individual, and that is attributable to mental retardation or to related conditions, including cerebral palsy, epilepsy, autism, or other neurological conditions, when such conditions result in impairment of general intellectual functioning or adaptive behavior similar to that of a person with mental retardation. The book focuses on the phenomenon of pain, a phenomenon that is fundamental to the human experience. Although interest in pain has been long-standing and the advances brought by scientific inquiry in the past 100 years have been remarkable, comparatively little attention has been paid to the unique problems posed by developmental disabilities. Contemporary research programs in pain represent a stunning example of our progress in understanding the structure of the nervous system and its function in relation to a universal human condition. In turn, a forum to discuss unmet clinical and research needs on pain in developmental disability should provide a venue to organize a discussion of what we know and do not know about an underacknowledged topic in the pain field and to map future strategies for policy and practice that will lead to improved outcomes.

Why did we choose to compile an edited volume on pain in developmental disabilities? The primary reason is the urgent need for a cross-disciplinary approach to the problem. In the area of developmental disability, the construct of pain does not reside in one domain of knowledge or field alone. Furthermore, because no one individual or research group is considered to be authoritative with respect to the topic of pain in developmental disability, an edited volume provides a forum for multiple perspectives on the full range of issues inherent in the phenomenon of pain. The contributors review a range of conceptual issues and our empirical knowledge concerning those issues germane to pain in developmental disabilities. Although the importance of technical precision required for effective communication about theory and research cannot be overstated, it is our hope that the chapters are not overly technical or laden with jargon. Our purpose was not to communicate with our own professional peers per se but to cut across traditional professional or knowledge boundaries and write for a wide audience of professional educators and others in the biomedical and behavioral sciences. We are confident that the authors have accomplished this task.

There are three major sections to this book. The first section (Pain: Foundational Issues) provides an overview and background to the conceptual, definitional, and ethical issues inherent in any discussion of pain experienced by individuals with developmental disabilities. We believe that interested readers must begin from a common understanding of the historical and contemporary conceptual and definitional issues in pain research. Accordingly, Chapter 2 brings to focus the history and changing definition of pain in general and in relation to developmental disabilities. Chapter 3 provides an essential forum on ethical issues raised by historical problems created by the conventional definition of pain, including a discussion of research participation and health care implications. Chapter 4 is a primer laying out the detailed phenomenology of pain in relation to underlying brain mechanisms.

The second section (Pain: Epidemiological, Developmental, and Functional Issues) discusses what is known about the prevalence and nature of pain conditions in developmental disabilities and provides a review of developmental and functional issues posed by chronic pain and disability. Our poor understanding of the epidemiology of pain across the spectrum of disabilities continues to limit research and clinical care. What is known suggests that pain is common and poorly treated among adults and children with disabilities. There is good reason to believe that pain is much more a part of the daily lives of most of these individuals than is the case for people without disabilities. At present, there are no satisfactory epidemiological data regarding the incidence or prevalence of chronic or acute pain in children with disabilities. Although the etiologies of the underlying conditions vary, making this a heterogeneous population, the additive effects of pain in the presence of a disability are common to many of the conditions associated with a developmental disability. Therefore, even by crude, indirect methods, it might be reasonable to estimate that pain is more common in children with developmental disabilities than among children in general, highlighting this as an area for urgent discussion and future study. Similarly, efforts to understand pain require an evaluation of the functional impact of the pain, its role in quality of life, and its compounding interaction with the disability itself. Studies of pain typically focus on describing symptoms, duration, and intensity of pain without accounting for the functional consequences of the symptom, even though pain is likely to have a major impact on the individual. The measurement of functional disability related to adult pain outcomes has received considerable attention because of issues related to work and cost-related effects; however, analogous research in pediatric and adolescent populations with developmental disabilities is limited, further highlighting the urgent need for a critical evaluation of what we know and what we need to know.

The third section (Pain: Assessment and Treatment Issues) focuses on the myriad research and clinical complexities in reliably and validly assessing pain in developmental disabilities and in the delivery of efficacious and effective treatment. Typically the "afferent component" of pain is perceived or experienced before "efferent responses" such as self-report or behavior changes occur. Feeling and reporting pain are often parallel and related phenomena, but self-report, nonverbal expression, and evidence of tissue damage can be highly discordant, particularly among individuals with disabilities. Many developmental disabilities are associated with painful conditions that require recurrent noxious and invasive procedures, resulting in increased pain during daily life. This is compounded by difficulties in communicating distress and by motor impairments inhibiting actions needed to solicit help, which in turn may lead to increased incidence, severity, and duration of pain. Thus, current knowledge about measurement of pain in developmental disability, including a critical examination of state-of-the-art assessment technologies, is reviewed for pediatric and adult populations. Finally, there is evidence that individuals may be denied appropriate and timely pain management because caregivers may not accept that the pain is real when the ability to communicate the experience with discrete words and motor movements is limited. Consequently, detailed information has been included to provide a balanced review of available treatment and pain management options and their corresponding empirical support.

In sum, this book aims to raise topics and review current knowledge to stimulate further discussion about, recognition of, and research into the problem of pain in individuals with developmental disability. If this volume improves clinical practice, then we will have accomplished our goal. The chapters were written by recognized international authorities, many of whom have pioneered work in the assessment and management of pain in pediatric and other populations. We believe this edited volume addresses one of the most profound aspects of developmental human experience, and it is our hope that it will be a valuable addition to a growing literature.

I

FOUNDATIONAL
ISSUES

2

THE CONSTRUCT
AND DEFINITION OF PAIN
IN DEVELOPMENTAL DISABILITY

Kenneth D. Craig

Is it necessary to debate whether people with developmental disabilities experience pain? Those who have observed the behavioral reactions to injury, disease, or invasive clinical procedures of the diverse population described by this term usually have little doubt. The reactions typically are not appreciably different from those that signify pain among people in general. A growing list of sound studies also supports this. Nevertheless, specific disabilities often are associated with important variations in pain experience and expression that demand attention in the delivery of care. Congenital insensitivity to pain, a rarity, represents but one of the possible variations (e.g., Biersdorff, 1994); in these cases, an absence of pain is of major importance because the individual does not have the protection from physical danger provided by pain. In other cases, there is evidence of increased painful distress despite beliefs in diminished sensitivity—for example, in children with autism (Nader, Oberlander, Chambers, & Craig, 2004). Understanding these differences directs attention to the unique needs of people with disabilities and reduces risks associated with failure to recognize, inadequate assessment, underestimation, and mistreatment of or failure to treat pain (e.g., Malviya et al., 2001; Stallard, Williams, Lenton, & Velleman, 2001).

The argument that pain is a significant reality in the lives of people with developmental disabilities must be supported by careful conceptualization about the nature of pain and by substantial evidence. Well-meaning advocates could be wrong. Contrary claims for insensitivity or indifference to pain are often made (Biersdorff, 1991; Terstegen, Koot, De Boer, & Tibboel, 2003). Also, pain control may be demanding for people suffering from pain, it may pose risks for adverse outcomes, and it may be onerous for those delivering care. However, failure to provide adequate pain control is increasingly associated with serious short- and long-term deleterious health, psychological, and social consequences (Brennan & Cousins, 2004). This chapter examines how the concept of pain must be adapted to accommodate special characteristics of the populations to which the term *developmental disability* refers. In addition, the social communication model of pain is presented to encourage an appreciation of pain inclusive of the social contexts in which people with developmental disabilities live and should receive care.

ON THE NATURE OF DEVELOPMENTAL DISABILITIES

The impairments associated with developmental disabilities could affect the subjective experience of pain, the ability to communicate subjective distress to others, or both. The term *developmental disabilities* refers to mental or physical disabilities evident in childhood and continuing throughout life. The scope, therefore, is broad and inclusive of people with diverse attributes and capabilities.

To illustrate the importance of attending to specific features of developmental disabilities, people with cerebral palsy invariably experience muscular impairment characterized by uncoordinated movement and posturing, but the condition may not include intellectual disability (Hadden & von Baeyer, 2002, 2005; Oberlander, O'Donnell, & Montgomery, 1999; Schwartz, Engel, & Jensen, 1999). If cognitive impairment were associated with the condition, thoughts and feelings during the painful experience would likely be affected. If there were no intellectual disability, the primary neuromotor functional limitations associated with cerebral palsy could lead to difficulties in verbally or nonverbally articulating painful distress; hence, for pain management, it may be important to understand communication limitations rather than cognitive or affective differences.

In contrast, many people with intellectual disabilities, or cognitive impairments leading to difficulties in learning, do not experience physical limitations. Cognitive impairment could affect both the subjective experience and effective use of verbal or nonverbal communication of pain. People with moderate to profound intellectual disabilities often share with people who have communication limitations arising from other impairments the requirement that pain should be recognized by attending to information other than self-report. Nonverbal behavior captured through observation can provide vital information (Hadjistavropoulos & Craig, 2002). Automatic protective reflexes and affective reactions largely remain intact despite loss of higher-level executive functions such as memory, planning, problem solving, or skills in role-based behavior (Breau, MacLaren, McGrath, Camfield, & Finley, 2003). Thus, in understanding the unique pain of a particular individual with developmental disability, attention could be focused on either the potential for differences in the experience of pain or the ability to communicate painful distress.

THE CONCEPT OF PAIN

Characteristics of pain that are unique to special populations are best understood through contrast with accounts of pain in the population at large. Over time, there have been debates concerning how best to conceptualize pain. Some have suggested that pain should be conceptualized as a sensation, an emotion, or a multidimensional experience that includes thoughts and feelings as well as sensory features (Chapman, 2004; Craig, 2005; Melzack & Casey, 1968). Reconstructing these arguments is not necessary because the multidimensional perspective is in ascendancy, as reflected in the definition of pain developed and promulgated by the International Association for the Study of Pain (IASP). This definition has enjoyed widespread popularity and usage for several decades. IASP defines pain as "an unpleasant sensory and emotional experience associated with actual or potential tissue damage, or described in terms of such damage" (Merskey & Bogduk, 1994). The definition has important declarative features. It is clear that pain is always a subjective experience. As such, pain cannot be observed directly by others but must be inferred through use of overt cues, with the multidimensional nature of the experience adding to the complexities of this task. Use of the term *unpleasant* in the definition clearly signifies noxious emotional qualities but understates the potential for extremes of severe or excruciating pain.

There are some notable omissions in the definition:

1. Thoughts, or cognitive features of the experience, are ignored. Thus, capabilities for thinking, memory, integrating current and past experiences, or problem solving are not recognized as required to be able to experience pain. This seems reasonable for people with or without intellectual disabilities. Still, current conceptualizations of emotional processes emphasize the role of thoughts as elicitors of emotions, adverse or constructive (e.g., Sullivan et al., 2001), and cognition ordinarily plays an important role in the pain experience (Bruehl & Chung, 2004). Hence, cognitive impairments could contribute to suffering because coping skills or a sense of self-efficacy or the ability to predict an end to a painful event could be missing in people with disabilities.

2. The definition excludes the requirement that tissue damage must be present. It only requires that the experience should be "associated with actual or potential tissue damage." Physical damage is recognized as playing a modest role and is not a necessary causal condition for pain. This has important implications in providing care. One must be alert to the presence of pain in people with developmental disabilities even when there is no evidence of physical pathology.

3. Finally, the phrase "or described in terms of such damage" takes this conceptualization further and emphasizes the reality of pain in people who complain of pain but for whom the best diagnostic assessment cannot provide clear evidence of tissue damage. This proviso is important because the majority of people with chronic pain have "medically unexplained pain" (Kirmayer, Groleau, Looper, & Dao, 2004). In these individuals, no organic pathology is evident that could provide a causal basis for the pain. This includes many conditions such as forms of headache, abdominal pain, considerable musculoskeletal pain including neck and lower back pain, and fibromyalgia. Neither the best research nor the finest diagnostic skills have been able to identify a pathophysiological basis for pain in the majority of people suffering from these conditions. There is no reason to believe that people with developmental disabilities could not also suffer from these same painful conditions.

Complicating the challenge of understanding pain that does not have a clear basis in injury or disease is the increased likelihood that people with developmental disabilities may not have the verbal capability to describe their pain, as the phrase "or described in terms of such damage" implies would be necessary. The focus in the definition on self-report as a means of communicating subjective distress does not include a provision for people without verbal self-report capabilities, but who nevertheless are suffering as a result of pain (Anand & Craig, 1996). Of course, these cases represent the most difficult assessment and diagnostic situations for clinicians and other observers. One is challenged to recognize pain when the person cannot verbally complain of it. Painful distress then must be evident in nonverbal expression, with the onus upon the observer to recognize this (McGrath, Rosmus, Camfield, Campbell, & Hennigar, 1998). The problem is familiar to those interested in caring for or understanding pain in infants and young children (Craig, 1998). It seems likely that the increased risk of serious medical problems arising from conditions such as unrecognized bowel obstruction would be diminished if greater attention were devoted to nonverbal expression of pain.

Fortunately, IASP has recognized the importance of nonverbal communication in people with language communication limitations. A note was added to the published definition in 2002 indicating that "the inability to communicate verbally does not negate the possibility that an individual is experiencing pain and is in need of appropriate pain-relieving treatment" (http://www.iasp-pain.org/terms-p.html). Nevertheless, there remains unfortunate resistance to acknowledging pain in people who have difficulty verbally expressing their distress. A notable example would be the European Federation of IASP Chapters, which declares on its web site that "when the individual is unable to report on his/her conscious percept, . . . the word 'nociception' is used instead of the word 'pain' to express that the nervous system has detected the noxious stimulus without necessarily implying that a pain percept was evoked" (http://www.efic.org/about_pain.htm#efic_declaration). This is regrettable opposition to accepting the importance of other communication modalities in the ability of people with developmental disabilities, as well as infants and young children, people suffering from acquired brain damage, or seniors with dementia and other brain impairments, to convey pain.

ON THE NATURE OF PAIN IN PEOPLE WITH DEVELOPMENTAL DISABILITIES

With the foregoing perspective on the nature of pain as a foundation, it is worthwhile to consider further the construct of pain as it applies to people with developmental disabilities. Cognitive impairments could have an impact on qualities of the pain experience, although not necessarily by limiting the capacity to experience pain. The impact is most likely to be observed in the individual's ability to deploy skills needed to understand, predict, and control circumstances associated with the painful event and to self-manage emotional distress and painful discomfort (Engel, Schwartz, Jensen, & Johnson, 2000). Limitations in the capacity to understand the meaning of the event, to predict its ultimate resolution, or to exercise behavioral or cognitive coping skills would seem to make the sensory and emotional distress associated with pain perceptually preeminent, thereby accelerating the severity of the experience.

Although there is ample behavioral and biological evidence of pain in the course of phylogenetic development, and pain is clearly regulated in noncerebral regions of the brain, there is also evidence that the human cerebral cortex plays an important role in pain perception and in modulating pain experiences. Activity in those regions of the brain epitomizing the highest evolved capabilities is involved in regulating the primitive qualities of pain that were conserved in the course of evolution. Jasmin, Rabkin, Granato, Boudah, and O'Hara (2003) observed that activity in the cortex can inhibit ascending pain afferent input. Enhancing activity in key regions of the cerebral cortex appears to diminish pain, whereas blocking transmission of signals from this region of the brain through the descending pain inhibitory system incites great pain. It seems likely that dysregulation of this system would contribute to pain in response to ordinarily innocuous events and facilitate the severity of emotional distress associated with pain, which would lead to increased fear associated with the pain experience. Loss of the capacity for abstract, goal-directed behavior need not have an impact on spontaneous or automatic, undirected experience.

Although deficits in sensory or affective processing are also possible, they seem less likely to be influenced by neurophysiological impairments arising from genetic diseases, injuries, anoxia, inflammation, and other congenital sources of brain damage. Sensory sensitivity and emotional response represent features of older evolutionary development and are instantiated biologically by brain mechanisms less dependent upon neocortical control. Hence, they appear less likely to be influenced by cerebral impairment associated with developmental disabilities. It is the higher levels of executive processing, memory, reasoning, or decision making that are more likely to be diminished by cortical impairment. Nevertheless, there is a paucity of research on the potential for the neurophysiological impairments associated with developmental disabilities to influence sensory and affective features of the pain experience. A number of adolescents suffering from significant neurological impairments displayed minimal behavioral and autonomic reactivity to skin needle puncture, suggesting they had become relatively insensitive to pain (Oberlander, Gilbert, Chambers, O'Donnell, & Craig, 1999). However, Symons (2002) has associated self-injurious behavior with altered pain mechanisms. Thus, it would appear important to continue pursuit of the relationship between the neurological status of people with developmental disabilities and qualities of the pain experience.

Language also plays a complex role in the experience of pain. It provides the major source of access to understanding the nature of experience in people able to introspect on their personal lives. The importance attached to self-report by clinicians and researchers is reflected in assertions that "pain is what people say it is," or "the patient's verbal report is the only way to determine the presence, intensity, and quality of pain" (Meinhart & McCaffery, 1983). This has led to self-report of pain being described as the gold standard for assessing pain. However, this overstates the case. Self-report can be "fool's gold" if those using it neglect such limitations as the need for substantial cognitive and social competence or the risk of self-serving biases. Additionally, reliance on self-report access to conscious experience may be misleading because nonconscious experience exists without higher order self-awareness or the self-reflective capabilities necessary to verbally report the event (Wilson & Dunn, 2004). Use of language in conceptualizing pain only slowly emerges in infancy and early childhood (Stanford, Chambers, & Craig, 2005) and is not a necessary feature of pain in young children and other populations who clearly do not use sophisticated verbal language to express pain in response to injury and disease (Hadjistavropoulos & Craig, 2002).

Nonverbal assessment tools have proven valuable in understanding pain in people with developmental disabilities (Breau, Finley, McGrath, & Camfield, 2002; Hadjistavropoulos, von Baeyer, & Craig, 2001; Hunt, Mastroyannopoulou, Goldman, & Seers, 2003; LaChapelle, Hadjistavropoulos, & Craig, 1999; Oberlander & Craig, 2003). Painful experiences could be devoid of linguistic or semantic qualities, as would be the case in newborns and young infants. When the capacity for speech is restricted or absent, characterization of the nature of subjective experiences becomes more speculative. Language does not appear necessary for phenomenal experience, with nonverbal communication the primary inferential resource that establishes basic capabilities for experiencing pain.

The rapidly developing literature on the nature of consciousness (Kurthen, Grunwald, & Elger, 1998; Searle, 2000; Zelazo, 2004) provides insight into the likely nature of pain experience in people for whom there are cognitive limitations. There currently is no consensus concerning characteristics of consciousness in people with developmental disabilities, in part because of the variability encountered, but certain features seem important. At a minimum, there must be some capacity for sentience or conscious awareness, even if this only represents consciousness of present sensations. This capacity perhaps is most easily recognized when people move through cycles of sleep/waking behavioral states. Deep sleep and coma states fully illustrate loss of consciousness. When awake and alert, people encounter a tremendous diversity of qualitatively varying experiences ranging from the most rudimentary of feeling states to highly complex intellectual, social, spiritual, and aesthetic experiences. It does not appear necessary that varying qualities of experience always should have explicit thoughts or memories attached to them, although some minimal capacity for memory would be required for experiences to have an organized and sustained impact on the individual. It is the deficits in features of conscious experience that are of importance to understanding pain in people with developmental disabilities.

Simply stated, the subjective experience of pain should change qualitatively when the brain is functioning at less than optimal levels. The irreducible level would be some "primal" form of sentience that includes only a capacity to appreciate that there is a certain way that the event or situation feels. With pain, this could be an ability to recognize that one situation is noxious and another is not. Zelazo described "minimal consciousness" in newborn babies as the simplest, but still conceptually coherent, form of consciousness and recognized it as motivating approach and avoidance based on pleasure and pain. Furthermore, it is "unreflective, present-oriented, and makes no reference to a concept of self" (2004, p. 13). Most people would agree this form of pain in people with developmental disabilities warrants care or intervention. An ability to shift moods from those that are colored by unhappiness and dissatisfaction to those signifying pleasure reflects a level of conscious appreciation needed to experience pain and its absence. This minimal state of consciousness perhaps is the primordial state of being that organized the experiences of ancient hominid ancestors before capacities for complex cognition evolved, with self-consciousness, consciousness of others' experiences, and the ability to act deliberately arising later in evolution.

Subsequent levels of consciousness are characterized by Zelazo (2004) as emerging ontogenetically. This provides a useful metaphor for characterizing different capacities of consciousness associated with different magnitudes of developmental disability. One would expect emergence of a capacity to shift attention and to learn from personal experience. People with developmental disabilities may display an impaired capacity to learn, but this rarely is complete. Distinctions are often made between explicit and implicit memory, the former concerning an ability to process the memory in focal attention or to overtly articulate the memory. The latter is evident in demonstrations that experience has produced changes in behavior, even though there may be no explicit recall of the antecedent events. People with intact cognitive functions would have a capacity to remember and recount events explicitly, but implicit memory reflects a continuing capacity for learning.

THE SOCIAL COMMUNICATION PERSPECTIVE ON PAIN APPLIED TO PEOPLE WITH DEVELOPMENTAL DISABILITIES

The issues discussed previously focus on the nature of the personal pain experience in people with developmental disabilities. The massive research enterprise focusing on neurobiological substrates of this experience and traditional approaches to medical management of pain using drugs, surgery, and other physical interventions reflect this emphasis on inner qualities of the experience and their biological origins. However, an inclusive theoretical and practical perspective on pain would also examine the overt and public manifestations of pain, the reactions of others to the person in pain, and the complex social systems engaged for the delivery of health services when people experience pain. After all, assessment and delivery of care to people suffering from pain are fundamentally social actions that require understanding and explanation if health services are to be optimized. The vulnerabilities of people with developmental disabilities to painful conditions and their extraordinary dependence on caregivers to palliate pain further accentuate the importance of attending to interpersonal parameters.

The social communication model of pain (Craig, Lilley, & Gilbert, 1996; Hadjistavropoulos & Craig, 2002, 2004; Prkachin & Craig, 1995) has potential to assist in understanding the challenges of controlling pain in people with developmental disabilities (see Figure 2.1). This perspective has proven useful in addressing pain in other vulnerable and dependent individuals, namely infants and children (Craig, 2002; Craig, Korol, & Pillai, 2002). The model argues that efforts to control another's episode of pain require an understanding of the nature and determinants of each of the following in the full sequence of events: 1) the painful experience associated with tissue damage, 2) overt expressions of distress, 3) others' assessments of the person's pain, and 4) decisions about whether and how to intervene. At each stage, intrapersonal and interpersonal events and processes would shape reactions of the person in pain, as well as the reactions of observers. Thus, the subjective experience of pain following actual or imminent tissue injury would be determined by those biological processes responsible for the pain experience, as determined and influenced by genetic inheritance, personal history, and social factors, the latter including the setting in which pain is experienced and the presence of others. The self-report or nonverbal expression of pain would similarly be subject to

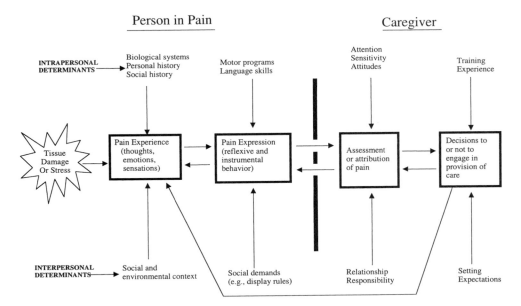

Figure 2.1. The social communication model of pain. An inclusive understanding of any person's pain must focus on more than the painful experience and its relationship to tissue damage. Consideration must also be directed to how the experience is encoded in expressive behavior, how observers judge pain on the strength of available information, and how inferences are related to decisions to intervene. At all stages, both intrapersonal and interpersonal factors will be important determinants, as illustrated in the model.

evolved genetic inheritance influencing motor expression and the use of language, as influenced by personal history, including social and cultural factors, and setting events, including those signaling what pattern of expression would be most socially appropriate. In a parallel manner, the judgments and decisions of caregivers (or antagonists) would be influenced by their personal and social history, including their relationship to the person in pain, such as kinship. Factors influencing biases as opposed to accurate judgments would be powerful determinants of the quality of care provided. As described in these brief terms, this linear sequence is idealized and oversimplified. It ignores the dynamic and recursive feedback loops and reciprocal influences that reflect how the caregiver and the person in pain interact with each other, but it does capture features of the social complexities of episodes of pain that must be considered if care is to be optimal.

The following discussion attempts to illustrate further some of the interpersonal complexities of pain that require consideration in understanding pain in people with developmental disabilities.

The Suffering Person

The potential for transformations in the nature of the pain experience arising from specific neurophysiological impairments has already been addressed. It is conceivable that specific cognitive impairments or generalized intellectual disabilities would leave the person less able to comprehend the nature of the experience, for example, its probable duration or his or her ability to control the source or features of the experience. As noted previously, this would not necessarily be associated with diminished pain distress or severity. People may have difficulty learning how one should respond to the pain experience to optimize receiving care. Acquisition of these skills is a feature of the prolonged socialization of young children. These skills are usually a product of people's long histories of painful events, adult and peer efforts to train adaptive personal and social coping skills, and observational learning of the requisite skills (Craig, 1986). People with developmental disabilities may have atypical histories in any of these domains; for example, medical necessities during early life can dictate frequent invasive and surgical interventions that could have lasting impact. The ability to benefit from social instruction and observational learning might also be limited. We note, for example, that children with Down syndrome are delayed in acquiring the language used by typically developing children to describe painful distress (Job, Chambers, Craig, & Oberlander, 2004). Slower socialization in sick-role behavior or difficulties comprehending the appropriate verbal and behavioral display of pain could also serve as impediments for caregivers. Being able to effectively communicate information about painful distress to others is often essential to effectively engage the health care delivery system. When attending to the needs of people with a diminished capacity to exercise language or social skills, it is imperative that caregivers attend to more reflexive and spontaneous expressions of distress.

The Response of Observers

Because people with developmental disabilities may be less able to engage in self-care during episodes of pain, there is added importance to the sensitivity and willingness of others to be prepared to intercede on their behalf. Despite the importance of the task, parents and other caregivers appear to have more difficulty assessing pain in children with developmental disabilities than in typically developing children (Breau et al., 2003; Fanurik, Koh, Schmitz, Harrison, & Conrad, 1998; Hennequin, Faulks, & Allison, 2003). Perhaps this is because adults are less able to accurately judge non-noxious social signals in young children with developmental delays (Walden, 1996).

The challenges for observers appear to go beyond the level of decoding the subjective states of people with developmental disabilities and encompass the ability to empathize with these individuals. Although personal experiences of pain tend to be vivid and highly meaningful, people have greater difficulty appreciating the nature of pain in other people. Sometimes there is powerful empathy, accurate understanding, and commitment to providing relief. In other situations, people appear capable of ignoring, minimizing, or even fostering the pain of others. Sympathetic understanding of another's pain is often determined by the relationship between the observing person and the person in pain. People likely to be sensitive to painful distress in another often have close attachments to the party in pain. Kinship, friendship, professional commitment, or even personal dispositions to being caring and concerned about the plight of others can enhance attention and concern when others experience pain. In contrast, intimate concern for the well-being of others is less likely when there is no personal attachment or commitment. It is important to appreciate that too often people characterized in this manner have been undervalued. The inequities associated with the social hierarchies characterizing human culture and society leave people with developmental disabilities at risk for inadequate understanding and care. Efforts to rectify risks of inadequate care require careful reflection on the nature of pain in these populations and the necessity of attending to uncommon patterns of pain display (e.g., Gilbert-MacLeod, Craig, Rocha, & Mathias, 2000). Examination of pain as a human phenomenon requires broad consideration of the risk factors to which people with developmental disabilities are exposed; the nature of the pain they experience and how they express it; and the reactions of others, including caregivers, who would be in a position to deliver care if they were to understand the distress the person is experiencing and had the resources available to diminish painful distress.

THE NEED FOR AN INTEGRATIVE APPROACH TO PAIN IN PEOPLE WITH DEVELOPMENTAL DISABILITIES

An integrative approach that considers not only intrapersonal features of pain (e.g., biological mechanisms, the experience of pain) but also the social contexts that shape the experience and expression of pain and the actions of other people who are in a position to deliver care is essential for optimal caregiving with people with developmental disabilities. Pain cannot be understood without an appreciation of the interpersonal nature of the experience. The social communication model bears some similarities to concepts proposed by the World Health Organization to generate a standard language to describe health and health-related states (http://www3.who.int/icf/icftemplate.cfm) (Oberlander & Craig, in press). Disability and functioning are viewed reasonably as outcomes of interactions between health conditions (diseases, disorders, and injuries), contextual factors (external environmental factors, social attitudes, architectural characteristics, legal and social structures), and internal personal factors (gender, age, coping styles, social background, education, past and current experience, behavioral patterns) that influence how disability is experienced by the individual. The model recognizes the necessity of including all of these factors in understanding the pain a person is experiencing and its consequences but also provides an understanding of how the social environment can have a major impact.

There then remains a considerable need for a better understanding of the many phenomena described. At the level of the person, we need a more intimate and detailed understanding of how specific developmental disabilities affect the conscious experience of pain, including sensory, cognitive, and affective features. The more exact this is with respect to the individual, the better the match can be with pain-controlling interventions. Appreciating the nature of the experience will require better measures of pain, psychometrically validated for the individual. The potential for personal and systemic social biases and attitudes to diminish the quality of care delivered appears a continuous risk and also needs to be better appreciated. The urgency for embarking on this research agenda appears considerable because often people with disabilities have been excluded from research studies because of the differences, which dictates a need to understand pain in these populations better.

In conclusion, it is now well accepted that respect for the human dignity of all people includes a universal right to prevention and control of pain (Brennan & Cousins, 2004; Fanurick et al., 1999; Savage, 1998). It is important that health care professionals, family members, and others able to provide care to individuals with developmental disabilities recognize, assess, and act to control and diminish pain the individual may be experiencing.

REFERENCES

Anand, K.J.S., & Craig, K.D. (1996). New perspectives on the definition of pain. *Pain, 67,* 3–6.

Biersdorff, K.K. (1991). Pain insensitivity and indifference: Alternative explanations for some medical catastrophes. *Mental Retardation, 29,* 359–362.

Biersdorff, K.K. (1994). Incidence of significantly altered pain experience among individuals with developmental disabilities. *American Journal on Mental Retardation, 98,* 619–631.

Breau, L.M., Finley, G.A., McGrath, P.J., & Camfield, C.S. (2002). Validation of the Non-Communicating Children's Pain Checklist–Postoperative Version. *Anesthesiology, 96,* 528–535.

Breau, L.M., MacLaren, J., McGrath, P.J., Camfield, C.S., & Finley, G.A. (2003). Caregivers' beliefs regarding pain in children with cognitive impairment: Relation between pain sensation and reaction increases with severity of impairment. *Clinical Journal of Pain, 19,* 335–344.

Brennan, F., & Cousins, M.J. (2004). Pain relief as a human right. *Pain: Clinical Updates, XII*(5), 1–4.

Bruehl, S., & Chung, I.Y. (2004). Psychological interventions for acute pain. In T. Hadjistavropoulos & K.D. Craig (Eds.), *Pain: Psychological perspectives* (pp. 245–269). Mahwah, NJ: Lawrence Erlbaum Associates.

Chapman, C.R. (2004). Pain perception, affective mechanisms, and conscious experience. In T. Hadjistavropoulos & K.D. Craig (Eds.), *Pain: Psychological perspectives* (pp. 59–85). Mahwah, NJ: Lawrence Erlbaum Associates.

Craig, K.D. (1986). Social modeling influences: Pain in context. In R.A. Sternbach (Ed.), *The psychology of pain* (2nd ed., pp. 67–96). New York: Raven Press.

Craig, K.D. (1998). The facial display of pain. In G.A. Finley & P.J. McGrath (Eds.), *Measurement of pain in infants and children* (pp. 103–122). Seattle, WA: IASP Press.

Craig, K.D. (2002). Pain in infants and children: Sociodevelopmental variations on the theme. In M.A. Giamberardino (Ed.), *Pain 2002—an updated review (refresher course syllabus, 10th World Congress on Pain, San Diego, CA)* (pp. 305–314). Seattle, WA: IASP Press.

Craig, K.D. (2005). Emotions and psychobiology. In S. McMahon & M. Koltzenburg, (Eds.), *Melzack and Wall's textbook of pain* (5th ed., pp. 231-239). Edinburgh: Churchill-Livingstone.

Craig, K.D., Korol, C.T., & Pillai, R.R. (2002). Challenges of judging pain in vulnerable infants. *Clinics in Perinatology, 29,* 445–458.

Craig, K.D., Lilley, C.M., & Gilbert, C.A. (1996). Social barriers to optimal pain management in infants and children. *Clinical Journal of Pain, 12,* 232–242.

Engel, J.M., Schwartz, L., Jensen, M.P., & Johnson, D.R. (2000). Pain in cerebral palsy: The relation of coping strategies to adjustment. *Pain, 88,* 225–230.

Fanurik, D., Koh, J.L., Schmitz, M.L., Harrison, R.D., & Conrad, T.M. (1998). Children with cognitive impairment: Parent report of pain and coping. *Journal of Developmental and Behavioral Pediatrics, 20,* 228–234.

Fanurik, D., Koh, J., Schmitz, M.L., Harrison, R.D., Roberston, P.K., & Killebrew, P. (1999). Pain assessment and treatment in children with cognitive impairment: A survey of nurses' and physicians' beliefs. *Clinical Journal of Pain, 15,* 304–312.

Gilbert-MacLeod, C.A., Craig, K.D., Rocha, E.M., & Mathias, M.D. (2000). Everyday pain responses in children with and without developmental delays. *Journal of Pediatric Psychology, 25,* 301–308.

Hadden, K.L., & von Baeyer, C.L. (2002). Pain in children with cerebral palsy: Common triggers and expressive behaviors. *Pain, 99,* 281–288.

Hadden, K.L., & von Baeyer, C.L. (2005). Global and specific behavioral measures of pain in children with cerebral palsy. *Clinical Journal of Pain, 21,* 140–146.

Hadjistavropoulos, T., & Craig, K.D. (2002). A theoretical framework for understanding self-report and observational measures of pain: A Communications Model. *Behaviour Research and Therapy, 40,* 551–570.

Hadjistavropoulos, T., & Craig, K.D. (2004). Social influences and the communication of pain. In T. Hadjistavropoulos & K.D. Craig (Eds.), *Pain: Psychological perspectives* (pp. 87–112). Mahwah, NJ: Lawrence Erlbaum Associates.

Hadjistavropoulos, T., von Baeyer, C., & Craig, K.D. (2001). Pain assessment in persons with limited ability to communicate. In D.C. Turk & R. Melzack (Eds.), *Handbook of pain assessment* (2nd ed., pp. 134–149). New York: The Guilford Press.

Hennequin, M., Faulks, D., & Allison, P.J. (2003). Parents' ability to perceive pain experienced by their child with Down syndrome. *Journal of Orofacial Pain, 17,* 347–333.

Hunt, A., Mastroyannopoulou, K., Goldman, A., & Seers, K. (2003). Not knowing—the problem of pain in children with severe neurological impairment. *International Journal of Nursing Studies, 40,* 171–183.

Jasmin, L., Rabkin, S.D., Granato, A., Boudah, A., & O'Hara, P.T. (2003). Analgesia and hyperalgesia from GABA-mediated modulation of the cerebral cortex. *Nature, 424,* 316–320.

Job, E.A., Chambers, C.T., Craig, K.D., & Oberlander, T.F. (2004). *Verbal pain expression among children with Down Syndrome.*

Kirmayer, L.J., Groleau, D., Looper, K.J., & Dao, M.D. (2004). Explaining medically unexplained symptoms. *Canadian Journal of Psychiatry, 49,* 663–672.

Kurthen, M., Grunwald, T., & Elger, C.E. (1998). Will there be a neuroscientific theory of consciousness? *Trends in Cognitive Sciences, 2,* 229–234.

LaChapelle, D.L., Hadjistavropoulos, T., & Craig, K.D. (1999). Pain measurement in persons with intellectual disabilities. *Clinical Journal of Pain, 15,* 213–231.

Malviya, S., Voepel-Lewis, T., Tait, A.R., Merkel, S., Lauer, A., Munro, H., et al. (2001). Pain management in children with and without cognitive impairment following spine fusion surgery. *Paediatric Anaesthesia, 11,* 453.

McGrath, P.J., Rosmus, C., Camfield, C., Campbell, M.A., & Hennigar, A. (1998). Behaviors caregivers use to determine pain in non-verbal cognitively impaired individuals. *Developmental Medicine and Clinical Neurology, 40,* 340–343.

Meinhart, N.T., & McCaffery, M. (1983). *Pain: A nursing approach to assessment and analysis.* Norwalk, CT: Appleton-Century-Crofts.

Melzack, R., & Casey, K.L. (1968). Sensory, motivational and central control determinants of pain: A new conceptual model. In D.L. Kenshalo (Ed.), *The skin senses* (p. 423). Springfield, IL: Charles C Thomas.

Merskey, H., & Bogduk, N. (Eds.). (1994). *Classification of chronic pain: Descriptions of chronic pain syndromes and definition of pain terms* (2nd ed). Seattle, WA: IASP Press.

Nader, R., Oberlander, T.F., Chambers, C.T., & Craig, K.D. (2004). The expression of pain in children with autism. *Clinical Journal of Pain, 20,* 88–97.

Oberlander, T.F., & Craig, K.D. (2003). Pain and children with developmental disabilities. In N.M. Schechter, C.B. Berde, & M. Yaster (Eds.), *Pain in infants, children and adolescents* (2nd ed., pp. 599–619). Baltimore: Williams & Wilkins.

Oberlander, T.F., & Craig, K.D. (in press). Pain and children with disabilities. In R.F. Schmidt & W.D. Willis (Eds.), *The encyclopedic reference of pain.* Berlin: Springer-Verlag.

Oberlander, T.F., Gilbert, C.A., Chambers, C.T., O'Donnell, M.E., & Craig, K.D. (1999). Biobehavioral responses to acute pain in adolescents with a significant neurological impairment. *Clinical Journal of Pain, 15,* 201–209.

Oberlander, T.F., O'Donnell, M.E., & Montgomery, C.J. (1999). Pain in children with significant neurological impairment. *Journal of Developmental and Behavioral Pediatrics, 20,* 235–243.

Prkachin, K.M., & Craig, K.D. (1995). Expressing pain: The communication and interpretation of facial pain signals. *Journal of Nonverbal Behavior, 19,* 191–205.

Savage, T.A. (1998). Children with severe and profound disabilities and the issue of social justice. *Advances in the Practice of Nursing Quarterly, 4,* 53-58.

Schwartz, L., Engel, J.M., & Jensen, M.P. (1999). Pain in persons with cerebral palsy. *Archives of Physical Medicine and Rehabilitation, 80,* 1243–1246.

Searle, J.R. (2000). *Mind, language and society.* New York: Basic Books.

Stallard, P., Williams, L., Lenton, S., & Velleman, R. (2001). Pain in cognitively impaired, non-communicating children. *Archives of Disease in Childhood, 85,* 460–462.

Stanford, E.A., Chambers, C.T., & Craig, K.D. (2005). A normative analysis of the development of pain-related vocabulary in children. *Pain, 114,* 278–284.

Sullivan, M.J., Thorn, B., Haythornthwaite, J.A., Keefe, F., Martin, M., Bradley, L.A., et al. (2001). Theoretical perspectives on the relation between catastrophizing and pain. *Clinical Journal of Pain, 17,* 52–64.

Symons, F.J. (2002). Pain and self-injury: Mechanisms and models. In S. Schroeder, T. Thompson, & M.L. Oster-Granite (Eds.), *Self-injurious behavior: Genes, brain and behavior* (pp. 223–234). Washington: American Psychological Association.

Terstegen, C.M., Koot, H.M., De Boer, J.B., & Tibboel, D. (2003). Measuring pain in children with cognitive impairment: Pain response to surgical procedures. *Pain, 103,* 187–198.

Walden, T.A. (1996). Social responsivity: Judging signals of young children with and without developmental delays. *Child Development, 67,* 2074–2085.

Wilson, T.D., & Dunn, E.W. (2004). Self-knowledge: Its limits, value and potential for improvement. *Annual Review of Psychology, 55,* 17.1–17.26.

Zelazo, P.D. (2004). The development of conscious control in childhood. *Trends in Cognitive Sciences, 8,* 12–17.

3

PAIN AND DISABILITY IN AN ETHICAL AND SOCIAL CONTEXT

Dick Sobsey

Much of this book is devoted to the developing field of assessing and treating pain in people with developmental disabilities. This chapter addresses a very different set of issues. It explores some of our previous assumptions and beliefs about the relationship of pain and suffering to developmental disabilities, and it speculates on some of the reasons for those assumptions. This chapter is based on the premise that our understanding of the ways that society has constructed its attitudes and beliefs about pain and developmental disabilities is important for our current understanding of pain in people with developmental disabilities. Post, Blustein, Gordon, and Dubler suggested, "If the perception of and response to pain are to be understood in a useful way, they must be examined in the context of culture, gender, imbalances of power, morality, and myth" (1996, p. 348). They are among the many experts who remind us of the essential role of the social context in understanding pain.

Our observations and interpretations of how people with developmental disabilities experience pain and suffering typically have been exaggerated and mythologized in both the distant and recent past. At times, it has been suggested that people with disabilities are incapable of experiencing pain or suffering from it. At other times, it has been suggested that they experience pain and suffering that is so extreme, constant, and unmanageable that death is the only humane alternative. Most incredibly it has been suggested that people with developmental disabilities are at once incapable of experiencing pain or suffering and tortured beyond endurance by pain and suffering. It also has been suggested that pain is a legitimate and beneficial teaching tool for people with developmental disabilities. Inflicting pain has been suggested as necessary for people with developmental disabilities to benefit from therapy or undergo meaningful behavior change.

The extremes expressed in these constructs of pain among people with severe developmental disabilities reveal something about how deeply hidden their actual feelings have been from most other members of society. These feelings have been hidden by impaired communication, by physical and social segregation, and by society's disinterest and, at times, active unwillingness to understand. To examine our ways of thinking about our constructs of pain and people with disabilities, we need to consider some history of the ways that people have spoken and written about them. We need to consider not only the meaning of these constructs but also their pragmatics. Such a pragmatic analysis asks, *What is the social purpose of our attitudes and beliefs about pain and developmental disabilities?*

INSENSITIVITY AND INDIFFERENCE TO PAIN

One of the most frequent and enduring beliefs about how people with developmental disabilities experience pain has been the belief that they do not feel pain or that they are much less sensitive to pain than people without disabilities. A variation on this belief asserts that they do perceive pain, but that they are indifferent to it. Therefore, pain is not viewed as a source of suffering.

Twentieth-Century Constructs

Before discussing insensitivity and indifference to pain as a construct applied to people with developmental disabilities, it should be acknowledged that pain insensitivity and indifference do exist as genuine phenomena in some very rare medical disorders. Some individuals lack any pain sensation or at least have greatly reduced sensation of pain. Some individuals have a sensation of pain but do not experience it as unpleasant or distressing (Nagasako, Oaklander, & Dworkin, 2003). Some of the older material reviewed in this chapter uses the term *insensible to pain* (e.g., Cather, 1919; "Insensibility of a Maori," 1888), which appears to have broadly encompassed the notions of both insensitivity and indifference. The use of the concept of insensibility further blurred the distinction between intellectual, emotional, and sensory impairments because multiple definitions of insensibility could imply any or all of these.

Nagasako et al. (2003) listed five distinct syndromes of pain insensitivity and one of pain indifference. In addition, they identified one additional distinct condition, *asymbolia for pain,* in which individuals cannot process information about their pain sensations. Some people who have syndromes that produce pain insensitivity and pain indifference also have intellectual disabilities, but many do not. The conditions of true pain insensitivity and pain indifference in people with intellectual disabilities are extremely rare, so rare that actual studies of people with disabilities and their pain reactions have typically failed to identify even a single case (e.g., Breau, Camfield, McGrath, & Finley, 2003; Stengel, Oldham, & Ehernberg, 1958).

More important, experimental and epidemiological studies have long demonstrated clearly that the vast majority of people with intellectual disabilities have normal pain perception and that pain and pain management are all too frequent issues for many people with developmental disabilities. Stengel, Oldham, and Ehernberg (1955, 1958) tested the pain reactions of 97 individuals with severe intellectual disabilities using standardized measures of pain response. The participants in their study responded to 11 different pain-inducing sensations (e.g., pressure, pinpricks) in a typical fashion. The researchers reported,

> This investigation clearly demonstrated that the average low-grade mental defective reacted to pain inflicted from the outside in the same way as other subjects . . . . Possibly, some of the conditions reported by earlier physicians were institutional artefacts [sic] . . . . The most striking result of this investigation was the finding that mental defectives who indulge in self injuries tended to react to pain inflicted on them from the outside only slightly less than other subjects . . . . Insensitivity to pain was not observed in any of the patients of this series. (Stengel et al., 1958, p. 438)

Although it would be difficult to conduct a similar study today because of the ethical issues regarding inflicting pain and informed consent, this finding has not been seriously challenged and remains consistent with findings from more recent research. Breau et al. (2003), for example, reported on the pain experiences of 94 children and adolescents with severe and profound intellectual disabilities. They did not report a single individual with pain insensitivity or pain indifference. Overall, although the number of actual scientific studies is small and the studies that are available have some weaknesses, as all studies do, the available scientific evidence clearly refutes the notion that there is any widespread insensitivity or indifference to pain specific to people with intellectual or developmental disabilities. Nevertheless, this notion has remained widespread and persistent for centuries. The existence of these rare disorders of pain perception was commonly cited as indirect evidence that large numbers of people with developmental disabilities may have similar absent or greatly reduced sensations of pain (Biersdorff, 1991, 1994; Couston, 1954), and anecdotal reports of institutionalized individuals who were apparently immune to pain have surfaced long before and long after the Stengel, Oldham, and Ehernberg study.

One of the earliest and most influential examples in the modern scientific literature comes from Francis Galton, the originator of the first intelligence test, influential contributor to the foundations of inferential statistics, and acknowledged primary founder of the eugenics movement:

> The discriminative faculty of idiots is curiously low; they hardly distinguish between heat and cold, and their sense of pain is so obtuse that some of the more idiotic seem hardly to know what it is. In their dull lives, such pain as can be excited in them may literally be accepted with a welcome surprise. During a visit to Earlswood Asylum I saw two boys whose toe-nails had grown into the flesh and had been excised by the surgeon. This is a horrible torture to ordinary persons, but the idiot lads were said to have shown no distress during the operation; it was not necessary to hold them, and they looked rather interested at what was being done. (1907)

Before considering a more general interpretation of Galton's statement, take note of his use of the word *idiot*. It might be tempting to assign a stigmatizing value to its use or simply dismiss it as simply a representation of the terminology used a century ago. There are two important aspects of the meaning of this term, however, that require consideration. First, the term *idiot* was coined to refer to the most severe intellectual disabilities. It does not precisely conform to any current category commonly used but comes closest to what would today be referred to as a profound intellectual disability. Second, the condition of idiocy was defined primarily as an intellectual disability that was so severe that the individual lacked the use of speech or other productive language. Idiots were originally defined as those who lived in their separate, personal, and private worlds because they could not communicate their observations, thoughts, or feelings to others. Galton and his contemporaries shared this notion. For example, his fellow eugenicist Davenport stated "at one extreme is the idiot, without language and incapable of attending to his bodily needs" (1911, p. 66). In fact the term *idiocy* (previously *idiosy*) comes from the Greek *idios,* meaning personal, private, separate, or distinct (*Oxford English Dictionary,* 1989). Thus, the critical defining attribute was severe impairment of communication. Therefore, Galton's focus was on how others can understand the pain experiences of people who cannot tell us what they are feeling through conventional means.

Regardless of the changes in terminology, this inherent communication issue remains important for two reasons. First, because people with severe developmental disabilities had extremely limited abilities to communicate about their pain, there were limited objective data upon which to base understanding. This lack of information made it easy to characterize their feelings and behavior in almost any manner. The lack of an overt response to apparently painful circumstances could be viewed as bravery, stoicism, or self-control as easily as insensitivity and indifference. As discussed later in this chapter, it was typically described as insensitivity or indifference when observed in marginalized people and as bravery when observed among more privileged classes. Second, this same limitation on communication meant that people with developmental disabilities, once characterized as insensitive or indifferent to pain, could do little to correct this impression.

Galton's comment on the insensitivity of people with severe intellectual disabilities to pain appears in a more general discussion of sensation and its relationship to intelligence. Galton believed that sensation was one of about 10 measures of intelligence. When Galton first established his intelligence testing clinic in 1882, tactile sensitivity and reaction time were included as essential measures of intelligence. In his model, those members of groups Galton considered to have greater intelligence would also be expected to have greater sensitivity to pain and all other stimuli. Galton equates lesser sensitivity with lesser intelligence; applying this paradigm freely reflected his views on race and gender as well as disabilities. For example, he assures his readers that men have more acute senses than women, offering as indisputable evidence the proposition that if women had senses that were as keen as men they would be more successful in securing employment in skilled professions. He explains that social custom forces men to drink the coffee and tea that women prepare for them, even though women lack the sensitivity required to brew drinks of better quality. In a similar manner, he assures readers that commonly held beliefs that nonwhites had keener senses were myths and misinterpretations: "My own experience, so far as it goes, of Hottentots, Damaras, and some other wild races, went to show that their sense discrimination was not superior to those of white men, even as regards keenness of eyesight" (Galton, 1907).

Galton's reasoning and presentation of information applied to people with disabilities, women, and "wild races" is uniform. It reflects the eugenic reasoning that runs through all of his work: All social problems can be attributed to inherent (genetically transmitted) flaws in those who suffer from them. If women are disadvantaged in employment, it must be due to some inherent inferiority. If people with developmental disabilities submit to what is "horrible torture to ordinary persons," it must be due to an inherent problem on their part. From this perspective, trying to protect "idiots" from torturous procedures would be as absurd as trying to establish employment equity for women. In Galton's own words, "The general intention of this chapter has been to show that a delicate power of sense discrimination is an attribute of a high race" (1907). In Galton's mind, this high race was white, male, and nondisabled. This conceptualization conformed nicely to the existing power structure, and helped provide a "scientific" rationale for the system of class and privilege.

Galton's work was influential in many respects, particularly in the developing conceptions of intellect and intellectual disability. For example, James Cattell, after working with Galton, conducted research at the University of Pennsylvania and Columbia University, further developed the idea of testing intelligence, and was the first to refer to intelligence tests as *mental tests* and *mental measurements.* These included tests of when pressure, heat, and cold were interpreted as pain as well as when loud sounds became painful. If women, nonwhites, and people with disabilities were to be constructed as less intelligent, they would also be constructed as less sensitive to pain and other stimuli. Galton was not the first or last to present these ideas. For example, late 19th-century articles in the *New York Times* reported that science has proved that women are only about half as sensitive to pain as men are ("Physical Sensibility," 1892) and presented information that "appear(s) to prove that Maories are less sensible to pain than Europeans" ("Insensibility of a Maori," 1888). Whereas the apparent ability of women, nonwhites, and people with disabilities to withstand pain was interpreted as evidence of insensibility, the ability of nondisabled, white men to withstand pain was interpreted as stoicism and bravery (e.g., "Affairs at Gettysburgh," 1863). In this manner, withstanding pain was constructed as an ability and a virtue when observed among the more empowered members of society but a deficit when observed among the disempowered. Considering this reasoning, it is not surprising that newborn babies and infants were also considered insensitive and indifferent to pain until fairly recently. As pointed out by Anand and Hickey (1987), "One result of the pervasive view of neonatal pain is that newborns are frequently not given analgesic or anesthetic during invasive procedures including surgery" (p. 1321).

Although later intelligence tests eliminated pain thresholds as a measure of intelligence for ethical, practical, and technical reasons, the inclusion of pain sensitivity as a measure of intelligence in these early assessments had continuing influence. Although there was very little scientific support, the insensitivity legend continued to be repeated, typically accompanied by anecdotal reports of people with severe disabilities who seemed to tolerate extreme pain, usually from people who lived in institutions. Couston's (1954) article on pain indifference was another collection of anecdotes from institutionalized individuals with developmental disabilities. Nevertheless, it was extremely influential because it helped legitimize the notion of pain insensitivity and indifference as it attempted to bolster the writer's interpretations of a few observations with the trappings of science: "In these mentally defective patients there was a marked indifference to pain although some discomfort was felt in a few cases" (Couston, 1954, p. 1129). Although Couston interpreted his observations as indicating that the seven individuals whom he describes are indifferent to pain, his descriptions seem to tell a different story. One "showed some resentment on movement" of a broken hip, and another displayed "annoyance" on being sutured without being given an anesthetic. Couston described other typical signs of pain among other so-called indifferent individuals. However, he assured us that these individuals felt no pain or remained indifferent to it, if they did. The presumed indifference to pain justifies what otherwise would be an unethical failure to protect the patient from painful procedures or to treat pain that cannot be prevented.

This notion of the insensitivity of the victim justifying the behavior of the perpetrator is hardly new. Ryan and Thomas (1987) provided a historical reference from Coxe's 1779 description of Swiss "imbeciles [who were] almost insensitive to blows" (p. 89). One can only speculate on the circumstances under which this remarkable insensitivity to blows revealed itself. Deutsch (1949) suggested that this idea of people with developmental disabilities or mental health disorders being insensitive to heat, cold, pain, and other stimuli was predominant in the United States from the days of the earliest European settlers through the middle to late 1800s. He suggested that this premise made their harsh treatment (e.g., unheated cells, beatings) not just excusable but also seemingly necessary. Because caregivers could not depend on normal consequences to control the behavior of their charges, extreme force would be required. In this manner, the construct of pain insensitivity or indifference provides a particularly dangerous form of dehumanization (Sobsey, 1994). If the casual observer was horrified by the cruelty and indifference directed toward the most vulnerable of people, it could be explained that this was not the result of the cruelty of the apparent perpetrators of the violence and neglect but rather the result of the insensitivity of the apparent victims.

Dehumanization, Depersonalization, and Insensitivity

Dehumanization has been widely discussed as a process by which people with developmental disabilities have been stigmatized as something other than and less than fully human (e.g., Deutsch, 1949; Vail, 1967; Wolfensberger, 1969). Wolfensberger explored the construct of people with intellectual disabilities as subhuman organisms and the process of dehumanization concisely in his classic essay "The Origin and Nature of Our Institutional Models" (1969), and his response to the lingering influence of this construct has been a major influence on his subsequent work that focused on re-humanizing people with disabilities and restoring their personal dignity.

Portraying people with disabilities (or any other groups or individuals) as lacking fundamental human feelings is critical to dehumanizing them. Hauerwas succinctly reminded us, "To be human is to suffer" (1986, p. 62). Indeed, it is difficult to imagine any human being whose life is free of pain and suffering, or even of any sensation or feelings. Certainly, if such an alien entity exists, there is no point in compassion for it. After all, we cannot be expected to share hurt feelings that do not exist. Of course, people with developmental disabilities have not been the only victims of dehumanization. It is a process by which many groups have been deprived of their most basic human rights. By simply altering our definition of who is human or who qualifies as a person, it becomes possible for a society simultaneously to maintain its status as fully egalitarian and to deny fundamental rights to broad categories of individuals (e.g., slaves, women, non–property owners) at various times in history.

The establishment of explicit definitions, rules, and laws that dehumanize specific groups of people can be classified as formal dehumanization. For example, bioethicist Joseph Fletcher (1972) attempted to define who was human and who was not human by IQ test scores. He proposed that a score of 40 or above might be required to be considered human and that a score of 20 or above must be required to be considered human. Bioethicist Peter Singer (2000) used somewhat different terminology. After pointing out that all offspring of human beings are undeniably human, he changed the critical variable to *personhood,* a status necessary for ethical consideration and personal rights. He considers sentience or self-consciousness as a critical criterion for personhood. In his view, not all humans qualify as persons, but some nonhumans do. Therefore, he proposed his own set of commandments to replace the original ten. In place of the old commandment,

"Thou shalt not kill," Singer suggested "Recognize that the worth of human life varies" (2000, p. 212). However, Singer's construct of human nonpersons does not merely allow for their destruction, it requires it. His replaceability principle suggests that because social and material resources are limited, destruction of nonpersons and of persons whose disabilities interfere with their achievement of happiness is ethically required to provide room for and direct resources to persons without any such limitations.

The shift from humanhood to personhood in ethical discussions adds a number of ethical complications. Despite Fletcher's previously cited assertion to the contrary, the notion of humanhood logically requires only human origin and living status to qualify for all human rights, whereas personhood suggests that other qualifications may be required. A naturalistic concept of personhood may define it in terms of humanhood (Ohlin, 2004); everyone who is biologically a living human is also a person. Non-naturalistic concepts, however, base personhood on other qualities such as sentience (the ability to feel), rationality (the ability to reason), or spirituality (the incorporation of a soul). Being human, therefore, can be seen as insufficient or even irrelevant to personhood. Some humans may fail to qualify, and some nonhumans may qualify. For example, in the law, corporations and political entities, such as nations, may be considered to be persons for some purposes. Singer suggested that some nonhuman animals be accorded rights as persons, while humans with severe cognitive disabilities be denied those rights as nonpersons (e.g., Singer, 2000).

The three additional requirements for personhood (i.e., sentience, rationality, and spirituality) might be seen as separate and independent from each other. However, they are closely related in their origin. Descartes is credited as one of the chief philosophers who defined persons as union between body and soul. He viewed the body as a machine or vehicle piloted by the soul (Ohlin, 2004). The soul was divine, connected to God, and was characterized by feelings and rationality (Descartes, 1641/1968). These feelings and rationality were to be viewed as part of the soul rather than the body. Nonhuman animals were viewed as mere machines lacking souls and were therefore incapable of true rationality or genuine feelings. Although other animals showed evidence of pleasure and pain, and of rational thinking, these were to be disregarded as lower order processes, mere bodily reflexes, in creatures that were believed to lack the soul that would be required for genuine thoughts and feelings. Similarly, people with severe developmental disabilities were viewed as lacking the critical component required for genuine thoughts and feelings. They were seen as comprising only *res extensa* (bodies) lacking the *res cogitans* (divine soul) necessary to be considered a complete person.

Insensitivity as Dehumanization in Earlier Times

These notions of personhood and insensitivity to pain were prevalent long before modern times. Wolfensberger (1969) traced the construct of the person with a developmental disability as a subhuman to Martin Luther's notion of "changelings." It is important to remember that the mythology of changelings was established centuries before Luther and that there were many different myths and legends that evolved over time. Changelings were believed to be the offspring of elves, leprechauns, or other mythical beings, and were often substituted for human babies when the parents were not watching. The characteristic of changelings varied from myth to myth, but they were commonly described as very slow to develop, highly demanding of their parents, and insensitive to all but the most severe brutality (Sobsey, 1994). In many cases, they were described as savants with hidden talents and were sometimes exposed by their talent when a parent or passerby found them exercising this skill (e.g., playing the bagpipes). With the spread of Christianity, these myths incorporated new elements. Changelings were increasingly viewed as offspring of the Devil and as having no soul.

Various editions of Luther's (1652/1886) Tabletalks provide similar accounts of his pronouncements about changelings as well as his claim of personal experience with a changeling. He described the child as normal in appearance, eating as much as four men, drooling, inarticulate, and incontinent. Luther recommended killing the child, and, when this recommendation is refused, he recommended praying for the child's death, which subsequently follows. When asked if killing the child was sinful, he replied that it is not a sin because the changeling had no soul and existed only as a *massa carnis* or lump of flesh.

Goodey and Stainton (2001) raised some important objections to the notion that Luther played a significant role in advocating the death of children with developmental disabilities. They pointed out that several different accounts of the Tabletalks exist in which the so-called instruction to kill is more ambiguous, and that Luther's use of the changeling myth probably was intended to address other religious and philosophical issues. Although their well-researched and cogently presented argument makes it clear that placing a great deal of blame on Martin Luther (1483–1546) is, at best, an oversimplification, the subsequent influence of the ideas attributed to Luther is undeniable. Descartes's (1596–1650) previously discussed notion that a body without a divine soul was not a real person reflected similar ideas. The ideas expressed by Luther and Descartes were enduring and influenced the development of more modern thinking about people with developmental disabilities.

Sammuel Howe (1848/1976), who is credited as a pioneer in the education and care of people with developmental disabilities, explained that "idiots of the lowest class are mere organisms, masses of flesh and bone in human shape, without any manifestation of intellectual or affective faculties" (p. 37). In turn, Howe credited another pioneer in the field, Seguin, for this idea: " [Seguin] finds, even in our fair commonwealth, breathing masses of flesh, but shorn of all human attributes" (p. 37). With the coming of our so-called scientific age, science and logic replaced religion and doctrine as our primary frameworks for constructing and understanding phenomena. Although it may be tempting to assume that the scientific view is inherently immune to the biases of the past, in many cases this scientific framework simply replaced the old religious framework to support the same constructs with new rationales. For example, in the religious framework, the dominant class deserved a disproportionate share of wealth and power because of divine right, but, with the coming of the scientific age, a science of eugenics developed that rationalized the same class structure on the basis of genetic differences. The duality of body and soul was transformed into the duality of body and mind, and the permission to kill human bodies that lacked *souls* was echoed in the bioethicists' assurance that we can kill human bodies who lack *potential quality of life.*

The dehumanized individual with developmental disabilities is constructed as incapable of meaningful feelings as well as rational thought. Burleigh (1994) followed this logic in the writing of psychiatrist Alfred Hoche in 1920. According to

Burleigh, Hoche believed that "full idiots" were "mentally dead," without human personality or self-consciousness, "on the intellectual level which we only encounter way down in the animal kingdom." Pity was a totally displaced emotion in these cases because "where there is no suffering, there can also be no pity" (Burleigh, 1994, pp. 18–19). This statement is explicit. Pity is wasted on beings that are not to be viewed as either living or human. Sympathy and empathy are impossible because these would require the individual to have feelings in order for others to share in those feelings.

These notions of dehumanization and depersonalization were connected strongly to the developing notion of people with developmental disabilities as insensitive or indifferent to pain. In order to view people with developmental disabilities as nonhuman, it was necessary to strip them of human feelings. Conversely, the belief that these individuals were less than human supported the view that they were incapable of having human feelings.

Disinhibiting Violence Through Dehumanization and Depersonalization

Although the preceding discussion is focused on formal dehumanization in a social context, it is important to understand the informal process of dehumanization that occurs within individuals on a personal level. Grossman's (1995) classic book on the process of disinhibiting violence discussed this issue in terms of social distancing. Grossman suggested that most individuals have an instinctive aversion to committing violence and are further socialized not to harm others throughout their childhood. Grossman presented the techniques of social distancing from his perspective as a military psychologist. Military methods commonly employ social distancing, which allow the individual to see his or her prospective target as less than fully human. Stereotyping the enemy as inhuman and lacking human feelings allows people to overcome their natural aversion to doing harm.

Ressler and Schactman (1992) explored the phenomenon of depersonalization and social distancing from the perspective of a criminal profiler. They described how many violent criminals cover the faces of their victims, stop their victims from telling their names or relating other simple personal details, and take other steps to assist themselves in viewing their victims as anonymous objects rather than fellow human beings. Thus, depersonalization and denial of the victims' suffering are critical steps in constructing the belief system necessary to permit their crimes. In turn, the actual crime and brutalization of the victims may further transform the victims into dehumanized objects and further reduce inhibition.

Bioethicist Peter Singer, in raising the proposition that "killing a defective infant is not morally equivalent to killing a person" (1979, p. 138), appears to be making a limited statement about medical ethics. It is important to note, however, that this statement bases the denial of the most fundamental human right, the right to life, on a presumption of nonpersonhood based on the infant's defect or disability. Thus, any crime committed against such an individual would also be a lesser crime or conceivably not a crime at all. If we accept Singer's statement about infants with severe disabilities, we implicitly accept that torturing a child or an adult with severe disabilities is also a lesser offense.

By the 1960s, the notion that pain insensitivity and indifference was widespread among people with severe developmental disabilities was clearly being threatened by growing scientific evidence. The growing human rights and advocacy movements that followed World War II also challenged these beliefs. The old beliefs would not die easily, but the statements became more restrained and qualified. Penrose provides a typical example:

> On the whole, psychophysical tests show rather low correspondence with scholastic capacity. For example, Bagley (1900) found the quickness of motor reaction had a negative relationship to success in school. Sensitivity to pain, however, showed a positive correlation to intelligence. This observation agrees with the finding that some idiots, though by no means all, seem to take pleasure in hitting their heads or limbs against hard objects or even in having their teeth extracted. (1963, p. 36)

The notion of pain insensitivity in people with developmental disabilities was an integral part of dehumanizing them and of rationalizing their abuse and neglect. It displaced the blame for brutality from the perpetrators to the victims. For example, in 1912, when a nurse at the much-lauded Vineland Home for Feeble-Minded Children scalded a 17-year-old to death in the shower, she was "exonerated" and kept her job because it was determined that "the fact that the youth was scalded escaped attention because the boy suffered from chronic anesthesia and was not susceptible to pain" ("Nurse's Error Kills Boy," 1912, p. 6). Whether the young man who was scalded to death actually had some rare pain insensitivity, of course, is irrelevant to the issue of neglect. If he did, it certainly would have been known by the time that he was 17; the simplest and most basic safety procedures require only that the person giving the shower tries the water on her or his own skin, and skin color changes associated with being scalded to death are typically obvious. Nevertheless, this explanation places the problem on the pathology of the victim rather than the behavior of the staff.

DISABILITY AS EXTREME SUFFERING

The prevalence of the notion of pain insensitivity among people with developmental disabilities has not precluded other constructs of pain in this population. People with developmental disabilities also have been portrayed as experiencing extreme pain and suffering. These constructs were less dehumanizing because they attributed human feelings to people with disabilities, but they were often equally unrealistic to the other extreme, attributing unbearable suffering to individuals with severe disabilities. These individuals were—and sometimes are—still viewed as humans, but such miserable and suffering humans that they would be better off dead:

> The boy whom Greenfield, a 45-year-old milliner, killed last Jan 12, had deteriorated into an imbecile who could not walk, talk, or feed himself. He suffered constant pain and frequent convulsions and Greenfield said that the "voice of God" came to him during one of his many troubled nights and told him to end the boy's suffering. ("Mercy Killers Freed," 1939, p. 5)

Although this notion of incredible pain and suffering seems clearly mutually exclusive with the previous description of insensitivity or indifference to pain, these two ideas have been combined in some descriptions:

> Here we have a young creature who is unable to feed herself, or to carry out the natural functions, who for all intents was a vegetable. But a vegetable which is in continual pain. (Hardin, 1994, p. A9)

In this view, people with developmental disabilities are seen as vegetative, by definition demonstrating only reflexive response to stimuli and having no conscious perception of pain, and at the same time as suffering excessively from pain. This construct has commonly been associated with calls for mercy killing or euthanasia of people with developmental disabilities, but the rationale is distinctly different from Hoche's or Singer's previously cited views that these people can be killed with impunity because they are not really alive or not really persons. Whereas Hoche argued that we must not pity them, the excessive suffering view demands pity for them and creates from that pity a foundation for their death. This humanitarian or altruistic rationale for killing people with developmental disabilities probably represents a greater threat than the utilitarian arguments. Whereas the utilitarian argument professes that it is permissible to hurt or kill because nothing of value is lost, the humanitarian argument professes that it is both heroic and morally necessary to kill to eliminate suffering.

Considering this view, it is not surprising that there was a considerable outpouring of popular support for the freeing of Greenfield, or that other parents might be influenced by Greenfield's act and the public response. Louis Repouille, who killed his 13-year-old son who had severe developmental disabilities shortly thereafter, also claimed he did so to end the pain of his "long suffering son" ("Turns against husband," 1939, p. 13), citing Greenfield as his inspiration and expressing anger that he was not so quickly exonerated. Repouille's wife claimed that the killing was actually her husband's way of punishing her for defying his demand that she stop drinking beer ("Turns against husband," 1939, p. 13). Nevertheless, the popular media generally ignored this possibility and reported the story as "a new test of a father's right to slay his imbecilic son" ("Slays imbecile son," 1939, p. 4), inviting readers to consider such acts as altruistic. In the end, the court provided a strong negative opinion about the notion of killing one's child to end suffering. Judge Jonah Goldstein spoke of the "grave danger" associated with this kind of killing, which "has become associated in the public mind with that, on certain occasions, it is an act of mercy" ("Father goes free," 1941, p. 44). In spite of Judge Goldstein's stern words, however, he gave Repouille a suspended sentence.

Although the construct of killing one's own child as an act of altruism or beneficence has been linked closely to so-called mercy killings of children with disabilities, this rationale is a construct that is actually employed by a much larger group of homicidal parents. Resnick (1969) was among the first to explore the motivations of parents who killed their children. He found that approximately half of parents claimed—and appeared to actually believe, at least to some extent—that they killed their children for altruistic reasons, sparing them from "greater harm." Subsequent studies (e.g., Marleau, Poulin, Webanck, Roy, & Laporte, 1999) have generally supported the belief that this motivation is among the most common. These parents may kill their children after convincing themselves that they are protecting their offspring from poverty, discrimination, abuse, ostracism, communism, homosexuality, drug addiction, or the presumed negative influence of an estranged parent. Constructing the belief system that is required to generate the altruistic motivation appears to be a critical element in overcoming strong natural inhibitions against killing one's own child.

Although these altruistic rationales for killing one's own children appear to be the same in parents who kill children with and without disabilities, the public, professional, and legal responses to this common rationale seem strikingly different. For example, in the highly publicized drowning of her two sons by a South Carolina mother, the mother's confession stated that she felt that children suffered greatly from the breakdown of families. She knew this from personal experience because she had been sexually abused by her stepfather. To save her children from suffering through her own divorce, she killed them. In another high-profile Texas case, the mother who drowned her children claimed that she did so to save them from the miserable lives they would have growing up with a depressed, mentally unstable mother. The public and legal response to both these mothers was decisive. They were considered to be either delusional or dishonest and received harsh sentences. No ethicist debated whether these might have been heroic acts of compassion. No petitions were signed to change the law to allow parents like these discretion to determine when their children were better off dead.

There is little doubt that children typically do suffer when parents divorce and when parents have serious mental health problems, but no one seriously believes that the compassionate response to their suffering is death. Why is disability any different? On November 7, 1994, in a small courtroom in North Battleford, Saskatchewan, the murder trial commenced for a 41-year-old farmer accused of poisoning his 12-year-old daughter with carbon monoxide. In spite of considerable physical evidence and a confession, his plea was not guilty. The defense argued that Robert Latimer killed his daughter Tracy, who had severe physical and mental disabilities, because it was the only possible way he could end her constant and excruciating pain. Although the prosecution and defense agreed that Mr. Latimer ended his daughter's life, the focus of the trial shifted to a number of other questions. What was the quality of Tracy Latimer's life? Was she experiencing pain and suffering? Was the pain she experienced unbearable and unremitting? Were there more appropriate alternatives available to manage any pain that she experienced?

Ultimately, an endless parade of questions boiled down to two fundamental issues. First, was Tracy Latimer better off dead than continuing to live as an adolescent with severe physical disability and a partially dislocated hip? Second, could it be that the lives of some people with very severe and multiple disabilities are truly lives not worth living, or *lebensunwertes leben*, as it has sometimes been suggested (see Loewy & Loewy, 1999)? The 1994 trial was only the first in a series of trials, appeals, and retrials debating these questions that would finally end in the upholding of a second-degree murder conviction, after a second hearing of the case by the Supreme Court of Canada in 2000. Throughout the six sets of courtroom proceedings, judges and juries struggled to understand the pain experience of a child who never could describe her sensations or feelings in words.

The public and the mass media seemed anxious to provide their own opinions about Tracy Latimer's life and pain. During the more than 5 years of courtroom proceedings, more than 2,000 newspaper articles were published about the case, along with countless stories on radio and television. Although the courts decided that the killing of Tracy Latimer constituted murder and must be punished, at least by the minimal sentence for that crime, the general population was more inclined to see the actions of this father as justifiable, necessary, or even heroic. A poll of Canadians shortly after the final Supreme Court decision, for example, indicated that 75% believed that the mandatory minimum 10-year sentence was too harsh and that Mr. Latimer should be released (Parker, 2001). Missing from the trial was any scientific or clinical evidence about the assessment or treatment of pain in people with developmental disabilities.

Exaggerated portrayals of people with developmental disabilities as suffering excessively from pain or other unpleasant conditions continue today. Of course, they do suffer from pain, sometimes more than their share, but their pain can be assessed and managed with about the same effectiveness as anyone else's pain. These exaggerated portrayals of pain provoke pity, but this pity rarely results in meaningful efforts to address their needs and sometimes provides a rationale for their elimination. In part, the lack of meaningful efforts to assess and manage their pain stems from inherent issues in their communication skills. It also stems from their lack of empowerment and a general disinterest in meeting their needs. In part, it stems from our tendency to view their suffering as such an essential characteristic of the individual that it cannot be eliminated without eliminating them.

PAIN AS A TEACHING TOOL

"Thou did'st beat my back and the instructions went in my ear." Simmons and Lovaas (1969, p. 25) attributed this brief quotation to ancient Egyptian sources, demonstrating the long-standing knowledge that pain is a powerful tool for manipulating human behavior. In spite of this long-standing knowledge, the infliction of pain as a consequence for undesirable behavior (punishment) or an inducement for desirable behavior (negative reinforcement) is generally considered immoral in modern civilization. In contemporary Western society, inflicting pain on criminals, prisoners of war, children, and other vulnerable adults is generally considered immoral and illegal. At best, it is considered a "necessary evil" or "last resort" that may be used reluctantly to prevent some more catastrophic outcome. This notion of using the infliction of pain as a "last resort" in educating children is not entirely new; for example, it was clearly expressed by the 18th-century philosopher Immanuel Kant (1776/1995). Although there can be no doubt that violence and the infliction of pain remain common events in today's world, they are clearly considered immoral and frequently are hidden elements of our world (Turner, 2003).

The professional endorsement of the use of pain to modify the behavior of people with developmental disabilities represents a rare departure from the general trend. This endorsement can be followed from its early days in the 1960s through its peak in the 1970s, and its vestiges remain with us at the beginning of the 21st century. Although Lovaas, Schaeffer, and Simmons (1965) cited Solomon (1964) for the justification for inflicting pain on children and Risley (1968) for the development of electric shock procedures, their article, "Experimental Studies in Childhood Schizophrenia: Building Social Behavior in Autistic Children with Electric Shock," was a major influence endorsing the use of pain as a treatment tool for people with developmental disabilities. They described and presented examples of "three ways that pain can be used therapeutically" (p. 99). First, pain could be used as punishment. Second, by inflicting pain until the child did what the therapist wanted and then ceasing to inflict pain, the therapist could use pain as a negative reinforcer. Finally, pain could be associated with other stimuli, so that the other secondary stimuli took on some of the power of pain to control behavior. Although Lovaas and his colleagues recognized objections to the infliction of pain on children, they dismissed them as having "a moral rather than scientific basis" (1965, p. 99) and therefore having little merit:

> Obviously, the use of techniques such as this [inflicting pain] by care-taking personnel are contrary to the basic concepts of care-taking, and, thus, make it im-

possible for some people to utilize it, since it presents a considerable conflict. This conflict alone, however, should not be the determining factor in whether pain is or is not used, rather one should rely on the experimental evidence which shows the uses and limitations of the technique. (Simmons & Lovaas, 1969, p. 34)

Although the academic publications on the use of pain as a teaching tool had some significant appeal, mass media coverage of this technique undoubtedly increased public interest. *Life* magazine's ("Screams, Slaps and Love," 1965) feature story described "a surprising, shocking treatment," with photos of a young boy with autism receiving a sharp slap in the face for not paying attention to his therapist. The article explains that, when yelling, shaking, and slapping were not sufficient to produce the required level of anxiety to gain compliance, more severe measures were taken. The article includes pictures of a child named Pamela in her bare feet. "To give her something to be anxious about, she was taken to the shock room, where the floor is laced with metallic strips. Two electrodes were placed on her bare back, and her shoes were removed" (p. 90). The shock room was described as the "last resort" for changing the behavior of "mentally crippled children" (p. 87). The apparent success of these techniques with children with autism was accompanied by the application of similar techniques to others. For example, electric shock was reported as a useful tool for teaching people with intellectual disabilities to name pictures and to eliminate rocking behavior. Occasionally, these electric shock and other aversive procedures were applied to people without developmental disabilities. For example, Cotter (1967) acknowledged Lovaas's work with autistic children as the essential influence in the development of his program using contingent electric shock and food deprivation on inmates of a Vietnamese mental hospital.

Interestingly, some of the proponents of using contingent shock reported that a significant obstacle was that some therapists found it difficult or even impossible to inflict pain on children. Risley (1968), for example, noted that the therapists who were required to administer shocks to children were reported to flush and tremble. In some cases, therapists overcame their reluctance to inflict pain on children; others had to be replaced by therapists who were less reluctant to hurt children. Risley stated that the child who received the shock "recovered from the shock episodes much faster than the experimenter" (1968, p. 25). Lichtstein and Schreibman (1976) agreed that we needed to be more concerned about the effects on those inflicting the pain than the effects on those on whom the pain was inflicted. They felt that this strong reluctance on the part of staff to hurt the people that they worked with might make it more difficult to provide effective programs. They did, however, discuss the alternative. If the successful implementation of shock programs required the employment of staff who were less reluctant to inflict pain or the modification of staff attitudes and behavior to make them more willing to inflict pain, how would that affect the welfare of children or adults who were the recipients of these services? How would the modeling of professional staff inflicting pain on clients affect the interactions of other caregivers with these clients? In fact, a later study systematically compared the happiness and job satisfaction of therapists who inflicted pain and applied other aversive stimuli to people with developmental disabilities. The authors concluded that staff members permitted to slap, pinch, pull the hair of, administer noxious odors and liquids to, and apply electric shocks to people with developmental disabilities enjoyed their work and experienced less stress than those who were not allowed to do so (Harris, Handleman, Gill, & Fong, 1991).

Although the use of pain as a teaching tool was always the subject of controversy, the open endorsement of the practice by professionals and the popular media continued in the 1970s. In a 1974 interview accompanied by a laudatory sidebar describing him as a "poet with a cattle prod" (p. 77), Lovaas continued to describe electric shock and slapping as essential treatment tools. He and his colleagues (Lovaas, Schreibman, & Koegel, 1974) continued to support these methods in the professional literature, providing the rationale that inflicting pain was absolutely necessary to saving children from self-injury, meaningless lives, or some other greater harm.

This argument of necessity or *force majeure* is one that permits acts that might otherwise be inappropriate or criminal in situations in which they are committed to prevent a greater harm. Breaking into a neighbor's home would ordinarily be a crime, but breaking into the same home if it is necessary to save the neighbor because the home is burning is a *force majeure* exception that is legally permitted because it prevents a greater harm. Similarly, although inflicting pain upon a child is generally considered immoral and in some cases criminal, it may be permitted if it prevents greater harm and there is no less harmful alternative available. Inflicting pain as a treatment tool thus requires two elements to be considered acceptable. First, there must be a reasonable expectation that it produces a benefit or prevents a harm that is greater than the harm it produces. Second, there must be no reasonable alternative to inflicting pain that would accomplish the same benefit or avoidance of harm. Whether these standards can be met in the case of slapping and shocking children or adults with developmental disabilities has been and remains a highly contested issue. Although many researchers and clinicians have repudiated the use of pain as a teaching tool (e.g., Stainton, 1988), others continued to defend its use as a necessary evil that does more good than harm. It is important to keep in mind that the purpose of this chapter is not to attempt to determine whether inflicting pain is necessary, but rather to explore the ways people have thought and written about pain in people with developmental disabilities.

In this regard, it is sufficient to point out that the use of pain and other aversive stimuli was always the subject of controversy and criticism, but by the middle to late 1970s, the weight of public opinion was increasingly critical of the use of inflicting pain. This growing rejection of the legitimacy of pain as a teaching tool came from two distinct perspectives. One perspective raised ethical and human rights issues about the use of painful procedures. The widespread influence of the normalization principle, which suggested that people with developmental disabilities be viewed and treated like other citizens, was a powerful force in raising these issues. Stanley Kubrick's (1971) award winning film, *A Clockwork Orange*, brought Anthony Burgess's (1963) powerful statement against aversive treatments into mainstream public consciousness. While the human rights and ethical perspectives frequently viewed all behavioral therapy, not just aversive treatments, as problematic, another critical perspective against aversives was developing within the heart of behavioral psychology. A group of leading figures in behaviorism was raising questions about whether inflicting pain was necessary and whether inflicting pain did more harm than good.

As early as the 1963, for example, Azrin, Hutchinson, and Hake demonstrated that using electric shock as an aversive stimulus produced aggression in previously nonaggressive animals. By 1977, Hutchinson's review of the harm done by the use of aversives provided a much longer list of problems, such as the unintended suppression of desirable responses and the reduced power of other forms of correction to influence behavior. By the 1980s, many researchers and clinicians were reaching a consensus that inflicting pain was rarely if ever justified and usually did more harm than good (e.g., Sobsey, 1987; The Association for the Severely Handicapped [TASH], 1981). TASH, a large international organization advocating for people with severe disabilities, passed a resolution in October of 1981 "to affirm the rights of people with disabilities to receive interventions that are respectful, free of pain and produce positive change for the individuals" and condemning the use of methods considered inappropriate when applied to other members of society. Of course, this did not mean that everyone rejected the use of pain as a teaching tool, but most who continued to advocate the use of aversive treatments changed the way that they communicated about treatments. Where the use of painful stimuli was often emphasized in the 1960s and 1970s, it seemed to be decidedly deemphasized in the 1980s and 1990s through the use of positive behavioral supports.

In this regard, it is clear that the ways we have discussed inflicting pain on people with disabilities changed substantially in the 1980s and 1990s. One of the clearest examples of this change has been demonstrated in the retrospective interest in the original Lovaas studies. Lovaas (1987) and McEachin, Smith, and Lovaas (1993) both provided long-term follow-up data of the children treated in "Lovaas programs." These long-term outcome studies suggested dramatic improvements in the children, but provided remarkably little information about what treatment they received. The article by McEachin et al. (1993) tells readers only that the treatment was "40 or more hours per week of one-to-one behavioral treatment" (p. 361). If readers want to know more exactly what the treatment consisted of, they are referred to Lovaas's (1987) description. However, there are no details of the treatment included in this article either. Instead, readers are referred to yet another source, *Teaching Developmentally Disabled Children: The ME Book* (Lovaas, 1981), which is described as a procedure manual for the early intensive behavioral intervention (EIBI) program. However, *The ME Book* also fails to identify specific procedures. It is rather written as a general guide for parents and other caregivers of children with developmental disabilities, including but not limited to autism. More surprisingly, although the book does suggest that aversives may occasionally be required, it takes a much softer position than Lovaas espoused in the 1970s, the period in which this book is supposed to have acted as a kind of procedure book and the period in which the children included in the outcome study were treated. According to *The ME Book*, "if milder aversives don't work, try a swat on the rear" (p. 26), and "as for spankings and swats, only use as much force as is necessary to hurt a little bit and to cause some apprehension in the child" (p. 17). In contrast to his 1970s clear endorsement of electric shock to eliminate such behavior as failing to pay attention, Lovaas clearly advised against electric shock "unless the child's life is in danger" (1981, p. 27). By the time *The ME Book* was published in the early 1980s, the images of the "poet with a cattle prod" and the open endorsement of "inflicting pain" were no longer presented.

This should not be interpreted to say that Lovaas, other professionals, or society in general had necessarily abandoned the belief in pain as a teaching tool for children with developmental disabilities. Lovaas stated, "In the within subject studies that were reported, contingent aversives were isolated as one significant variable. It is therefore unlikely that treatment effects could be replicated without this component" (1987, p. 8). In fact, Lovaas (1987) noted that, without slapping and other aversive interventions, EIBI did not produce significant improvements, but even without the other components of EIBI, slapping and other aversives rapidly reduced inappropriate behaviors and rapidly increased appropriate behaviors. However, the bold pronouncement that pain is a legitimate teaching tool had disappeared. Phrases such as "inflicting pain" and "contingent electric shock" have almost vanished, and the role of inflicting pain has clearly been recast from a critical feature of the program description to something so minor and incidental that it can be omitted entirely from the articles describing the effects of the program.

In her essay, "The Misbehaviour of Behaviourists," Dawson (n.d.) raised serious questions about ethics of behavior modification as applied to children and adults with autism. Writing from the perspective of an autistic woman who asserts her choice to be autistic, her concerns are much more broad than the use of aversives. One of the questions that she raised, however, is central to the way that we have discussed inflicting pain on people with autism and other developmental disabilities. Dawson (n.d.) asked, "Do autistics deserve ethics?" In asking this question, she invites us to examine how we have been able to consider them as somehow outside the ethical framework that we apply to other human beings. If the use of electric shock to coerce or punish the behavior of criminals or political prisoners is viewed as an unacceptable violation of human rights, why should the rights of adults or children with developmental disabilities have less protection? The arguments of necessity and the greater good can be made in every case. Might it be better to inflict some pain on criminals than to allow them to go on to commit greater crimes against innocent persons? Might not a few well-placed and well-timed electric shocks retrieve the cooperation of some enemy of the state that might prevent grave harm to thousands of others? The notion that it is in the best interest of the individual, or that the individual will later realize that it is in his or her best interest, might also be extended equally to all groups. Might not the criminal be thankful one day for the inflicted pain that set him or her on a better path? Might not the fascist once tortured into adopting democratic principles later express gratitude? Such arguments have been and will be made and occasionally acted upon in the future, but, as a society, we have found them unacceptable. As Dawson pointed out, the fact that there has been a double standard with which we have aggressively applied pain to people with developmental disabilities at a time in which it was considered unethical and immoral to apply it to others points to our failure to view people with developmental disabilities as human.

RETHINKING PAIN

As we entered the 21st century, we began to view people with developmental disabilities fully as human beings, complete with human feelings and human rights. This view is not entirely new, and it is not entirely complete. It has evolved over time, and vestiges of our old constructs remain. They include portrayals of people with developmental disabilities as subhuman creatures incapable of feelings, as victims of extreme suffering, or as potential humans who require us to inflict pain upon them to transform them to fully human status.

Even when these notions were predominant, there have always been a few people among us who questioned these dehumanizing characterizations. The classic American author, Willa Cather, for example, invoked the stereotype of people with developmental disabilities as insensitive to pain in developing her fictional character Marek. At the same time that she presented the insensitivity stereotype, however, she disputed its validity:

The crazy boy went with them, because he did not feel the cold. I believed he felt cold as much as anyone else, but he liked to be thought insensible to it. He was always coveting distinction, poor Marek! (Excerpt from MY ANTONIA by Willa Cather. Copyright 1918, 1926 by Willa Silbert Cather, renewed 1946 by Willa Cather Silbert; copyright © renewed 1954 by Edith Lewis. Reprinted by permission of Houghton Mifflin Company. All rights reserved.)

This chapter has attempted to pick up where Cather left off many years ago, considering and questioning some of the common ways that we as a society and as a group of professionals have constructed notions about pain in general and pain in people with developmental disabilities in particular.

Pain is one of the most fundamental and most private of human experiences. It is fundamental for at least four distinct but closely related reasons. First, pain is unique. It is a basic sensation that cannot be constructed by combining other sensory experiences. Second, pain is extremely influential. It shapes both individual behavior and the history of nations. Third, pain is virtually a universal experience. It is an element of life from cradle to grave. An individual who lacked any experience of pain throughout his or her life would be highly exceptional. Finally, pain, along with the closely related concept of suffering, has been frequently identified as a necessary component that defines the human experience.

Despite its universality and influence, however, pain remains intensely private. We cannot see, hear, feel, or otherwise sense another person's pain directly; although we may see its causes or effects, hear what others tell us about their pain, and imagine what it must feel like. One might say that as a society, we demonstrate a remarkable ability to tolerate pain and suffering, as long as it is not our own. A number of studies have demonstrated that professionals tend to deny or disregard pain and suffering of members of racial and ethnic minorities (e.g., Todd, Deaton, D'Adamo, & Goe, 2000). Bonham suggested that this constitutes a form of health care racism:

> The studies [reviewed in this paper] as a body of research paint the clear picture that one's race and ethnicity matter in the treatment of pain. The common thread is that there are empirical data indicating differences in pain treatment based on the patient's racial and ethnic background. (2001, p. 60)

> The experience of racism in the every day lives of people is pervasive. It is a part of our unconscious and conscious lives to treat people who look or speak differently as in fact different from those who look or speak like ourselves. The majority of the time, the disparity in how we treat people is only a demonstration of our ignorance. However, health care is an area where this ignorance can cause potentially life-threatening outcomes. (p. 65)

This book is a testament to the new scientific interest in assessing and treating pain in people with developmental disabilities. It would be unfair and inaccurate to view these new developments as solely the result of our social attitudes and beliefs about people with developmental disabilities. Nevertheless, it would be equally misleading to see these developments as solely the outcomes of science and somehow outside the social context. The last half of the 20th century produced a growing trend toward empowerment, normalization, and inclusion. As we began to view people with disabilities as fellow humans with feelings and needs similar to our own, we could no longer maintain the fictions of insensitivity to pain or exaggerated suffering. We also found it much more difficult to justify pain as a teaching tool for people with disabilities when we had rejected its use as a teaching tool for others on moral grounds.

Science is a tool, never an end in itself. It can be powerful. It can be used for the betterment or detriment of mankind, and even for the betterment or detriment of specific groups and individuals within society. How we use it is a matter of choice, and our choices are always based in our values and beliefs. We have only recently embarked on the scientific quest to identify and treat pain more effectively. How we will accomplish this is a scientific issue. Why we have chosen this quest is an ethical one. In part, this quest became possible and became necessary when we began to see people with disabilities as fellow human beings, as "us" rather than "them." As we made that transition, legends such as insensitivity and indifference to pain were no longer viable as we were forced to ask, *whose insensitivity, whose indifference, and whose pain?* Looking back, it seems obvious it was all of us who were insensitive and indifferent to the pain of people with developmental disabilities. Looking forward, we can change that.

REFERENCES

Affairs at Gettysburgh. (1863, July 18). *New York Times,* p. 2.

Anand, K.J.S., & Hickey, P.R. (1987). Pain and its effects in the human neonate and fetus. *New England Journal of Medicine, 317,* 1321–1329.

Azrin, N., Hutchinson, R.R., & Hake, D.F. (1963). Pain induced fighting in the squirrel monkey. *Journal of Experimental Analysis of Behavior, 6,* 620.

Bagley, W.C. (1900). On the correlation of mental and motor ability in children. *American Journal of Psychology, 12,* 193.

Biersdorff, K.K. (1991). Pain insensitivity and indifference: Alternative explanations for some medical catastrophes. *Mental Retardation, 29,* 359–362.

Biersdorff, K.K. (1994). Incidence of significantly altered pain experience among individuals with developmental disabilities. *American Journal of Mental Retardation, 98,* 619–631.

Bonham, V.L. (2001). Race, ethnicity, and pain treatment: Striving to understand the causes and solutions to the disparities in pain treatment. *Journal of Law, Medicine & Ethics, 24,* 52–68.

Breau, L.M., Camfield, C.S., McGrath, P.J., & Finley, G.A. (2003). The incidence of pain in children with severe cognitive impairments. *Archives of Pediatric and Adolescent Medicine, 157,* 1219–1226.

Burgess, A. (1963). *A clockwork orange.* New York: Norton.

Burleigh, M. (1994). *Death and deliverance: 'Euthanasia' in Germany 1900–1945.* Cambridge, UK: University of Cambridge Press.

Cather, W.S. (1919). *My Ántonia.* London: William Heinemann.

Cotter, L.H. (1967). Operant conditioning in a Vietnamese mental hospital. *American Journal of Psychiatry, 124,* 23-28.

Couston, T.A. (1954). Indifference to pain in low-grade mental defectives. *British Medical Journal, 1,* 1128-1129.

Davenport, C.B. (1911). *Heredity in relationship to eugenics.* New York: Henry Holt.

Dawson, M. (n.d.). *The misbehaviour of behaviourists.* Retrieved May 28, 2005, from http://www.sentex.net/~nexus23/naa_aba.html

Descartes, R. (1968). *Discourse on methods and meditations.* London: Penguin Books. (Original work published 1641)

Deutsch, A. (1949). *The mentally ill in America: A history of their care and treatment from colonial times.* New York: Columbia University Press.

Father goes free in mercy slaying. (1941, December 25). *New York Times,* p. 44.

Fletcher, J. (1972). Indicators of humanhood: A tentative profile of man. *Hastings Center Report, 2*(5), 1–4.

Galton, F. (1907). *Inquiries into human faculty and its development* (2nd ed.). London: J.M. Dent & Son. (Retrieved December 15, 2004, from Project Gutenberg, http://www.gutenberg.org/dirs/1/1/5/6/11562/11562-h/11562-h.htm)

Goodey, C., & Stainton, C.F. (2001). Intellectual disability and the myth of the changeling myth. *Journal of the History of the Behavioral Sciences, 37*, 223–240.

Grossman, D. (1995). *On killing.* Boston: Little, Brown.

Hardin, S.J. (1994, November 26). Case cries out for mercy. *Edmonton Journal*, p. A9.

Harris, S.L., Handleman, J.S., Gill, M.J., & Fong, P.L. (1991). Does punishment hurt? The impact of aversives on the clinician. *Research in Developmental Disabilities, 12*, 17–24.

Hauerwas, S. (1986). Suffering the retarded: Should we prevent retardation? In P. Dokecki & R. Zaner (Eds.), *Ethics of dealing with persons with severe handicaps* (pp. 53–70). Baltimore: Paul H. Brookes Publishing.

Howe, S.G. (1848/1976). On the causes of idiocy: Report of Commission to Inquire into the Conditions of Idiots of the Commonwealth of Massachusetts. Boston: State Senate Document No. 51. Reprinted in M. Rosen, G.R. Clark, & M.S Kivitz. The history of mental retardation: Collected papers (vol 1, pp. 31-60). Baltimore: University Park Press.

Hutchinson, R.R. (1977). By products of aversive control. In W.K. Honig & J.E.R. Staddon (Eds.), *Handbook of operant behavior* (pp. 415–431). Englewood Cliffs, NJ: Prentice Hall.

Insensibility of a Maori to pain. (1888, December 9). *New York Times*, p. 19.

Kant, I. (1995). Education (A. Churton, Trans.). In H. Ozman & S. Carver (Eds.), *Philosophical foundations of education* (6th ed., pp. 45-48). Upper Saddle River, NJ: Merrill. (Original published in 1776)

Kubrick, S. (Producer & Director). (1971). *A clockwork orange* [Motion picture]. United States: Warner Bothers.

Lichtstein, K.I., & Schreibman, L. (1976). Employing electric shock with autistic children: A review of side effects. *Journal of Autism and Developmental Disability, 6*, 163–173.

Loewy, E.H., & Loewy, R.S. (1999). Lebensunwertes leben and the obligation to die: Does the obligation to die rest on a misunderstanding of community? *Health Care Analysis, 7*(1), 23–36.

Lovaas, I. (Interviewed by P. Chance). (1974, January). "After you hit a child, you can't just get up and leave him; you are hooked on that kid": A conversation with Ivar Lovaas about self-mutilating children and how their parents make it worse. *Psychology Today*, pp. 76–84.

Lovaas, I. (1981). *Teaching developmentally disabled children: The ME book.* Baltimore: University Park Press.

Lovaas, O.I. (1987). Behavioral treatment and normal educational and intellectual functioning in young autistic children. *Journal of Consulting and Clinical Psychology, 55*, 3–9.

Lovaas, O.I., Schaeffer, B., & Simmons, J.Q. (1965). Experimental studies in childhood schizophrenia: Building social behaviors in autistic children with electric shock. *Journal of Experimental Research in Personality, 1*, 99–109.

Lovaas, O.I., Schreibman, L., & Koegel, R.L. (1974). A behavior modification approach to the treatment of autistic children. *Journal of Autism and Child Schizophrenia, 4*, 111–129.

Luther, M. (1886). *Colloquia mensalia: Dr. Martin Luther's divine discourses at his table.* London: Cassell & Co. (Original published in 1652)

Marleau, J.D., Poulin, B., Webanck, T., Roy, R., & Laporte, L. (1999). Paternal filicide: A study of 10 men. *Canadian Journal of Psychiatry, 44*, 57–63.

McEachin, J.J., Smith, T., & Lovaas, O.I. (1993). Long-term outcome for children with autism who received early intensive behavioral treatment. *American Journal of Mental Retardation, 97*, 359–372.

Mercy killers freed by jury; To adopt child. (1939, May 12). *The Freeport Journal Standard*, p. 5.

Nagasako, E.M., Oaklander, A.L., & Dworkin, A.H. (2003). Congenital insensitivity to pain: An update. *Pain, 101,* 213–219.

Nurse's error kills boy. (1912, May 24). *New York Times,* p. 6.

Ohlin, J.D. (2004). Is the concept of the person necessary for human rights? *Columbia Law Review, 105,* 208–249.

Parker, J. (2001, January 19). Lawyer appeals to justice minister for pardon: Latimer the victim of a terrible injustice, Brayford says. *Star-Phoenix* [Saskatoon, Saskatchewan, Final Edition], p. A3.

Penrose, L.S. (1963). *The biology of mental defect.* London: Sidgwick and Jackson.

Physical sensibility in women. (1892, March 20). *New York Times,* p. 4

Post, L.F., Blustein, J., Gordon, E., & Dubler, N.N. (1996). Pain: Ethics, culture, and informed consent to relief. *Journal of Law, Medicine & Ethics, 24,* 348–359.

Resnick, P.J. (1969). Child murder by parents: A psychiatric review of filicide. *American Journal of Psychiatry, 126,* 325–334.

Ressler, R.K. & Schactman, T. (1992). Whoever fights monsters. New York: St. Martin's Press.

Risley, T. (1968). The effects and "side effects" of the use of punishment with an autistic child. *Journal of Applied Behavior Analysis, 1,* 21–34.

Ryan, J., & Thomas, F. (1987). *The politics of mental handicap* (Rev. ed.). London: Free Association Books.

Screams, slaps and love: A surprising, shocking treatment that helps far gone mental cripples. (1965, May 7). *Life,* pp. 87-97.

Simmons, J.Q., & Lovaas, O.I. (1969). The use of pain and punishment with childhood schizophrenics. *American Journal of Psychotherapy, 23,* 23–36.

Singer, P. (1979) *Practical ethics.* Cambridge, UK: Cambridge University Press.

Singer, P. (2000). *Writings on an ethical life.* New York: Harper Collins.

Slays imbecile son. (1939, October 19). *The Zanesville Signal,* p. 4.

Sobsey, D. (1987, November). Non-aversive behavior management: The verdict is in! *Newsletter of the American Association on Mental Retardation, 1*(2), 2, 6.

Sobsey, D. (1994). *Violence and abuse in the lives of people with disabilities: The end of silent acceptance?* Baltimore: Paul H. Brookes Publishing.

Solomon, R.L. (1964). Punishment. *American Psychologist, 19,* 239–253.

Stainton, T. (1988). Aversive conditioning: Necessity of failure? In The G. Allan Roeher Institute (Ed.), *The language of pain: Perspectives on behavior management* (pp. 15–34). Downsview, ON: The G. Allan Roeher Institute.

Stengel, E., Oldham, A.J., & Ehernberg, A.S.C. (1955). Reactions to pain in various abnormal mental states. *Journal of Mental Science, 101,* 52–69.

Stengel, E., Oldham, A.J., & Ehernberg, A.S.C. (1958). Reactions of low-grade mental defectives to pain. *Journal of Mental Science, 104,* 434–438.

The Association for Persons with Severe Handicaps (TASH). (1981). *TASH resolution on positive behavioral supports.* Retrieved September 7, 2005, from http://www.tash.org/resolutions

Todd, K.H., Deaton, C., D'Adamo, A.P., & Goe, L. (2000). Ethnicity and analgesic practice. *Annals of Emergency Medicine, 35,* 11–16.

Turner, S.M. (2003). Justifying corporal punishment loses its appeal. *The International Journal of Children's Rights, 11,* 219–233.

Turns against husband in 'mercy murder.' (1939, October 13). *Mansfield News Journal,* p. 13.

Vail, D.J. (1967). *Dehumanization and the institutional career.* Springfield, IL: Charles C Thomas.

Wolfensberger, W. (1969). The origin and nature of our institutional models. In R.B. Kugel & W. Wolfensberger (Eds.), *Changing patterns in residential services for the mentally retarded* (pp. 59–172). Washington, DC: The President's Committee on Mental Retardation.

4

OVERVIEW OF PAIN MECHANISMS

Neuroanatomical and Neurophysiological Processes

Lois J. Kehl and Gary Goldetsky

The purpose of this chapter is to provide an overview of current knowledge regarding basic neurobiological and neuropsychological processes involved in pain transmission and modulation at the cellular and systems levels. The majority of knowledge regarding mechanisms of pain transmission and modulation is derived from animal studies and research using *in vitro* preparations. Because of the difficulty involved in studying the physiology of pain processes in humans, fewer studies of this type exist. Methods used in human studies include quantitative sensory testing following administration of experimental pain (e.g., hot and cold temperatures, pressure, pinch), functional magnetic resonance imaging (fMRI) studies, and drug clinical trials. Studies to investigate pain perception have only recently begun with individuals with developmental disabilities. Consequently, little is currently known regarding alterations in physiological pain processes that may be associated with different forms of developmental disabilities.

The first part of this chapter provides a basic foundation in the neurobiology of pain mechanisms. The second part of the chapter integrates our knowledge regarding basic pain mechanisms into the context of current research findings that bear special significance to practitioners treating pain in individuals with developmental disabilities. Hopefully, this discussion will provide some appreciation for the connection and interaction of neuropsychological and neurobiological processes that contribute to pain perception. With new information continuing to emerge, the exact boundary between psychological factors and neurobiological factors is becoming blurred, causing the disciplines of pain management, neuroscience, and clinical psychology to evolve, mature, and perhaps eventually merge.

PAIN TRANSMISSION:
BASIC NEUROBIOLOGIC CONCEPTS, PATHWAYS, AND MODULATION

Primary Afferent Terminals

The sensory division of the somatic nervous system provides us with information about our internal and external environments. One important protective aspect of this role is to alert us to noxious stimuli in the environment that may harm or injure us. For the majority of people, noxious stimuli evoke the sensation of pain.

When we sense pain, reflex pathways are activated, and we instinctively withdraw from the painful stimulus. In this way we protect our tissues from further injury. *Nociception* is the term used to describe the perception of noxious or painful stimuli. In a few rare individuals with congenital insensitivity to pain, a mutation of the nerve growth factor receptor tyrosine kinase A results in repeated self-injury (Miranda et al., 2002). It is currently unknown whether this also contributes to self-injurious behavior in individuals with developmental disabilities.

Detection of all types of sensation, including pain, requires an intact nervous system linking the peripheral sensory nerve fibers that first detect stimuli to the somatosensory cortex and other cortical areas of the brain where this information is processed. Because peripheral sensory nerve fibers are the first link in the "chain" of nerves required for the transmission and perception of sensation, including pain, they are called *primary afferent* fibers. Primary afferent neurons have a bipolar morphology early in development that becomes unipolar with maturation. Unipolar neurons exhibit a short stem connecting the neuron's cell body to the main peripheral and central projections. Their cell bodies are located in the dorsal root ganglia at the level of the spinal cord and in the trigeminal (also called gasserion or semilunar) ganglia at the level of the head.

The first step in the process of detecting sensation is activation of specialized nerve endings, such as Pacinian corpuscles, which sense vibration, and Meissner corpuscles, which transmit tapping sensation, on the peripheral terminals of these fibers (Willis, 1985). Pain and temperature afferents do not have specialized receptors but rather have "free nerve endings" at their peripheral terminations (Byers & Bonica, 2001). *Free nerve endings* are unmyelinated and house vesicles containing neurotransmitters. When primary afferent neurons are depolarized as the result of tissue damage, these vesicles release neurotransmitters into the local area.

The pain that is perceived as the result of damage to free nerve endings is actually the consequence of substances released by damaged tissues, such as bradykinin, histamine, and nociceptive peptides. These activate receptor proteins (also called receptors) located on primary afferent fibers. *Receptors* are three-dimensional proteins embedded in the plasma membranes of sensory nerve fiber terminals in peripheral tissues such as skin, muscle, joints, and visceral organs. Many different receptor proteins exist. Each responds to specific stimulus modalities such as mechanical shearing forces, different temperature ranges, and various endogenous or exogenously applied chemicals. In the case of primary afferent nerve fibers that sense pain, the peripheral receptors are activated by noxious stimuli such as hard pressure or pinch, temperatures in the noxious hot or cold ranges, and certain chemicals. Noxious chemicals can be from the environment, such as acid or capsaicin (the compound that makes chili peppers hot), or can be substances released from damaged tissues. Examples of the latter include adenosine triphosphate (ATP) and excitatory amino acids, extruded from cytoplasm, and bradykinin, released from blood when blood vessels are torn by injury (Figure 4.1). Prostaglandins are quickly manufactured from cellular membranes as well. In response to activation by these noxious stimuli, a subset of primary afferent fibers called C fibers release the peptides substance P and calcitonin gene-related peptide (CGRP) from their peripheral terminals into the local area. Substance P and CGRP produce dilation and extravasation of the local vasculature that in turn promotes infiltration of inflammatory cells, mast cell degranulation, and release of histamine at the site of injury. The part of the inflammatory response initiated by substance P and CGRP release from primary afferent terminals is termed *neurogenic inflammation*.

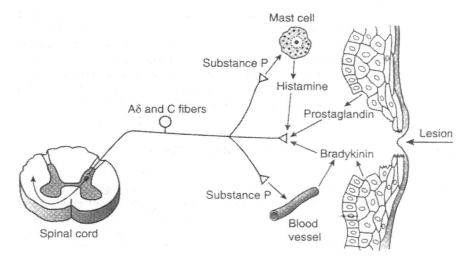

Figure 4.1. Peripheral sensitization. Tissue damage causes local cells to release bradykinin and prostaglandins, which excite nociceptive fibers and cause them to release substance P and other neuropeptides. Substance P causes histamine release and promotes vasodilation, effects that cause additional release of bradykinin. These chemical changes increase the sensitivity of nociceptive fibers to subsequent stimulation. (From Pritchard, T.C., & Alloway, K.D. [1999]. *Medical neuroscience* [p. 218]. Madison, CT: Fence Creek Publishing; reprinted by permission.)

Each receptor protein is associated with a membrane-spanning protein with a central pore that allows ions to move into or out of the cell. Under normal circumstances, the protein that forms the pore is configured in such a way as to prevent passage of ions into the cell from the extracellular space. When a stimulus that is able to activate the receptor is applied, the protein forming the pore deforms to allow positively charged ions such as Na^+ and Ca^{2+} into the cell, increasing the net charge inside the cell. The process whereby the pore opens and closes to allow ions to pass through is termed *gating*. Ion channels can be gated by changes in a cell's polarity (i.e., via voltage-gated ion channels) or by chemical compounds (i.e., via ligand-gated ion channels). The process whereby mechanical, thermal, and chemical stimuli are converted to electrical signals inside neurons is termed *transduction*.

Under normal circumstances, the inside of a neuron is electronegative (e.g., −70 mV), or *polarized*, with respect to the outside of the cell. When cations enter through peripheral terminal receptors, the polarity of the cell becomes electropositive (e.g., −25 mV), or *depolarized*, relative to the cell's resting membrane potential (−70 mV). Multiple receptors are typically activated when a stimulus is applied. If the depolarization that results from activation of these receptors exceeds a neuron's threshold for activation (e.g., typically in the range of −40 mV), action potentials can be generated, causing the electrical signal to be propagated along the length of the axon to the cell's body. When action potentials are generated in primary afferent neurons, their central terminals release neurochemicals from synaptic vesicles on presynaptic membranes into the synaptic cleft formed with second-order neurons in the spinal cord (Figure 4.2). These neurochemicals bind to and activate receptors on the postsynaptic membrane (i.e., the spinal cord neuron's membrane). The resulting ion flow into or out of the postsynaptic neuron results in excitation or inhibition. In this way, information is transmitted from the peripheral nervous system (PNS) to the central nervous system (CNS).

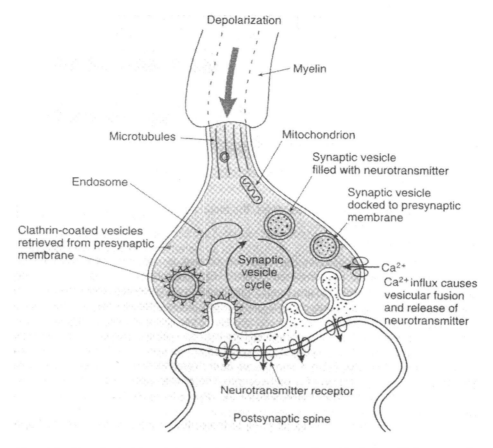

Figure 4.2. Neurochemical transmission. Depolarization causes synaptic vesicles to fuse with the presynaptic membrane and release their neurotransmitters. Although vesicles are originally produced in the soma and transported to the terminal by microtubules, segments of the presynaptic membrane are retrieved and recycled into synaptic vesicles by an endosome. (From Pritchard, T.C., & Alloway, K.D. [1999]. *Medical neuroscience* [p. 42]. Madison, CT: Fence Creek Publishing; reprinted by permission.)

Peripheral Sensory Nerve Types

Three types of sensory afferent nerve fibers are known to participate in pain transmission in the periphery. These are A-beta, A-delta, and C fibers. Under normal conditions, A-beta fibers are only activated by innocuous stimulation, but A-delta fibers are activated by both innocuous and noxious stimuli. Cell bodies associated with these two fiber types are generally considered to be large and light-staining when viewed through a microscope. Only noxious stimuli, such as those that produce pain, activate C fibers. The cell bodies for this type of sensory fiber are generally considered to be small and dark-staining when viewed microscopically. The best characterized type of C-nociceptive neurons are called C-polymodal nociceptors because they respond to more than one type of noxious stimulus (i.e., chemical, thermal, and mechanical).

Clinically and experimentally, these three fiber types are distinguished on the basis of their conduction velocities. Myelinated A-beta and thinly myelinated A-delta fibers have faster conduction velocities (A-beta: 30–70 m/sec; A-delta: 5–30 m/sec), whereas C fibers are unmyelinated and have slower conduction velocities (0.5–2.0 m/sec) (Byers & Bonica, 2001). The significance of these different primary afferent fiber types is that they are activated by and transmit different types of signals. For example, A-delta fibers signal "fast" pain, which is typically considered to have a sharp, prickly quality, whereas C fibers signal "slow pain" with a dull aching or burning quality (Chery-Croze, 1983).

Spinal and Trigeminal Organization

Second-order spinal cord neurons are organized into different layers called laminae. The significance of these layers of termination is that second-order neuronal cell bodies are organized into laminae according to certain characteristics such as function, the type or modality (i.e., mechanical, thermal) of input received, and the destination of their projection fibers. For example, the ventral (also called anterior) portion houses cell bodies of motor neurons that, when activated, cause muscle contraction, and the dorsal (also called posterior) half of the spinal cord receives primarily sensory input. Nociceptive primary afferent fibers (A-delta and C) from tissues at the spinal level enter the CNS via the dorsal roots (Figure 4.3). From there, they ascend a short distance in Lissauer's tract, the area of the white matter located between the dorsal horn and the spinal cord's surface. Many of these affer-

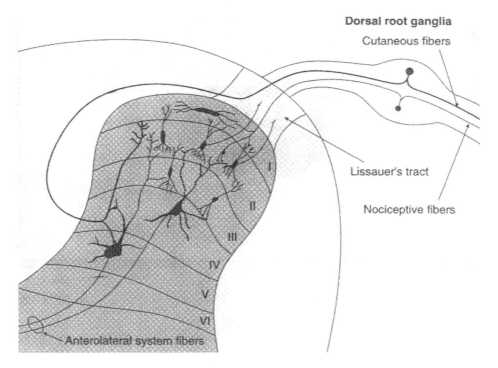

Figure 4.3. Cytoarchitecture of the dorsal horn. The dorsal horn is composed of Rexed laminae I–VI in which each layer is characterized by different types of neurons. Large- and small-diameter afferent fibers enter the cord through Lissauer's tract before diverging into medial and lateral groups. The larger fibers enter the medial side of the dorsal horn and terminate in laminae II, IV, and V, whereas the thin fibers enter laterally to terminate in laminae I, II, IV, and V. Laminae I, IV, and V contain projection neurons whose axons cross the midline before ascending into the lateral funiculus. (From Pritchard, T.C., & Alloway, K.D. [1999]. *Medical neuroscience* [p. 100]. Madison, CT: Fence Creek Publishing; reprinted by permission.)

ents branch extensively to terminate in multiple spinal laminae. Neurons located in the superficial dorsal horn (laminae I and II) are important players in the transmission of pain, whereas those in laminae III–IV function to transmit information about innocuous stimuli and proprioception. This organization can be seen when the tissue is prepared using specific histologic stains. For example, the most superficial laminae of spinal cord dorsal horn (laminae I and II) appear light and large motor neurons in the ventral horn appear dark in histologically stained tissue.

In the sensory nervous system, primary afferent fibers terminate in characteristic patterns on neurons in the spinal cord dorsal horn and the trigeminal nuclei. For example, A-delta fibers synapse on second-order neurons and interneurons in laminae I, IIo (the outer, or most dorsal, portion of lamina II), V, and X of the dorsal horn of the spinal cord. C nociceptors innervating somatic tissues (e.g., skin, joint, muscle) terminate primarily in lamina II. Visceral C fibers terminate in lamina V (Byers & Bonica, 2001). The larger A-beta fibers transmitting innocuous stimuli travel in the dorsal columns to synapse in laminae III–V of the spinal cord. Large sensory fibers that innervate specialized muscle-stretch receptors send collateral branches to laminae V–IX. The proximity of their central terminals to motor neurons in the ventral horn laminae VIII and IX allows for direct activation of muscles when stretch receptors are sufficiently activated. This pattern of connectivity forms the basis for monosynaptic reflexes such as the knee jerk reflex.

The trigeminal nerve provides the majority of sensation to the head and facial area, including the anterior two thirds of the tongue, the cornea, the teeth, the oral mucosa, and the dura mater of the anterior and middle cranial fossae. This nerve is divided into three branches that serve different regions of the skin: the ophthalmic (V1), maxillary (V2), and mandibular (V3) branches. The trigeminal nerve also has motor fibers that provide efferent activation of the muscles of mastication. Even though these sensory and motor peripheral fibers traverse the facial tissues together, they can serve both motor and sensory functions because they terminate in different areas of the brainstem.

The majority of trigeminal fibers entering the brainstem bifurcate into ascending and descending branches (Figure 4.4). The ascending branch synapses on neurons in the trigeminal main sensory nucleus. This nucleus mediates innocuous sensations such as touch from the face and oral structures. The descending branch travels in the spinal tract of the trigeminal nerve to terminate in the spinal nucleus of the trigeminal nerve. This nucleus is subdivided into three parts: the subnucleus oralis, subnucleus interpolaris, and subnucleus caudalis. Generally speaking, these laminae provide 1) intraoral and tactile inputs, 2) tactile and dental nociceptive inputs, and 3) nociception, respectively. Nociceptive A-delta and C fibers from the trigeminal ganglia terminate largely in the spinal subnucleus caudalis, but nociceptive afferents also terminate in the transition zone between interpolaris and caudalis.

Some central projections of cervical spinal afferents also ascend to terminate in the subnucleus caudalis. This overlapping of inputs from the cervical and trigeminal receptive fields provides an anatomical basis for the substantial interactions between these areas seen in clinical pain states. For example, pain is often referred from the neck to the head and vice versa. Like the spinal cord, the subnucleus caudalis is also organized in laminae. The spinal cord dorsal horn and subnucleus caudalis actually exist contiguously, with the former transitioning into the latter at the level of the second or third cervical segment. Given their similar-

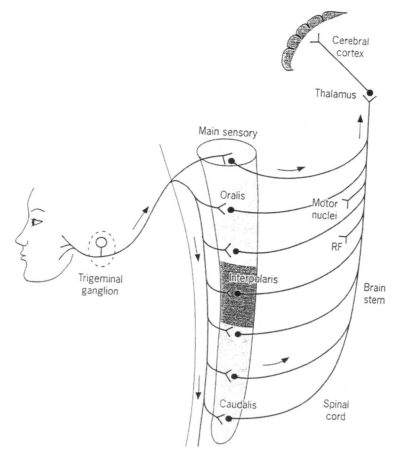

Figure 4.4. Major pathway transmitting sensory information from the face and mouth to the somatosensory areas of the cerebral cortex. The first synaptic relay of information from the face and mouth may conceivably occur on neurons at all levels of the trigeminal brainstem sensory nuclear complex. From the brainstem complex, sensory information may then be relayed directly to the thalamus and then to the cerebral cortex, or less directly by multisynaptic pathways involving, for example, the reticular formation (RF). The sensory information may also pass to other brainstem structures (e.g., cranial nerve motor nuclei involved in reflex responses to the sensory inputs from the face and mouth). (From Sessle, B.J. [1986]. Recent developments in pain research: Central mechanisms of orofacial pain and its control. *Journal of Endodontics, 12*, 435–444; copyright 1995; reprinted by permission from Elsevier.)

ities, the subnucleus caudalis (also called the medullary dorsal horn) and the spinal cord dorsal horn are considered to be homologous structures.

Individual neurons at all levels of the somatosensory nervous system are directly (i.e., dorsal root ganglia) or indirectly (i.e., spinal cord, thalamus, cortex) activated by stimulation from a discrete peripheral area (i.e., skin, muscle, joint, viscera). The specific area that is innervated by an individual neuron is called the *receptive field* for that neuron. Several areas of the nervous system important in pain transmission and modulation are organized topographically so that adjacent neurons have bordering receptive fields in the body. This topographic arrangement is called *somatotopic organization*. Somatotopic organization is an important feature of the nervous system that can be particularly important in understanding the presentation of certain clinical pain conditions. For example, second-order neurons in the subnucleus caudalis are somatotopically organized in such a way that those receiving innervation from the midline and around the mouth and nose are located in the most rostral part of the caudalis and those with progressively more lateral input are located more and more caudally. Consequently, a brainstem lesion affecting the rostral subnucleus caudalis could manifest itself as an area of altered pain sensation in the mouth, teeth, and nose. If an individual with this symptom presented clinically, the evaluating clinician would likely order a magnetic resonance imaging (MRI) scan to evaluate for this possibility. Somatotopic organization also exists in the dorsal column nuclei, ventral posterior lateral and medial thalamus, and somatosensory cortex. Generally speaking, very sensitive and densely innervated areas (e.g., mouth, hand) have disproportionately larger representations at higher levels (i.e., thalamus, cortex).

Spinal Cord and Trigeminal Pain Pathways

Second-order spinal cord neurons that participate in pain transmission and modulation have been classified into three types on the basis of the stimuli that they respond to and their apparent function. These types are nociceptive-specific neurons (NS), wide dynamic range neurons (WDR), and low-threshold (LT) neurons (Terman & Bonica, 2001). Nociceptive-specific neurons receive inputs mainly from primary afferent fibers that transmit pain (i.e., A-delta and C afferents). These neurons are located mainly in laminae I, IIo, V, and X. Collectively, laminae I and II are commonly referred to as the superficial dorsal horn. This region is considered to be very important in the transmission of pain at the spinal level. Lamina V contains primarily wide dynamic range neurons. These neurons respond more vigorously to nociceptive afferent inputs but are also activated in response to innocuous stimuli. Low-threshold neurons of the thermoreceptive type are activated by temperatures in the innocuous range and have cell bodies in the superficial dorsal horn as well. Low-threshold mechanoreceptive neurons respond to innocuous touch and are present thoughout the dorsal horn laminae with the exception of lamina I. Direct and indirect interactions among these different cell types both mediate and modulate pain transmission to supraspinal levels.

The *anterolateral system* is the name given to a group of ascending spinal pathways that conduct pain information. The most important and most widely studied of these is the *spinothalamic tract* (STT). The STT transmits pain and temperature as well as innocuous touch. This tract is composed principally of neurons with cell bodies located in laminae I, IV–VI, IX, and X (Terman & Bonica, 2001). Central projections of these cells cross to the other side of the spinal cord within one to two segments in the ventral white commissure, just ventral to the central canal, to ascend in the contralateral ventrolateral white matter (Figure 4.5).

Pain has both discriminative and arousal-emotional components. The discriminative and arousal-emotional aspects of these sensations are distinguished through the types of primary afferent fibers involved and the termination of the fibers carrying this information in different areas of the thalamus. The term *discriminative* refers to the ability of the affected individual to distinguish the type and nature of the injury, including localization of the painful stimulus. The discriminative component of pain is often referred to as "fast" pain because it occurs relatively quickly following a noxious stimulus. STT neurons carrying the discriminative

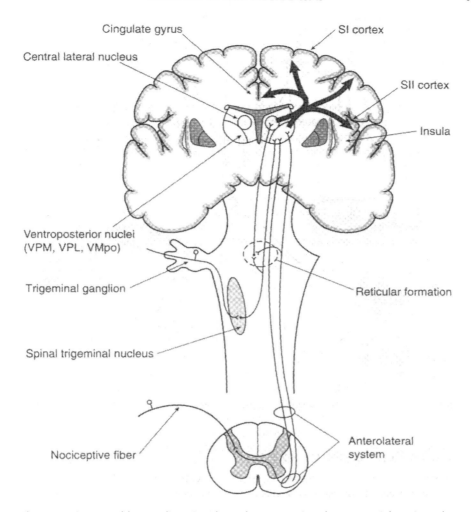

Cingulate gyrus

SI cortex

Central lateral nucleus

SII cortex

Insula

Ventroposterior nuclei
(VPM, VPL, VMpo)

Trigeminal ganglion

Reticular formation

Spinal trigeminal nucleus

Nociceptive fiber

Anterolateral
system

Figure 4.5. Summary of the ascending pain pathways that convey pain and temperature information to the brainstem, thalamus, and cerebral cortex. The fibers of the anterolateral system terminate in the ventrobasal complex (ventroposterolateral [VPL] and ventroposteromedial [VPM] nuclei) and the posterior part of the ventral medial nucleus (VMpo). Other fibers terminate in the reticular formation, which, in turn, sends ascending projections to the central lateral nucleus. Pain-sensitive regions in the thalamus project to a variety of cortical regions, including the anterior cingulate gyrus, the insula, and the primary (SI) and secondary (SII) somatosensory cortices. (From Pritchard, T.C., & Alloway, K.D. [1999]. *Medical neuroscience* [p. 219]. Madison, CT: Fence Creek Publishing; reprinted by permission.)

component of pain are thought to 1) receive input largely from A-delta primary afferents; 2) originate principally in laminae I and V; and 3) terminate in the posterior and ventrobasal thalamus, including the ventroposterolateral nucleus. In the thalamus, these axons synapse on third-order neurons that terminate in the somatosensory cortex. This part of the STT is referred to as the neospinothalamic tract (Terman & Bonica, 2001).

The arousal-emotional component of pain determines the unpleasantness and fear of further injury associated with the original trauma. The part of the STT that is thought to mediate the arousal-emotional component of pain originates in laminae IV–IX, with a contribution from lamina I. Some of these cells project directly to the central lateral and intralaminar nuclei of the thalamus and others connect indirectly via the reticular formation, the periaqueductal gray, the hypothalamus, and then the medial and intralaminar thalamic nuclei. Here they synapse with neurons projecting to the limbic forebrain through complex circuits and send projections to other diffuse areas of the brain. This part of the STT is referred to as the paleospinothalamic tract (Terman & Bonica, 2001) and is considered to be responsible for the "slow" component of pain.

One example of the differential effects that pathology may have on the sensory-discriminative and affective components of pain was reported by Benedetti and colleagues (2004). These investigators reviewed the impact of brain dysfunction on pain perception in a study involving patients with Alzheimer's disease. They found that the sensory and affective processes of pain perception became dissociated as the disease progressed, with little impact on the patients' pain thresholds and ability to detect stimuli.

In addition to the STT, second-order spinal nociceptive neurons also project to supraspinal areas through the spinomesencephalic, spinoreticular, spinocervical, and postsynaptic dorsal column pathways (Jessel & Kelly, 1991). At the level of the trigeminal system, nociceptive impulses are transmitted supraspinally from the subnucleus caudalis via the ventral trigeminothalamic tract pathway (Byers & Bonica, 2001).

Interruption of the STT and the ventral trigeminothalamic tract blocks the transmission of pain to supraspinal areas where cortical pain processing occurs. This fact is exploited in the treatment of severe pain that fails to respond to more conventional treatment through the surgical procedure called a cordotomy or tractotomy. In this procedure, the STT is lesioned to interrupt transmission of pain impulses supraspinally (Mayer, Price, & Becker, 1975). Because the STT ascends in the white matter contralateral to the side where afferent pain input occurs, this surgical procedure provides analgesia to pain from the contralateral side. However, in many cases pain returns within months to years (White & Sweet, 1969).

The Thalamus

The thalamus serves as a relay station between the spinal cord and the brain. STT projections ascend within the spinal cord and brainstem to synapse on third-order neurons in different areas of the thalamus. STT neurons mediating the discriminative component of pain terminate in the ventrobasal complex. This area is composed of the ventroposterolateral and ventroposteromedial nuclei. Neurons in the ventroposterolateral and ventroposteromedial nuclei are activated by both noxious and innocuous stimuli. Neurons in the ventral posterior thalamus are somatotopically organized and mediate the discriminative component of pain. Ventroposterolateral and ventroposteromedial neurons project to the somatosensory cortex (Chudler & Bonica, 2001). The ventral posterior part of the thalamus contains the posterior part of the ventral medial thalamic nuclei. These nuclei receive sensory input primarily from the STT and respond primarily to noxious stimuli. Many posterior ventral medial thalamic neurons project to the insular cortex, a region adjacent to but independent of the somatosensory cortex (Chudler & Bonica, 2001).

In contrast to the ventrobasal and posterior nuclei, intralaminar nuclei have large, divergent receptive fields and send projections to diffuse cortical areas, including the frontal, parietal, and limbic areas. The diffuse connectivity exhibited by these third-order neurons has led to the supposition that they are involved in the arousal-emotional component of pain (Chudler & Bonica, 2001).

Cortical Pain Processing

According to van der Kolk's (2002) organizational paradigm, the brain is organized into three interconnected anatomical divisions with different functions. The *brainstem and hypothalamus* contribute to maintaining appropriate internal homeostasis. The *limbic system* maintains or balances the connections with internal reality and external reality. The *neocortex* serves to provide additional processing and intention to external reality. No single area is involved in the perception of pain. Rather, multiple brain areas participate in the body's reaction to painful stimuli, although our understanding of cortical pain processing is relatively limited.

Noninvasive imaging studies have shown that the largest increases in cortical blood flow in response to painful stimuli occur in the anterior cingulate gyrus and the insula, areas of the limbic system (Pritchard & Alloway, 1999). These areas receive projections from the thalamus, including the ventrobasal (ventroposterolateral and ventroposteromedial) and intralaminar regions and the posterior part of the ventral medial nucleus (Pritchard & Alloway, 1999). These areas are thought to be involved in the affective component of pain (Hammond, 1986). Participation by the limbic system (i.e., amygdala, cingulate cortex) in pain transmission is thought to account for the analgesia associated with extreme stress, learned helplessness, and hypnosis (Chudler & Bonica, 2001; Terman & Bonica, 2001).

The discriminative component of pain perception is mediated by projections from the ventrobasal thalamus to the somatosensory cortical areas. More specifically, nociceptive stimuli activate 1) the somatosensory cortex area I (SI), 2) the somatosensory cortex area II (SII), 3) the retroinsular cortex, and 4) area 7b. The somatosensory cortex is somatotopically organized, with the most caudal regions of the body (i.e., feet, toes) represented most medially and the most rostral body areas (i.e., mouth, face) represented most laterally (Figure 4.6). Areas that are most densely innervated, such as the face, fingers, and feet, have a proportionately larger representation.

In addition to mediating motivational and cognitive aspects of pain perception, cortical areas also participate in modulation of incoming pain signals. For example, corticospinal tract fibers originating in the somatosensory cortex synapse in spinal cord laminae I–VII. In response to stimulation of SI and SII somatosensory cortex, the corticospinal and extrapyramidal pathways mediate inhibition of wide dynamic range neuronal activation by noxious stimuli (Terman & Bonica, 2001). SI and SII neurons also project to the mesencephalon, intralaminar thalamic nuclei, striatum, and reticular formation. These areas may also mediate analgesia (Terman & Bonica, 2001). Collectively, although comparatively little is currently known regarding the specifics of cortical influences on nociceptive transmission, these areas are considered to be important even though they are difficult to study systematically.

Modulation of Pain

The transmission of nociceptive impulses from primary afferent neurons to spinal dorsal horn neurons may be inhibited in two ways: 1) by descending pathways that terminate on these second-order neurons, and 2) by innocuous peripheral input. The former, which are referred to as descending inhibitory pathways, are described first. Descending inhibition of nociception involves four different levels of the CNS: 1) the

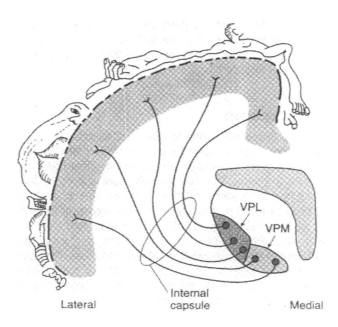

Figure 4.6. Map of the primary somatosensory (SI) cortex. The somatotopic organization of the SI cortex is determined by the pattern of projections from the ventroposteromedial (VPM) and ventroposterolateral (VPL) nuclei of the thalamus. (From Pritchard, T.C., & Alloway, K.D. [1999]. *Medical neuroscience* [p. 216]. Madison, CT: Fence Creek Publishing; reprinted by permission.)

cortex and diencephalon; 2) the periaqueductal gray (PAG) of the mesencephalon; 3) the nucleus raphe magnus (NRM) of the rostroventral medulla; and 4) the spinal and medullary dorsal horn, which receives inputs from the NRM (Figure 4.7).

Electrical activation of the PAG produces analgesia equipotent to that produced by high doses of morphine in laboratory animals that have been subjected to noxious stimuli such as heating of the skin, cutaneous and visceral injection of chemical irritants, and electrical stimulation of the tooth pulp (Cannon & Liebeskind, 1979). Analgesia begins within a few seconds and lasts for up to several hours. This "stimulation-produced analgesia" shares many characteristics with opioid analgesia in that 1) tolerance develops to repeated brain stimulation; 2) crosstolerance can occur between opiate analgesia and stimulation-produced analgesia; and 3) stimulation-produced analgesia can be reversed by opiate antagonists, such as naloxone (Akil, Mayer, & Liebeskind, 1976; Mayer & Hayes, 1975). Experimental evidence indicates that this type of analgesia is mediated at the level of the spinal cord and brainstem via activation of enkephalin-containing neurons in close proximity to neurons densely populated with opioid receptors in the superficial dorsal horn (Ruda, Bennett, & Dubner, 1986).

Projections from PAG neurons synapse on neurons in the NRM that, in turn, send serotonin-rich projections to the spinal cord and medullary dorsal horn. These serotonin-containing NRM nerve fibers terminate among nociceptive second-order neurons in laminae I, IIo, and V. Electrical stimulation of the NRM produces analgesia, and lesions of the NRM inhibit PAG stimulation–induced analgesia (Basbaum & Fields, 1984). These findings provide evidence that the NRM relays descending inhibitory information between the PAG and areas of the spinal and medullary dorsal horn important in transmitting nociception.

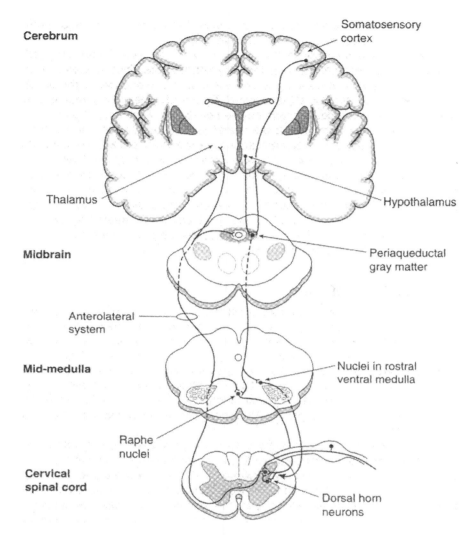

Cerebrum

Somatosensory
cortex

Thalamus

Hypothalamus

Midbrain

Periaqueductal
gray matter

Anterolateral
system

Mid-medulla

Nuclei in rostral
ventral medulla

Raphe
nuclei

Cervical
spinal cord

Dorsal horn
neurons

Figure 4.7. Pain-modulating pathways. The periaqueductal gray (PAG) region can be engaged by ascending fibers of the anterolateral system or by descending inputs from the hypothalamus and the cerebral cortex. Descending projections from the PAG region activate serotonergic neurons in the nucleus raphe magnus or noradrenergic neurons in the nucleus paragigantocellularis. Descending projections from these regions activate enkephalinergic neurons in the dorsal horn of the spinal cord and the spinal trigeminal nucleus. (From Pritchard, T.C., & Alloway, K.D. [1999]. *Medical neuroscience* [p. 224]. Madison, CT: Fence Creek Publishing; reprinted by permission.)

Projections from the PAG also synapse on the nucleus paragigantocellularis. Activation of paragigantocellularis neurons in turn activates neurons in the locus coeruleus (LC), a group of neurons located in the ventrolateral aspect of the PAG (Aston-Jones, Ennis, Pieribone, Nickell, & Shipley, 1986; Ennis & Aston-Jones, 1988). The LC has diffuse projections to all levels of the CNS from the spinal cord to the cerebral cortex. These noradrenergic neurons contribute to endogenous inhibition of pain, but whether this activation is direct or indirect remains uncertain (Svensson, 1987). In addition to responding to nociceptive stimuli, the LC is also activated in response to nonpainful stressors such as loud noises and light flashes (Rasmussen, Morilak, & Jacobs, 1986) as well as rectal, stomach, and bladder distention (Elam, Svensson, & Thoren, 1985). This stress response is subject to adaptation and learning. For example, pairing a stressor with a noxious stimulus increases LC firing, whereas pairing the former with a reward evokes no change in LC activation (Rasmussen et al., 1986). The LC has been shown to respond excessively to inescapable shock in animals (Weiss & Simson, 1986). In this experimental paradigm, animals demonstrate "learned helplessness" in that, as the shock becomes more persistent, behaviors directed at avoiding the noxious stimulus become less frequent (Seligman, Weiss, Weinraub, & Schulman, 1980). This experimental paradigm is considered to be a model for posttraumatic stress disorder (PTSD).

In addition to modulation by descending inhibitory pathways, local enkephalin-containing neurons in the dorsal horn (spinal cord laminae I, II, V, VII, and X) (Basbaum, 1985) also play an important role in pain modulation (Figure 4.8). Met- and leu-enkephalin are naturally occurring opioids manufactured by the body. Enkephalin-containing neurons inhibit activation of ascending nociceptive neurons (e.g., anterolateral system second-order neurons, including STT neurons) through both direct and indirect inhibition as follows. The central terminals of primary afferent fibers terminating in lamina I and the outer portion of lamina II (IIo) contain large dense-core vesicles. These vesicles contain peptides such as substance P and CGRP that are released into the synaptic cleft when the first-order neuron is depolarized. When sufficient peptide is released, the second-order neuron is depolarized and action potentials can be generated. In addition to containing

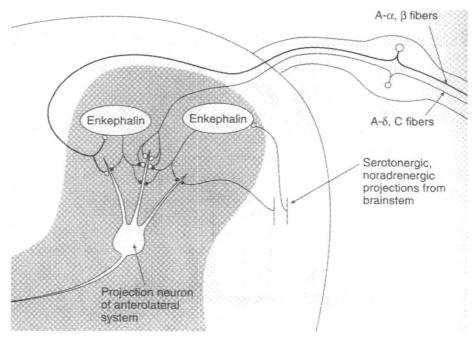

Figure 4.8. Pain control circuits in the posterior horn. A schematic illustration of the gate control mechanism for modulating nociception in the posterior horn. Inhibitory synapses are indicated by *filled terminals,* and excitatory synapses are indicated by *open terminals.* Enkephalinergic neurons in the substantia gelatinosa inhibit projection neurons directly and also inhibit the release of excitatory transmitters from the C fibers. Enkephalinergic neurons can be activated either by cutaneous stimulation (A-beta [A-β] fibers) or by serotonergic and noradrenergic fibers descending from the brainstem. Projection neurons in the anterolateral system exhibit wide dynamic responses because they receive inputs from both cutaneous and nociceptive afferents. (From Pritchard, T.C., & Alloway, K.D. [1999]. *Medical neuroscience* [p. 102]. Madison, CT: Fence Creek Publishing; reprinted by permission.)

pain-transmitting peptides, the central terminals of nociceptive primary afferent nerve fibers also contain receptors for enkephalin and other inhibitory compounds. Release of enkephalin by local inhibitory neurons (indicated by large white "enkephalin"-containing circles in Figure 4.8) activates the enkephalin receptors on primary afferent central terminals, resulting in inhibition of substance P and CGRP release. This is known as presynaptic inhibition. Postsynaptic inhibition occurs when enkephalin release directly activates opioid receptors on STT neurons, thereby inhibiting transmission of pain information through the affected neuron.

Enkephalin-containing neurons are activated by the descending noradrenergic (LC) and serotonergic (NRM) pathways described previously as well as by cutaneous stimulation. The theory that innocuous stimuli can inhibit nociceptive transmission was first postulated by Patrick Wall and Ronald Melzack in 1965 as the "gate control theory." This theory states that activation of large, myelinated A-beta nerve fibers that transmit innocuous sensation can reduce the sensitivity of dorsal horn neurons to painful stimuli mediated by A-delta and C fibers (Melzack & Wall, 1965). This theory has been implemented clinically through certain pain management strategies, including transcutaneous electrical nerve stimulation (TENS), vibration, and gentle massage. Following the acquisition of new information, this theory was modified to incorporate the effect of descending inhibitory pathways (Melzack & Wall, 1982). Newer findings, including the observation that under certain conditions, A-beta fibers can actually activate pain pathways (described in more detail later in this chapter), conflict with some aspects of the gate control theory. However, one cannot argue against the important contribution that this theory has made to the fields of pain research and management.

Basic research to elucidate mechanisms of pain modulation has demonstrated that, in addition to the inhibitory neuropeptides (i.e., the opioids beta-endorphin, met-enkephalin, and leu-enkephalin) and neurotransmitters (i.e., norepinephrine and serotonin) described earlier, other endogenous chemicals produced by the body also block pain transmission. Examples of these include gamma-aminobutyric acid (GABA), glycine, adenosine, and endocannabinoids (marijuana-like compounds). The chemical structures of inhibitory compounds such as these have been exploited by the pharmaceutical industry to synthesize structurally similar compounds that are also capable of producing analgesia. The goal in this type of research and development process is to develop highly effective and selective compounds with minimally adverse side effect profiles.

Sensitization and Neuroplasticity

Tissue injury within the distribution of the PNS results in anatomical and physiological changes in both the PNS and CNS. In the PNS, damaged cells release their intracellular contents, including K+ ions and ATP. Inflammatory cells recruited to the area release proinflammatory cytokines and growth factors (Levine & Reichling, 1999). The purpose of this inflammatory response is to assist with healing, protection of the damaged tissue, and adaptation. However, repeated application of noxious stimuli in the continued presence of inflammatory mediators such as bradykinin, histamine, prostaglandins, and serotonin leads to increased pain sensitivity. This phenomenon, which is called *hyperalgesia,* is characterized by a reduction in the activation threshold for peripheral nociceptive neurons, an increase in these neurons' responsiveness, and spontaneous pain. Release of these inflammatory mediators into the local area alters the responsiveness of pain-conducting primary afferent neurons (Perl, 1996) through changes in conduction velocity, action potential duration, and type and distribution of membrane ion channels (Djouhri & Lawson, 1999; Fjell, Cummins, Dib-Hajj, et al., 1999; Fjell, Cummins, Fried, Black, & Waxman, 1999). Hyperalgesia that occurs within the area of injury is called *primary hyperalgesia*.

In addition to increased sensitivity in A-delta and C fibers, inflammation can also alter A-beta fibers in such a way that they too respond to noxious stimuli (Neumann, Doubell, Leslie, & Woolf, 1996). This change in A-beta fibers is thought to contribute to the phenomenon termed *allodynia* in which nonpainful stimuli, such as vibration or light touch, evoke pain. A simple example of allodynia is the pain that one feels in response to light touch or warm water when the skin is sunburned. Allodynia is characteristic of neuropathic pain states such as diabetic neuropathy and trigeminal neuralgia. Changes in the "hard wiring" of A-beta fiber central terminals occur in which mechanoreceptors that previously mediated innocuous stimuli establish new synapses with dorsal horn neurons that normally receive nociceptive input (Neumann et al., 1996). As a result, activation of A-beta fibers by touch or vibration will subsequently activate pain pathways. The term coined for this phenomenon is *phenotypic switching* (Neumann et al., 1996).

In addition to these PNS changes, tissue injury can also lead to changes in the CNS. The most widely studied changes are those that occur in the spinal cord dorsal horn, where brief but intense noxious stimulation can evoke physiological, biochemical, and even morphological changes in primary afferent terminals and second-order neurons. The associated increased sensitivity of central neurons is called *central sensitization*. During the early phase following injury, these changes are initiated with the increased responsiveness of N-methyl D-aspartate (NMDA) receptors to the excitatory amino acid glutamate (Terman & Bonica, 2001). The resulting increased neuronal excitability leads to activation of pro-nociceptive second-order neurons by stimuli that ordinarily would not be painful. Increased pain and allodynia may also spread to uninjured tissue surrounding a site of injury. Hyperalgesia in the uninjured area is termed *secondary hyperalgesia*.

After the early changes in existing proteins, changes occur in the gene expression (e.g., c-*fos* and c-*jun*) of second-order dorsal horn neurons. These changes affect the type and quantity of enzymes, neuropeptides, and proteins produced by the spinal cord neurons involved. One example of such a change is the increased expression of cyclooxygenase-2 (COX-2) in CNS neurons within several hours following peripheral tissue injury (Samad et al., 2001). Resulting increases in prostaglandin E2 produce pre- and postsynaptic changes that facilitate synaptic transmission and increase neuronal excitability. These changes in gene expression constitute the late phase of central sensitization. In this way, a relatively brief but intense injury in the PNS can result in persistent changes in the dorsal horn, including increases in neural sensitivity, excitation, and receptive field size. Neuroplasticity of the CNS pain pathways is likely a major contributing factor in the development and perpetuation of *chronic pain*.

The complexity of the nervous system interconnections involved in the perception of pain along with its capacity for plasticity likely contribute to the poor clinical correlation between tissue damage, radiological findings, physical function, and reported pain (Bruyere et al., 2002; Sarzi-Puttini et al., 2002). It is helpful to keep in mind that the size of the lesion is not necessarily the most significant factor in chronic pain conditions. Hence, size may matter, but not in chronic pain. In addition, it must be noted that the size of the lesion is not part of the diagnostic criteria for a chronic pain disorder in the *Diagnostic and Statistical Manual of Mental Disorders, Fourth Edition, Text Revision* (*DSM-IV-TR;* American Psychiatric Association [APA], 2000). In some chronic pain conditions, such as chronic fatigue syndrome, irritable bowel syndrome, tension headache, and fibromyalgia, the pathophysiology of the lesion may not even be clearly identified or understood.

Limitations of Animal Models of Pain

Our current knowledge regarding neurobiological mechanisms of pain transmission and modulation is largely based on research done using animal models of pain. Although animal models of pain do provide valuable insights concerning the primary physiological mechanisms of pain, they lack clarification of motivational factors, politics, and secondary gain issues for pain in humans. Hence, the clinical presentation of pain and the laboratory approach to pain may differ at times. Generally, the animal model of pain does not highlight psychosocial factors associated with pain, including motivation for returning to work after injury; secondary gain from lawsuits or environmental response to injury; union work rules; anxiety, depression, and other comorbidities; prior family modeling of maladaptive pain behavior; drug seeking and drug abuse or dependency; and iatrogenic issues (doctor/treatment causes), among the many potential factors that affect chronic pain and disability. None has been seriously explored with respect to individuals with developmental disabilities.

A variety of concepts such as the biopsychosocial model, psychoneuroimmunology, and mind–body medicine have been utilized in an attempt to more accurately address the complexity of illness and pain behavior in humans (Flor & Hermann, 2004; Pert, 1999; Turk, 1996). For example, many researchers and clinicians support a biopsychosocial model with chronic pain patients. This model brings together the patient's physiological status, psychological response patterns, clinical dynamics, education, mind–body awareness, problem-solving skills, adaptive intelligence, affect, vocational interests, and local labor market realities to better understand and treat chronic pain and disability. The next section of this chapter seeks to put the previous information regarding neurobiologic mechanisms of pain into a clinical context with particular relevance to clinicians treating chronic pain in individuals with developmental disabilities.

NEUROBIOLOGY AND
COMORBIDITIES ASSOCIATED WITH CHRONIC PAIN

Chronic Pain Overview: Basic Neuropsychological Concepts of Pain

In the study of chronic pain, there are many significant questions concerning why and how an individual with chronic pain fails to adjust or return to physiological homeostasis following injury and the passage of an appropriate amount of time for healing. Many clinicians with experience in treating chronic pain stress the importance of multidisciplinary management for chronic pain patients because of the complexity of the interactions between the mind, the body, and behavior. The basis for this multidisciplinary focus with chronic pain is evident in the diagnostic criteria for a pain disorder according to the *DSM-IV-TR* (APA, 2000, p. 498):

A. Pain in one or more anatomical sites is the predominant focus of the clinical presentation and is of sufficient severity to warrant clinical attention.

B. The pain causes clinically significant distress or impairment in social, occupational, or other important areas of functioning.

C. Psychological factors are judged to have an important role in the onset, severity, exacerbation, or maintenance of the pain.

D. The symptom or deficit is not intentionally produced or feigned.

E. The pain is not better accounted for by a Mood, Anxiety, or Psychotic Disorder and does not meet criteria for Dyspareunia. (Reprinted by permission from *DSM-IV-TR.*)

For the purpose of this book, it is important to note that, although the diagnostic criteria do not rule out the likelihood that individuals with developmental disability may experience chronic pain, there is almost a complete absence of a clinical research base specific to chronic pain issues among populations with developmental disabilities (but see Chapter 7 for information on new work being conducted in individuals with cerebral palsy).

Hence, complexity and the interaction of physical and psychological factors are key issues with chronic pain. The definition of chronic pain as used in the DSM-IV is broad and inclusive, but not precise. The experience and impact of chronic pain in our society is enormous with respect to the financial costs, days lost from work, and number of medical visits attributed to chronic pain complaints. Gallagher and Verma (2004) reported that more than 50 million Americans suffer from chronic pain and that chronic pain is the most common complaint for seeking medical care. In clinical practice, there is often uncertainty and confusion regarding the exact percentage of the patient's reported pain that is attributed to "pure" psychological process, pure physical process, or both processes.

In addition to the sensory component of pain described in detail previously, the experience of pain also includes an important affective-emotional component. Processing of this affective component is done in cortical association areas that exist outside the primary somatosensory cortex. These cortical association areas play an important role in analyzing multiple inputs (e.g., sensation, auditory input, odor) and influencing associated behaviors. Anxiety, depression, emotions, pain, and pain modulation are intertwined, even sharing similar neurotransmitters, such as norepinephrine, serotonin, and GABA (Gallagher & Verma, 2004). This may account for the analgesic effects reported for selective serotonin reuptake inhibitors (SSRIs) and selective serotonin and norepinephrine reuptake inhibitors (SSNRIs).

Many studies document the positive relationship between pain and anxiety in both clinical and experimental settings (Kain, Sevarino, Alexander, Pincus, & Mayes, 2000; Melzack, 1973; Suls & Wan, 1989). Similar findings concerning the comorbidity of depression and chronic pain have been noted (Banks & Kerns, 1996; Krishnan et al., 1985; Lindsay & Wyckoff, 1981). The role of noradrenergic pathways in anxiety, stress, and PTSD has been recognized by many researchers (Bremner, Krystal, Southwick, & Charney, 1996a, 1996b; Charney & Deutch, 1996). Di Piero and colleagues (2001), using single-photon emission computed tomography (SPECT), demonstrated that diazepam, a drug used to treat anxiety, improved study participants' ability to handle pain from a cold stimulus test by blocking the emotional or affective component of the pain. They report that diazepam modified the temporal lobe activation pattern and modulated the study participants' emotional response to the induced pain from the cold stimulus.

Stress, Glucocorticoids, and Brain Morphology and Function

Any circumstances or situations that dramatically increase circulating glucocorticoids, especially during critical periods of neurodevelopment, may demonstrate long-lasting consequences on brain morphology and function. These effects appear to be particularly important with respect to hypothalamic-pituitary-adrenocortical axis sensitization and hippocampal neurogenesis. These changes may persist over the life span (Huot, Plotsky, Lenox, & McNamara, 2002). Van der Kolk (2004) noted similar hippocampal and other psychobiological interconnections with PTSD and related disorders. The impact of severe stress on learning, adaptation, and health is significant, especially in the case of children and quite likely in individuals with developmental disabilities who both may be at special risk with the experience of severe stress and trauma (van der Kolk, 2004).

Impact of the Limbic System on Chronic Pain

The amygdala and related limbic structures are involved in both chronic pain (Schneider et al., 2001; Wu et al., 1999) and PTSD because these structures are involved in the fear response. The amygdala and the limbic system transform sensory stimuli into emotional, hormonal, and fear responses. With chronic pain patients, the psychologist is often requested to evaluate the patient and assist him or her with stress management and relaxation. One of the common clinical manifestations of a chronic pain syndrome is the patient's fear and anxiety of increasing the pain symptoms through returning to work, increasing exercise and flexibility, and resuming more normal (preinjury) activities of daily living. The impact of depression on chronic pain patients concerns limited energy for rehabilitation efforts, hopelessness, and some risk of suicide, as is the case for depression generally. Work of this nature has not been conducted specific to populations with developmental disabilities, but the clinical parallels suggest that a search for common mechanisms may be important. From a clinical standpoint, it is often difficult to ascertain the precise boundary between chronic pain, depression, and poor stress management in many cases.

Practical Significance of the Hippocampus

The hippocampus is a brain structure involved with learning and memory. This structure has a high density of glucocorticoid receptors. Many researchers note that prolonged stress and high exposure to cortisol and related hypothalamic-pituitary-adrenocortical axis activations interfere with learning and memory (Lupien & McEwen, 1997; Lupien et al., 1998; McEwen & Sapolsky, 1995). Huot and colleagues (2002) reported that this result is even more pronounced during critical periods of neurodevelopment when it may result in long-term consequences for brain morphology and function. For example, maternal separation reduces hippocampal mossy fiber density in adult Long Evans rats. Although not specific to individuals with developmental disabilities, van der Kolk (2004) reported additional hippocampal findings using positron emission tomography (PET) scanning in PTSD patients. Given that memory and cognitive function are vital for individuals to understand rehabilitation program and treatment goals, it is likely

that this too is an underrecognized area of research and treatment among individuals with developmental disabilities and chronic pain. Cognitive functions assist individuals in recalling situations and behaviors that could cause a flare-up in
symptoms and must either be avoided or approached in a way that maximizes
safety. These cognitive functions also facilitate interpretation of the experience in
the context of either treatment procedures or the experience of pain. For example,
Ploghaus and colleagues (Ploghaus, Becerra, Borras, & Borsook, 2003; Ploghaus et
al., 2000) reported evidence that the hippocampus is "disengaged" when adequate
preparatory information and education occur prior to medical and dental procedures. Hence, there are many advantages for the treatment or surgical team to in-
vest in adequate preparatory efforts with patients and their families.

Given the important role of learning and memory in pain perception and
therapeutic intervention, any biopsychosocial factor that can interfere with con-
solidation of these functions needs to be addressed. This is especially true in the
case of severe or chronic stressors, either in the past or in the current circumstances. The clinical team needs to understand the impact of stress on the patient
and to suggest stress management strategies to facilitate the treatment of and adjustment to chronic pain.

Belief Systems Affecting Fear and the Anticipation of Pain

Psychologists have long known that belief and anticipation affect adaptive behavior, attention, emotional reactivity, perception, and psychopathology. Some authors suggest that chronic pain patients may even suffer more from the emotional
and cognitive features of pain than from the physical pain alone (Crombez, Vlaeyen,
Heuts, & Lysens, 1999).

Ploghaus and colleagues (2003) noted that fear and the anticipation of pain
are commonly seen in chronic pain patients. They reported that certain and uncertain expectations about the pain are mediated by different neural pathways, as
documented in functional MRI studies. For example, the rostral anterior cingulate
cortex and posterior cerebellum mediate certain expectations, whereas the ven-
tromedial prefrontal cortex, mid-cingulate cortex, and hippocampus mediate uncertain expectations. Hence, the level of certainty likely impacts both behavioral
and neural factors involved in the expectation of pain. Both human and animal
studies suggest that there may be a differential impact of fear and anxiety on pain
perception, with fear leading to decreased pain sensitivity and anxiety contributing to increased pain sensitivity (Ploghaus et al., 2003; Rhudy & Meagher, 2000).
Hence, the clinical importance of managing a patient's anxiety, especially concerning pain and treatment procedures, should not be underestimated.

Laboratory research with experimentally induced pain reveals the significant
impact of anticipation and expectation on the experience of pain. When humans
were studied using functional MRI scans, the anticipation of pain triggered increased activity in the primary somatosensory cortex even without a noxious pain
exposure (Porro et al., 2002). Hence, a major activity and goal of the psychologist
in working with patients with chronic pain is to clarify the patient's belief system
and how this facilitates or impedes adjustment and pain management.

Generally, clinical outcomes are improved when the individuals and their
families are appropriately educated and emotionally prepared for medical and rehabilitation procedures (Suls & Wan, 1989). Examples of areas in which education
is important include details of the treatment process, time of recovery, things to

avoid, types of medications to be used, and related details that help with calming the patient and removing uncertainty and anxiety. Hence, efforts to minimize the physical and emotional trauma and anxiety from medical procedures should be a priority of the treatment team and a "best practice" conceptualization. There is no reason to think that these issues are absent in the management of chronic pain among individuals with developmental disabilities. In short, the human experience with pain integrates the totality of experience involving physiological/genetic factors, cognition, emotion, memory, sensation, and perception.

PAIN: A MULTIDISCIPLINARY AND MULTISYSTEM TOPIC

Chronic pain and disability is a complex and multifaceted topic area. Hence, the study and appreciation of chronic pain and disability involves multiple academic disciplines such as medicine, dentistry, psychology, psychiatry, social work, nursing, physical therapy, occupational therapy, rehabilitation counseling, vocational placement, and in some cases biomedical engineering. Mogil and Devor (2004) highlighted the history of pain genetics and documented reasons that an expert in genomics will soon be a member of the chronic pain treatment team, if one is not already.

Many chronic pain programs employ a biopsychosocial treatment model with multidisciplinary staffing that attempts to work collaboratively with chronic pain patients. The comprehensive multidisciplinary chronic pain team includes medical specialists (e.g., neurologist, physical medicine and rehabilitation specialist, rheumatologist, anethesiologist, dentist) and a psychologist, physical therapist, occupational therapist, vocational counselor, and other allied medical staff. In addition, alternative and complementary therapies and health care providers may be utilized (e.g., biofeedback, Qi Gong, chiropractic, acupuncture/traditional Chinese medicine, homeopathy, therapeutic massage, yoga, aromatherapy). The multidisciplinary chronic pain team attempts to assist the patient to better understand the multifaceted features of his or her pain, such as the impact of mood, anxiety, treatment compliance, conditioning, and environmental obstacles to treatment or self-care. This can best be accomplished when all members of the treatment team have an appreciation for the way in which the multiple interconnected systems within the body contribute to the complete pain experience. Increasingly, the pathways and structures that interconnect systems within the body and that contribute to various pain syndromes are being elucidated. However, much remains unknown.

REFERENCES

Akil, H., Mayer, D.J., & Liebeskind, J.C. (1976). Antagonism of stimulation-produced analgesia by naloxone, a narcotic antagonist. *Science, 191,* 961–962.

American Psychiatric Association. (2000). *Diagnostic and statistical manual of mental disorders* (4th ed., Text rev.). Washington, DC: American Psychiatric Press.

Aston-Jones, G., Ennis, M., Pieribone, V.A., Nickell, W.T., & Shipley, M.T. (1986). The brain nucleus locus coeruleus: Restricted afferent control of a broad efferent network. *Science, 234,* 734–737.

Banks, S.M., & Kerns, R.D. (1996). Explaining high rates of depression in chronic pain: A diathesis-stress framework. *Psychological Bulletin, 119,* 95–110.

Basbaum, A.I. (1985). Functional analysis of the cytochemistry of the spinal dorsal horn. *Advances in Pain Research and Therapy, 9,* 149–175.

Basbaum, A.I., & Fields, H.L. (1984). Endogenous pain control systems: Brainstem spinal pathways and endorphin circuitry. *Annual Review of Neuroscience, 7,* 309–338.

Benedetti, F., Arduino, C., Vighetti, S., Asteggiano, G., Tarenzi, L., & Rainero, I. (2004). Pain reactivity in Alzheimer patients with different degrees of cognitive impairment and brain electrical activity deterioration. *Pain, 111*, 22–29.

Bremner, J.D., Krystal, J.H., Southwick, S.M., & Charney, D.S. (1996a). Noradrenergic mechanisms in stress and anxiety: I. Preclinical studies. *Synapse, 23*, 28–38.

Bremner, J.D., Krystal, J.H., Southwick, S.M., & Charney, D.S. (1996b). Noradrenergic mechanisms in stress and anxiety: II. Clinical studies. *Synapse, 23*, 39–51.

Bruyere, O., Honore, A., Rovati, L.C., Giacovelli, G., Henrotin, Y.E., Seidel, L., et al. (2002). Radiologic features poorly predict clinical outcomes in knee osteoarthritis. *Scandinavian Journal of Rheumatology, 31*, 13–16.

Byers, M.R., & Bonica, J.J. (2001). Peripheral pain mechanisms and nociceptor plasticity. In J.D. Loeser (Ed.), *Bonica's management of pain* (3rd ed., pp. 26–72). Philadelphia: Lippincott Williams & Wilkins.

Cannon, J., & Liebeskind, J. (1979). Descending control systems. In R. Beers & R. Bassett (Eds.), *Mechanisms of pain and analgesic compounds* (pp. 171–184). New York: Raven Press.

Charney, D.S., & Deutch, A. (1996). A functional neuroanatomy of anxiety and fear: Implications for the pathophysiology and treatment of anxiety disorders. *Critical Reviews in Neurobiology, 10*, 419–446.

Chery-Croze, S. (1983). Painful sensation induced by a thermal cutaneous stimulus. *Pain, 17*, 109–137.

Chudler, E.H., & Bonica, J.J. (2001). Supraspinal mechanisms of pain and nociception. In J. Loeser (Ed.), *Bonica's management of pain* (pp. 153–179). Philadelphia: Lippincott Williams & Wilkins.

Crombez, G., Vlaeyen, J.W., Heuts, P.H., & Lysens, R. (1999). Pain-related fear is more disabling than pain itself: Evidence on the role of pain-related fear in chronic back pain disability. *Pain, 80*, 329–339.

Di Piero, V., Ferracuti, S., Sabatini, U., Tombari, D., Di Legge, S., Pantano, P., et al. (2001). Diazepam effects on the cerebral responses to tonic pain: A sPET study. *Psychopharmacology (Berlin), 158*, 252–258.

Djouhri, L., & Lawson, S.N. (1999). Changes in somatic action potential shape in guinea-pig nociceptive primary afferent neurones during inflammation in vivo. *Journal of Physiology (London), 520*(Pt. 2), 565–576.

Elam, M., Svensson, T.H., & Thoren, P. (1985). Differentiated cardiovascular afferent regulation of locus coeruleus neurons and sympathetic nerves. *Brain Research, 358*, 77–84.

Ennis, M., & Aston-Jones, G. (1988). Activation of locus coeruleus from nucleus paragigantocellularis: A new excitatory amino acid pathway in brain. *Journal of Neuroscience, 8*, 3644–3657.

Fjell, J., Cummins, T.R., Dib-Hajj, S.D., Fried, K., Black, J.A., & Waxman, S.G. (1999). Differential role of GDNF and NGF in the maintenance of two TTX-resistant sodium channels in adult DRG neurons. *Brain Research: Molecular Brain Research, 67*, 267–282.

Fjell, J., Cummins, T.R., Fried, K., Black, J.A., & Waxman, S.G. (1999). In vivo NGF deprivation reduces SNS expression and TTX-R sodium currents in IB4-negative DRG neurons. *Journal of Neurophysiology, 81*, 803–810.

Flor, H., & Hermann, C. (2004). Biopsychosocial models of pain. In R.H. Dworkin & W.W. Breitbart (Eds.), *Psychosocial aspects of pain: A handbook for healthcare providers* (Progress in Pain Research and Management, Vol. 27, pp. 47–75). Seattle: IASP Press.

Gallagher, R.M., & Verma, S. (2004). Mood and anxiety disorders. In R.H. Dworkin & W.S. Breitbart (Eds.), *Psychosocial aspects of pain: A handbook for healthcare providers* (Progress in Pain Research and Management, Vol. 27, pp. 139–178). Seattle: IASP Press.

Hammond, D.L. (1986). Control systems for nociceptive afferent processing: The descending inhibitory pathway. In TL. Yaksh (Ed.), *Spinal afferent processing* (pp. 363–390). New York: Plenum Press.

Huot, R.L., Plotsky, P.M., Lenox, R.H., & McNamara, R.K. (2002). Neonatal maternal separation reduces hippocampal mossy fiber density in adult Long Evans rats. *Brain Research, 950,* 52–63.

Jessel, T.M., & Kelly, D.D. (1991). Pain and analgesia. In E.R. Kandel & J.H. Schwartz (Eds.), *Principles of neural sciences* (pp. 385–399). Norwalk, CT: Appleton & Lange.

Kain, Z.N., Sevarino, F., Alexander, G.M., Pincus, S., & Mayes, L.C. (2000). Preoperative anxiety and postoperative pain in women undergoing hysterectomy. A repeated-measures design. *Journal of Psychosomatic Research, 49,* 417–422.

Krishnan, K.R., France, R.D., Pelton, S., McCann, U.D., Davidson, J., & Urban, B.J. (1985). Chronic pain and depression. I. Classification of depression in chronic low back pain patients. *Pain, 22,* 279–287.

Levine, J.D., & Reichling, D.B. (1999). Peripheral mechanisms of inflammatory pain. In P.D. Wall & R. Melzack (Eds.), *Textbook of pain* (4th ed., pp. 59–84). Edinburgh: Churchill Livingstone.

Lindsay, P.G., & Wyckoff, M. (1981). The depression-pain syndrome and its response to antidepressants. *Psychosomatics, 22,* 571–573, 576–577.

Lupien, S.J., de Leon, M., de Santi, S., Convit, A., Tarshish, C., Nair, N.P., et al. (1998). Cortisol levels during human aging predict hippocampal atrophy and memory deficits. *Nature Neuroscience, 1,* 69–73.

Lupien, S.J., & McEwen, B.S. (1997). The acute effects of corticosteroids on cognition: Integration of animal and human model studies. *Brain Research: Brain Research Reviews, 24,* 1–27.

Mayer, D.J., & Hayes, R.L. (1975). Stimulation-produced analgesia: Development of tolerance and cross-tolerance to morphine. *Science, 188,* 941–943.

Mayer, D.J., Price, D.D., & Becker, D.P. (1975). Neurophysiological characterization of the anterolateral spinal cord neurons contributing to pain perception in man. *Pain, 1,* 51–58.

McEwen, B.S., & Sapolsky, R.M. (1995). Stress and cognitive function. *Current Opinion in Neurobiology, 5,* 205–216.

McGrath, P. (2004). Psychosocial and psychiatric aspects of pain in children. In R.H. Dworkin & W.S. Breitbart (Eds.), *Psychosocial aspects of pain: A handbook for healthcare providers* (Progress in Pain Research and Management, Vol. 27, pp. 479–494). Seattle: IASP Press.

Melzack, R. (1973). *The puzzle of pain.* New York: Basic Books.

Melzack, R., & Wall, P. (1982). *The challenge of pain.* New York: Basic Books.

Melzack, R., & Wall, P.D. (1965). Pain mechanisms: A new theory. *Science, 150,* 971–979.

Miranda, C., Di Virgilio, M., Selleri, S., Zanotti, G., Pagliardini, S., Pierotti, M.A., et al. (2002). Novel pathogenic mechanisms of congenital insensitivity to pain with anhidrosis genetic disorder unveiled by functional analysis of neurotrophic tyrosine receptor kinase type 1/nerve growth factor receptor mutations. *Journal of Biological Chemistry, 277,* 6455–6462.

Mogil, J.S., & Devor, M. (2004). Introduction to pain genetics. In J.S. Mogil (Ed.), *The genetics of pain* (Progress in Pain Research and Management, Vol. 28, pp. 1–20). Seattle: IASP Press.

Neumann, S., Doubell, T.P., Leslie, T., & Woolf, C.J. (1996). Inflammatory pain hypersensitivity mediated by phenotypic switch in myelinated primary sensory neurons. *Nature, 384,* 360–364.

Perl, E.R. (1996). Cutaneous polymodal receptors: Characteristics and plasticity. *Progress in Brain Research, 113,* 21–37.

Pert, C.B. (1999). *Molecules of emotion: The science behind mind-body medicine.* New York: Touchstone.

Ploghaus, A., Becerra, L., Borras, C., & Borsook, D. (2003). Neural circuitry underlying pain modulation: Expectation, hypnosis, placebo. *Trends in Cognitive Sciences, 7,* 197–200.

Ploghaus, A., Tracey, I., Clare, S., Gati, J.S., Rawlins, J.N., & Matthews, P.M. (2000). Learning about pain: The neural substrate of the prediction error for aversive events. *Proceedings of the National Academy of Sciences of the United States of America, 97,* 9281–9286.

Porro, C.A., Baraldi, P., Pagnoni, G., Serafini, M., Facchin, P., Maieron, M., et al. (2002). Does anticipation of pain affect cortical nociceptive systems? *Journal of Neuroscience, 22,* 3206–3214.

Pritchard, T.C., & Alloway, K.D. (1999). *Medical neuroscience.* Madison, CT: Fence Creek Publishing.

Rasmussen, K., Morilak, D.A., & Jacobs, B.L. (1986). Single unit activity of locus coeruleus neurons in the freely moving cat. I. During naturalistic behaviors and in response to simple and complex stimuli. *Brain Research, 371,* 324–334.

Rhudy, J.L., & Meagher, M.W. (2000). Fear and anxiety: Divergent effects on human pain thresholds. *Pain, 84,* 65–75.

Ruda, M.A., Bennett, G.J., & Dubner, R. (1986). Neurochemistry and neural circuitry in the dorsal horn. *Progress in Brain Research, 66,* 219–268.

Samad, T.A., Moore, K.A., Sapirstein, A., Billet, S., Allchorne, A., Poole, S., et al. (2001). Interleukin-1beta-mediated induction of COX-2 in the CNS contributes to inflammatory pain hypersensitivity. *Nature, 410,* 471–475.

Sarzi-Puttini, P., Fiorini, T., Panni, B., Turiel, M., Cazzola, M., & Atzeni, F. (2002). Correlation of the score for subjective pain with physical disability, clinical and radiographic scores in recent onset rheumatoid arthritis. *BMC Musculoskeletal Disorders, 3*(1), 18.

Schneider, F., Habel, U., Holthusen, H., Kessler, C., Posse, S., Muller-Gartner, H.W., et al. (2001). Subjective ratings of pain correlate with subcortical-limbic blood flow: An fMRI study. *Neuropsychobiology, 43,* 175–185.

Seligman, M.E., Weiss, J., Weinraub, M., & Schulman, A. (1980). Coping behavior: Learned helplessness, physiological change and learned inactivity. *Behaviour Research and Therapy, 18,* 459–512.

Suls, J., & Wan, C.K. (1989). Effects of sensory and procedural information on coping with stressful medical procedures and pain: A meta-analysis. *Journal of Consulting and Clinical Psychology, 57,* 372–379.

Svensson, T.H. (1987). Peripheral, autonomic regulation of locus coeruleus noradrenergic neurons in brain: Putative implications for psychiatry and psychopharmacology. *Psychopharmacology (Berlin), 92,* 1–7.

Terman, G.W., & Bonica, J.J. (2001). Spinal mechanisms and their modulation. In J.D. Loeser (Ed.), *Bonica's management of pain* (pp. 73–152). Philadelphia: Lippincott Williams & Wilkins.

Turk, D.C. (1996). Biopsychosocial perspective on chronic pain. In R.J. Gatchel & D.C. Turk (Eds.), *Psychological approaches to pain management: A practitioner's handbook* (pp. 3–32). New York: The Guilford Press.

van der Kolk, B.A. (2002). Beyond the talking cure: Somatic experience and subcortical imprints in the treatment of trauma. In F. Shapiro (Ed.), *EMDR: promises for a paradigm shift* (pp. 3–29). New York: APA Press.

van der Kolk, B.A. (2004). Psychobiology of posttraumatic stress disorder. In J. Panksepp (Ed.), *Textbook of biological psychiatry* (pp. 30–54). New York: John Wiley & Sons.

Weiss, J.M., & Simson, P.G. (1986). Depression in an animal model: Focus on the locus coeruleus. *Ciba Foundation Symposium, 123,* 191–215.

White, J.C., & Sweet, W.H. (1969). Pain and the neurosurgeon. Springfield, IL: Charles C Thomas.

Willis, W.D. (1985). Evidence for nociceptive transmission systems. In P.L. Gildenberg (Ed.), *The pain system* (pp. 7–21). Basel: Karger.

Wu, M.T., Hsieh, J.C., Xiong, J., Yang, C.F., Pan, H.B., Chen, Y.C., et al. (1999). Central nervous pathway for acupuncture stimulation: Localization of processing with functional MR imaging of the brain—preliminary experience. *Radiology, 212,* 133–141.

II

EPIDEMIOLOGICAL, DEVELOPMENTAL, AND FUNCTIONAL ISSUES

5

THE EPIDEMIOLOGY OF PAIN IN DEVELOPMENTAL DISABILITIES

Shauna Bottos and Christine T. Chambers

For many years, it was believed that individuals with developmental disabilities were incapable of experiencing or expressing pain. Although it is now generally accepted that this belief was false and unfounded, epidemiological studies examining pain in individuals with developmental disabilities have only very recently begun to emerge in the scientific literature. These studies are necessary in order to determine the distribution of pain among individuals with developmental disabilities, as well as to provide data on the prevalence (i.e., the percentage of the population that exhibits pain during a specified time period) and incidence (i.e., the percentage of new cases within a population exhibiting pain during a defined period of time) of their pain. Epidemiological studies also provide information that is critical to understanding the etiology, risk factors, natural history, and aggregation of pain among those with developmental disabilities (Goodman & McGrath, 1991). Epidemiological research in this area remains vital because there is mounting evidence suggesting that these individuals may be at greater risk for experiencing pain compared to the general population. These individuals may be particularly vulnerable to both acute and chronic forms of pain because they frequently have comorbid painful medical conditions and are likely to be exposed to more surgical and other medical procedures that are painful than are individuals without disabilities (P.J. McGrath, Rosmus, Camfield, Campbell, & Hennigar, 1998; Schwartz, Engel, & Jensen, 1999; Turk, Geremski, Rosenbaum, & Weber, 1997). Epidemiological research has the potential to provide invaluable insights into the nature and scope of pain in children and adults with developmental disabilities and has important implications for prevention efforts and treatment strategies.

This chapter not only examines the status of epidemiological research on pain in children with developmental disabilities but also provides a brief overview of pain in children who do not have developmental disabilities in order to establish a comparison against which the painful experiences of children with developmental disabilities can be best understood. As this chapter illustrates, children with developmental disabilities often experience more pain on a daily basis than do children without developmental disabilities; and, because of communication limitations, it is often more difficult for them to verbally express their pain, which makes pain assessment a particular challenge. Although our knowledge regarding the epidemi-

S. Bottos was supported by a doctoral award from the Nova Scotia Health Research Foundation, and C.T. Chambers was supported by a Canada Research Chair during the preparation of this chapter.

The authors are grateful to Dr. Ken Craig for his helpful comments on a previous draft of this chapter, Ms. Sarah Peddle for her assistance with revisions, and Ms. Kelly Hayton for her editorial input.

ology of pain in children without developmental disability has increased, the dearth of research on individuals with developmental disabilities has limited our understanding of the prevalence and experience of pain in these populations.

In addition, this chapter highlights the unique challenges researchers and health care providers confront when assessing the pain experiences of people with developmental disabilities. The difficulties in obtaining adequate pain assessment are particularly pertinent to epidemiological research, in which accurate prevalence rates of pain are sought. Although the majority of research on pain in people with developmental disabilities has focused on children, many of the same issues and challenges in assessing and understanding pain among such individuals are encountered across the life span (Gibson & Chambers, 2004; Hadjistavropoulos, von Baeyer, & Craig, 2001). In particular, access to the subjective experience of pain is particularly difficult in people with developmental disabilities because their cognitive impairments diminish their ability to communicate verbally. Prevailing assumptions about the experience of pain in individuals with developmental disabilities are also discussed as they influence the recognition and treatment of pain among these populations. However, the majority of this chapter is devoted to providing a comprehensive analysis of contemporary research on the prevalence and types of pain seen across the spectrum of developmental disabilities, including those disabilities in which cognitive impairment is the defining feature (e.g., mental retardation, Down syndrome), pervasive developmental disorders, and cerebral palsy. Although the focus is on children, the prevalence of pain among adults with disabilities is given where available. Finally, gaps in the current knowledge base and directions for future epidemiological research on pain in populations with developmental disability are highlighted.

PAIN IN CHILDREN WITHOUT DEVELOPMENTAL DISABILITY

Pain is a common experience in children and adolescents without disabilities. The different forms of pain most commonly experienced by children are listed in Table 5.1. Pain can be experienced in the form of bumps and bruises obtained from everyday activities or caused by accidents and, more specifically, acute pain incidents (i.e., pain produced by noxious stimuli with relatively short durations, such as the pain associated with a needle injection or other medical procedures). The pain intensity associated with acute pains diminishes over a short period of time (days to weeks) in comparison to the persistence of chronic pain conditions. However, pain originating in injuries and diseases that persists beyond the span of time when tissue healing is expected to have occurred often can turn into chronic pain (see Chapter 4). It has been found that young children experience incidents of everyday pain, on average, once every 3 hours (Fearon, McGrath, & Achat, 1996; von Baeyer, Baskerville, & McGrath, 1998), most of which are relatively minor in nature, resulting in minimal damage to bodily tissue (Fearon et al., 1996). Over the normal course of growing up, a significant number of children may also experience pain from needles used for immunizations or blood collection procedures (Goodenough, Perrot, Champion, & Thomas, 2000; Goodman & McGrath, 1991), with younger children describing needle procedures to be more painful than their older counterparts (Fradet, McGrath, Kay, Adams, & Luke, 1990; Goodenough et al., 1997). Using validated pain measurement techniques, one study reported prevalence rates of pain during blood-drawing procedures to be between 36% and 64%

Table 5.1. Pain types and examples

Type of pain	Examples	Related terms	Pain intensity
Acute	Bumps, bruises, needle procedure pain, surgery, burns, fractures	Accidental, everyday pains, procedural	Diminishes steadily over time (minutes, days, or weeks)
Chronic	Recurrent abdominal pain, headaches, chest pains, limb pains	Persistent, recurrent, constant	Lasts 3 months or longer

for children 3–6 years of age, depending on the pain measurement technique used, compared with 52% for children 7–17 years of age (Fradet et al., 1990).

Although all children experience acute pain at many points in their development, a smaller proportion will develop or are born with chronic pain conditions. Chronic pains have been defined as repeated or persistent episodes of acute pain (e.g., headache, abdominal pain) that are either experienced as a component of a medical disorder, or experienced by otherwise healthy children in the absence of a well-defined organic etiology (P.A. McGrath, 1990). In order for pain to be classified as chronic, it must be constant over a period of 3 months or longer (Schechter, Berde, & Yaster, 2003). In a large-scale study of pain in children and adolescents, 54% were reported to have experienced pain within the previous 3 months, with up to 25% of these children documented to have experienced chronic pain, defined as recurrent or continuous pain for more than a 3-month period (Perquin et al., 2000). The most common types of chronic pain reported were headache (23%), abdominal pain (22%), and limb pain (22%), trends that are consistent with the results of other investigations (Goodman & McGrath, 1991; Hyams, Burke, Davis, Rzepski, & Andrologis, 1996).

The prevalence and incidence of pain in populations without developmental disabilities has been well documented through research. Although only a few large-scale studies are available for reference (e.g., Perquin et al., 2000), it is widely accepted that pain is a normal experience in childhood in the form of everyday bumps and bruises. A less universal but still common experience is recurrent or persistent pain or, more specifically, chronic pain conditions. Reliable pain assessment becomes imperative in pain management, especially when communication is challenging. The following section addresses the plethora of challenges involved in pain assessment, especially with children who cannot communicate their pain verbally.

PAIN IN CHILDREN WITH DEVELOPMENTAL DISABILITIES

Challenges in Pain Assessment

The assessment of pain, even in children without developmental disabilities, is challenging because pain is an inherently subjective phenomenon (Merskey, 1986; Merskey & Bogduk, 1994). With young children, it may be difficult to obtain reliable measures of pain because of their cognitive immaturity and their inability to separate pain from feelings of fear and anxiety (Franck, Greenberg, & Stevens, 2000; St.-Laurent-Gagnon, Bernard-Bonnin, & Villeneuve, 1999). For example, Stanford, Chambers, and Craig (2005) found that the word *pain* was not commonly used by young children, emerging as late as 6 years of age.

The recognition and assessment of pain in individuals with disability is hindered by their limited expressive repertoire, resulting from any of a number of cognitive, verbal, and motor impairments, as well as by uncertainty surrounding the meaning of available behavior as a sign or expression of pain (Fanurik, Koh, Schmitz, Harrison, & Conrad, 1999; Hadjistavropoulos et al., 2001; Oberlander, O'Donnell, & Montgomery, 1999). Although the "gold standard" in pain measurement is often said to be self-report (Merskey & Bogduk, 1994), those individuals with severe neurological or cognitive impairments who are without speech are unable to report their pain verbally and, consequently, may be particularly vulnerable to having their pain underestimated and undertreated (Donovan, 1997; Fanurik et al., 1999; Oberlander, O'Donnell, et al., 1999).

Even though several researchers have identified what appears to be a core set of behavioral cues that indicate when children with cognitive impairment are in pain (McGrath et al., 1998; Terstegen, Koot, de Boer, & Tibboel, 2003), accurate observational assessment of pain may be difficult among this population owing to idiosyncratic behaviors such as vocal abnormalities (e.g., moaning, grunting) and atypical facial expressions (e.g., grimacing) that may result in overestimates by people unfamiliar with the individual's usual behavioral tendencies (Fanurik et al., 1999). At the same time, the lack of "normal" responses to pain among these individuals may lead to underrecognition and poor management of their pain. Given the potential for misinterpretation of vocal and facial actions in adults with a developmental disability, LaChapelle, Hadjistavropoulos, and Craig (1999) conducted an important research study that looked at typical facial expressions that related to the experience of pain using the Facial Action Coding System (FACS; Ekman & Friesen, 1978). They found that when people with a developmental disability experienced low levels of pain, there was a marked increase in both the frequency and intensity of chin raising and in the intensity of brow lowering.

Because of the communication impairments commonly observed in children with developmental disabilities, researchers and clinicians often rely on the observations of third parties, most notably the child's caregivers. The use of third-party assessment necessarily presumes that these children express pain in a reasonably consistent manner, albeit sometimes idiosyncratically, and that the cues they use are accurately interpreted (Stallard, Williams, Velleman, Lenton, & McGrath, 2002b). Unfortunately, there is a lack of agreement between studies examining caregivers' ability to accurately assess pain even among children without disability (Chambers, Reid, Craig, McGrath, & Finley, 1998). Whereas some studies have found caregivers' assessments of pain-related behaviors in their child with cognitive impairment to be relatively consistent with the child's own responses (Benini et al., 2004; Breau, Camfield, McGrath, Rosmus, & Finley, 2001), others have noted that parents tend to underestimate or unreliably estimate their child's pain (Doherty, Yanni, Conroy, & Bresnihan, 1993; Manne, Jacobsen, & Redd, 1992). The relationship is likely complex because evidence suggests that the degree of cognitive impairment may influence caregivers' ratings (Fanurik et al., 1999). Indeed, parents of children with mild to moderate cognitive impairment have been documented to rely on direct expressions of pain in their child (e.g., verbal reports); given that expressive speech has been found to be present in the majority of people who have mild to moderate impairment, this is not surprising (Fanurik et al., 1999). Parents of children with mild to moderate cognitive impairment have also been found to exhibit a tendency to report that their child experienced less pain (Breau, MacLaren, McGrath, Camfield, & Finley, 2003). In contrast, parents of children with severe cognitive impairments were only able to determine the presence of pain by their child's indirect behaviors (e.g., crying) or behavioral or emotional changes (Fanurik et al., 1999), and judged their child to experience pain more frequently (Breau, Camfield, McGrath, & Finley, 2003). Although intriguing, these findings are preliminary. As noted by Breau, Camfield, et al. (2003), caregivers' preconceived beliefs regarding individuals with cognitive impairment may play an important role in their perception of the individuals' pain, and may be a fruitful avenue for future research. Nevertheless, given the intimate knowledge caregivers have of their child's typical behavior, they remain an important resource for gathering information on their child's experience of pain.

The Pain Insensitivity Hypothesis

The underrecognition and undertreatment of pain in people with cognitive impairments by both caregivers and health care professionals may largely be based on the erroneous assumption that these individuals have a lower sensitivity to or are indifferent to pain. Malviya et al. (2001) demonstrated that fewer children with cognitive impairment were assessed for postoperative pain, and they were prescribed and administered significantly fewer analgesic medications, compared to their peers without disabilities, corroborating findings reported among adults with disabilities (Feldt, Ryden, & Miles, 1998; Kaasalainen et al., 1998).

The long-believed notion that individuals with developmental disabilities have a higher pain threshold or a reduced sensitivity to pain has largely been based on anecdotal studies and case reports. Children and adults with significant neurological or cognitive impairments may fail to display the pain behaviors one would expect when in contact with a noxious stimulus or when a painful chronic condition is present. This has led to the belief that these individuals have an increased likelihood of pain insensitivity (i.e., a decreased sensory experience of pain) or pain indifference (i.e., a decreased emotional response to pain) (Biersdorff, 1991, 1994). In an observational study of individuals with developmental disability, Biersdorff (1994) asked a number of service providers and family members to remember a time when the person was injured or ill in a way that was expected to be painful and to describe that person's behavior. It was found that the frequency of pain behaviors (e.g., facial expressions, body postures) following injury or illness was reported to be low, with 37% concluded to be hyporesponsive to pain, of whom 25% were deemed to have a high pain threshold. The implications of these findings are hindered by the questionable validity of retrospective accounts (e.g., recall biases, memory distortion) and the fact that there was no control group for comparison. Indeed, a disrupted *expression* of pain does not necessarily imply that these individuals are pain insensitive. Instead, a number of authors have proposed that they may process information and respond more slowly to painful incidents, or they may express their pain in a manner different from those without disabilities (Breau et al., 2001; Defrin, Pick, Peretz, & Carmeli, 2004; Gilbert-MacLeod, Craig, Rocha, & Mathias, 2000; Hennequin, Morin, & Feine, 2000).

Studies that have examined behavioral responses to laboratory-induced acute pain incidents among populations with disabilities have typically used methods that are reaction-time dependent (Defrin et al., 2004). However, the cognitive or motor impairments, or both, that are common among individuals with developmental disabilities may hinder their ability to effectively communicate that they are experiencing pain, either verbally or nonverbally. For example, Hennequin, Morin, et al. (2000) sought to measure the cold-pain threshold of a group of individuals with Down syndrome by measuring the time elapsed from the application of an ice cube on the skin to the first verbal or behavioral expression of pain. The authors found that patients with Down syndrome exhibited significantly longer pain latencies relative to controls, suggesting that, although individuals with disabilities are not insensitive to pain, they may have a higher pain threshold. Because a reaction-time deficit is a well-documented characteristic of this population, it is quite possible, and perhaps more likely, that this may account for delayed response to sensory stimulation (Hennequin, Morin, et al., 2000). However, in research by Defrin and colleagues (2004), although reaction time was found to be slower in adults with intellectual disability, including those diagnosed with Down syndrome, compared to controls, both groups performed comparably on a reaction time–dependent measure. When employing a measure that is dependent on the subject's reaction time, a slow reaction time should induce an artificial elevation in the pain threshold (Defrin et al., 2004). The lack of elevation in the heat-pain threshold among people with cognitive impairments, despite their slower reaction time, implies that this group may actually have a lower heat-pain threshold (i.e., a greater sensitivity to heat pain) compared to normal. Although the studies by Hennequin and colleagues and by Defrin et al. yielded somewhat contradictory findings, direct comparisons of these two studies is difficult because of differences in the methodology employed, as well as the nature of the pain (i.e., cold pain versus heat pain) studied. Nevertheless, their findings add to the growing body of literature suggesting that the assumption of pain insensitivity among individuals with disabilities is erroneous at best and may be detrimental to the comfort and well-being of these populations at worst. More research examining the reliability and validity of reaction time–dependent and reaction time–free measures among individuals with disabilities is clearly needed.

Beyond the perceived slower pain responses evident in some individuals with developmental disabilities, several investigations also highlight that the manner in which pain is expressed may be different for individuals with and without developmental disabilities. At this point, it is important to draw attention to the difference between the experience of pain and the expression of pain. Pain measurement strategies typically assess pain expression, that is, an individual's response to a noxious event or his or her pain behaviors. Such behaviors may provide insight into an individual's experience of pain, such as the severity of his or her discomfort, but experience and expression do not mirror each other. Given that the frequency and duration of pain would fall under the individual's pain experience, not only may individuals with developmental disabilities experience pain differently but their expression of pain may also differ. For instance, in a study examining everyday pain among children with developmental disabilities, Gilbert-MacLeod and colleagues (2000) found that these children tended to exhibit a moderated distress response to potentially painful incidents in a child care setting. Compared to their peers who do not have developmental disabilities, children with developmental disabilities were more likely to engage in no response, less likely to cry, and less likely to engage in help-seeking behaviors in response to everyday bumps and bruises. A dampened behavioral and physiological reaction to acute noxious stimuli (e.g., vaccinations) has also been recorded among both children and adults with developmental disabilities and may be particularly evident as the severity of cognitive impairment increases (Oberlander, Gilbert, Chambers, O'Donnell, & Craig, 1999; Porter et al., 1996).

In contrast to these studies, which suggest a moderated behavioral response to potentially painful stimuli (Gilbert-MacLeod et al., 2000; Oberlander, Gilbert, et al., 1999; Porter et al., 1996), Nader, Oberlander, Chambers, and Craig (2004) examined the expression of pain in children with autism. They found that these children exhibited a substantial facial pain reaction when undergoing venipuncture, suggesting that they may, in fact, be more sensitive to pain than their peers without autism. Direct comparisons between this study and the others previously discussed are difficult, however, because of the marked differences in their measures and sample composition. Whereas Nader and associates' (2004) sample comprised a rather homogeneous group of children with autism, the other investigations included children with an array of diagnoses and varying degrees of cognitive functioning. In addition, Nader et al. used facial expression as an index of pain, whereas other studies, such as that of Gilbert-MacLeod et al., used an observational measure that focused on the behavior context and the person's distress response.

In summary, despite the findings that individuals with cognitive impairment may exhibit an altered or attenuated pain response to acute noxious events and the presence of persisting pain, there is no conclusive evidence indicating that they are insensitive or indifferent to pain (Oberlander, O'Donnell, et al., 1999; Stallard, Williams, Lenton, & Velleman, 2001). In fact, not only is there evidence of intact pain sensitivity in a substantial proportion of individuals with disabilities (Gilbert-MacLeod et al., 2000; Hennequin, Morin, et al., 2000; Oberlander, O'Donnell, et al., 1999), but there is also evidence indicating that they may be more sensitive to various types of pain than are people without disabilities (Defrin et al., 2004; Nader et al., 2004).

PREVALENCE AND TYPES OF PAIN IN INDIVIDUALS WITH DEVELOPMENTAL DISABILITIES

Scant attention has been devoted to the epidemiology of pain in children and adults with developmental disabilities, in spite of the growing body of evidence that these individuals may be at heightened risk for experiencing pain. One study suggested that pain associated with injuries may differ for people with and without disabilities (Leland, Garrard, & Smith, 1994). Children with disabilities may also frequently experience pain from sources seldom encountered by children without disabilities, including pain caused by medical interventions such as intravenous line insertions, irritations caused by prostheses, and surgeries (Breau, McGrath, Camfield, Rosmus, & Finley, 2000; Oberlander, O'Donnell, et al., 1999). Pain associated with chronic conditions comorbid with their disorder (e.g., spasticity in cerebral palsy) is also common among individuals with developmental disabilities (Carter, McArthur, & Cunliffe, 2002; Hunt, Goldman, Seers, Crichton, & Mastroyannopoulou, 1999; Oberlander, O'Donnell, et al., 1999). Thus, in this section, what is currently known about the prevalence and correlation of these various types of pain among children and adolescents with developmental disabilities is presented, drawing on the adult literature where available. A summary of the common pains experienced among people with various developmental disabilities is summarized in Table 5.2. Comparisons are made between people with and without disabilities

Table 5.2. Common pains experienced by persons with developmental disabilities

Developmental disability	Painful comorbid conditions	Location/type of pains experienced as a result of painful conditions
Down syndrome	Cancer (leukemia)	Disease process Diagnostic procedures Treatment
	Oral health—diseases	Periodontal General dental Temporomandibular
	Drug toxicity	Mucositis Infection Peripheral neuropathy
	Congenital health defect	General locations: • Ear, nose, throat • Leg, abdomen, head, neck, and back
Autism	Epilepsy	Post-seizure
	Gastrointestinal disorder	Gastroesophageal reflux Reflux esophagitis Abdominal
Cerebral palsy	Gastrointestinal	Gastroesophageal reflux Constipation
	Musculoskeletal (including hip and back pain)	Muscle spasms Dislocated hips Joint problems Position/posture changes Spontaneous pain
ALL	Pain experienced more commonly than the general population	Medical procedure related pain Daily living Infection Gastrointestinal discomfort

when possible. However, the vast majority of studies to date have failed to include control groups of children or adults without disabilities, and direct comparison across studies is difficult because of differences in the methodology employed and the nature of the samples studied.

Children with Intellectual Disabilities

The population of individuals with cognitive impairment is a diverse group. These individuals may have an established diagnosis of mental retardation (a label only used in diagnostic terms) or Down syndrome, for example, or may simply be functioning below the intellectual level appropriate for their chronological age and may not hold a formal diagnosis per se. Intellectual disability is typically classified on the basis of an individual's deficits in adaptation, age, and IQ scores (Grossman, 1983): mild impairment is indicated by an IQ score of 50–70; moderate, 35–49; severe, 20–34; and profound, an IQ score below 20.

A substantial portion of the research on pain in children with intellectual disabilities comes from the work of Breau and colleagues (Breau, Camfield, et al.,

2003; Breau, Camfield, McGrath, & Finley, 2004). These studies with children and adolescents with intellectual disabilities are among the few to compare acute or everyday pains and recurrent or chronic pains experienced by this population. Breau et al. found children and adolescents with severe intellectual disabilities to exhibit high levels of pain persistently (Breau, Camfield, et al., 2003). During a 4-week period, an overwhelming 78% of the children in their sample were reported by caregivers to experience pain on at least one occasion, and between 35% and 52% experienced pain on a weekly basis. Stallard and associates (2001) reported a similarly high rate of pain among their sample of children with intellectual disabilities who have difficulties with communication, with nearly 75% experiencing pain at least once over a 2-week period and 84% experiencing pain on 5 or more days. In a report based on retrospective accounts regarding the frequency of pain among children with severe intellectual disability, Stallard, Williams, Velleman, Lenton, and McGrath (2002a) found that 41% of caregivers judged their child to experience pain almost every day, with a further 17% reporting their child to experience pain at least once a week. For nearly 40% of the children, their pain lasted longer than 24 hours.

As for the type of pain encountered among children with intellectual disability, it appears that nonaccidental pain may be particularly problematic for these youngsters because the occurrence of nonaccidental pain has been found to be approximately double that of pain related to accidents (62% versus 30%, respectively) (Breau, Camfield, et al., 2003). Breau, Camfield, et al. (2003) found that the most common types of nonaccidental pain in children with intellectual disabilities include gastrointestinal discomfort (reported by 22%), pain arising from infection (20%), and musculoskeletal pain (19%). Similarly, Hunt et al. (1999) found that 51% of pain reported was due to gastrointestinal discomfort and 48% was musculoskeletal pain. In addition, 13% of these children were documented to have recurrent pains (e.g., ear pain, diaper rash), and 11% everyday pains (e.g., teething, menstruation, headaches) (Breau, Camfield, et al., 2003). Although not as frequent as nonaccidental pain, 13% were reported to experience pain associated with medical procedures (e.g., needles, postoperative, feeding tube irritation). It is important to stress that the pain many children with intellectual disabilities endure is often substantial, with approximately 22%–67% reporting their pain to be moderate or severe (Hunt et al., 1999; Stallard et al., 2001). Furthermore, the most intense pain reported is nonaccidental pain, the most common type of pain among these children and the most enduring in nature (Breau, Camfield, et al., 2003; Hunt et al., 1999). Unfortunately, as noted in several studies (Breau, Camfield, et al., 2003; Fanurik et al., 1999; Oberlander, O'Donnell, et al., 1999), those who experience the most pain tend to be the children with greater physical and cognitive impairments, the very individuals who may have the most difficulty effectively communicating their discomfort.

Although methodologies vary dramatically among studies, if one compares the overall rates of pain experienced by children with intellectual disability in the aforementioned studies (i.e., Breau, Camfield, et al., 2003; Stallard et al., 2001) to those reported in studies of children without intellectual disability (e.g., Goodman & McGrath, 1991; Perquin et al., 2000), it is clearly evident that children with disabilities experience markedly higher rates of pain than their typically developing peers. For example, in the study by Perquin and associates (2000), the authors found that just over 50% of their otherwise healthy sample experienced pain during a 3-month period compared to the 75%–85% prevalence rates found among children with intellectual disability over a much shorter time span (i.e., 2–4 weeks) (Breau, Camfield, et al., 2003; Stallard et al., 2001). This finding is alarming because a great deal of the pain experienced by children with disabilities is not due to the more transient injuries and common childhood pains, such as headaches or medical procedures, but to enduring comorbid medical conditions or illnesses.

Relative to acute and chronic pain episodes, very few studies have documented the rates of everyday or accidental pain associated with injuries in children with intellectual disability, despite their rather frequent occurrence even among the population without disabilities (Fearon et al., 1996). In one of the few studies to compare injuries in children with and without disabilities, Leland and colleagues (1994) found that 72% of ambulatory children with cognitive impairments in a child care setting had at least one injury, compared to only 25% of children without intellectual disability. Furthermore, children with intellectual disabilities incurred approximately twice as many injuries as children without disabilities over the 1-year study period and were more likely to be injured by another child than those without disabilities (20% versus 1%, respectively). However, many children without disabilities were more likely to be injured while running (16%) or playing on playground equipment (15%), activities during which only 6% of the children with disabilities were injured. These findings taken together suggest that children with intellectual disabilities experience pain from diverse sources, pain that is more commonly chronic than episodic in nature. Beyond recognition that children with intellectual disabilities as a group experience multiple types of pain, research documenting and comparing the unique sources and types of pain among specific patient populations is virtually nonexistent. Knowledge of pain sources and the type of pain in individuals with intellectual disability is imperative in order to manage diagnosis-specific pain, and ultimately to reduce the disability associated with persistent painful conditions, as well as to improve an individual's mental and physical well-being.

Children with Down Syndrome

Down syndrome is a common chromosomal disorder, with an incidence of 1 in 700 live births (Torfs & Christianson, 1998), and is characterized by a trisomy of chromosome 21. Although Down syndrome is the most common congenital cause of cognitive impairment around the world (Hennequin, Faulks, & Allison, 2003), few studies have addressed the prevalence and incidence of pain in this population. The overwhelming majority of the research studies providing epidemiological data on pain in children with cognitive impairment discussed previously have comprised rather heterogeneous samples of children with developmental disabilities, including children diagnosed with mental retardation, autism, cerebral palsy (CP), and Down syndrome. It is not uncommon, however, for individuals with Down syndrome to have comorbid medical conditions at a greater frequency than that noted among the general population, including those with other developmental disabilities, thereby exposing them to several additional potential sources of pain. Three conditions that individuals with Down syndrome are particularly at risk for developing, and for which pain is a serious secondary problem, are cancer, oral health issues, and hip abnormalities. With each of these conditions is a dearth of research.

Several studies have highlighted that children with Down syndrome have a greater risk than the general population for certain types of cancer, particularly leukemia (e.g., acute lymphoblastic leukemia, acute myeloid leukemia) (Hasle, Clemmensen, & Mikkelsen, 2000; Hill et al., 2003). However, beyond documentation of the prevalence and incidence (approximately 1%–1.4% over a 1-year period) (Hill et al., 2003; Winell & Burke, 2003) of these diseases in this population, surprisingly little attention has been devoted to obtaining epidemiological data on acute or chronic pains among these individuals. Among children without developmental disabilities who have leukemia, it is well documented that numerous sources of pain exist, including pain from the disease process, diagnostic procedures, and treatment regimens (Ljungman, Gordh, Sorensen, & Krueger, 1999, 2000). In one study, approximately 95% of children without disabilities reported pain when receiving diagnostic procedures for leukemia; although the percentage reporting pain decreased somewhat over the course of treatment, pain continued to be reported by a substantial proportion of children, with the lowest rate evident after the institution of a pain management program (i.e., approximately 60% reporting pain) (Van Cleve et al., 2004). The most common locations of pain (i.e., leg pain, 27%; abdominal pain, 17%; head and neck pain, 16%; and back pain, 14%) are consistent with the effects of the disease process, side effects of chemotherapy, and lumbar and bone marrow aspirations (Ljungman & McGrath, 2003; Van Cleve et al., 2004). Drug toxicity among children treated for leukemia is also cause for concern because it often results in painful conditions, including mucositis (i.e., inflammation of a mucous membrane), infection, and peripheral neuropathy (Van Cleve et al., 2004). Therefore, given the breadth of sources and types of pain children with cancer experience, this is an area in urgent need of exploration.

In addition to being at risk for developing leukemia, it is well documented that children with Down syndrome have a high level of oral health problems (Hennequin, Allison, & Veyrune, 2000; Hennequin, Morin, et al., 2000). It has been proposed that children with Down syndrome may have a higher incidence of dental pain than their peers because of the higher frequency of chronic facial pain disorders (e.g., temporomandibular disorder, characterized by symptoms of pain in the temporomandibular joint; headache; earache; neck, back, or shoulder pain; limited jaw movement) or the higher incidence of periodontal disease among this population (Hennequin, Faulks, Veyrune, & Bourdiol, 1999). However, the only available study that compared the experience of dental pain in children with Down syndrome to that of their siblings without Down syndrome revealed that there were no significant differences between the two groups in the percentage reported to have ever experienced dental pain. Approximately 18% of the children with Down syndrome and 20% of their siblings were reported by parents to have experienced dental pain (Hennequin et al., 2003). These findings were described as preliminary and deserve replication in future research.

As noted by several authors (Hennequin, Morin, et al., 2000; Kioschos, Shaw, & Beals, 1999), hip abnormalities are also a frequent cause of discomfort and pain among individuals with Down syndrome, including hip instability or dislocation. The vast majority of research on hip disease in children with Down syndrome is unfortunately limited to case reports, thus making estimates of its prevalence difficult. In one study of 65 adults with Down syndrome, hip abnormalities were found in 28% (Hresko, McCarthy, & Goldberg, 1993). Left untreated, the subsequent natural history of hip instability is a progression from acute dislocation to fixed dislocation, often resulting in a painful arthritis and, ultimately, the cessation of ambulation (Winell & Burke, 2003). Early detection is therefore crucial in order to avoid potentially debilitating conditions.

In summary, children with Down syndrome may experience pain from a number of unique sources that children in the general population and those with other types of developmental disabilities are less likely to encounter. The medical diagnoses highlighted previously by no means provide an exhaustive list of conditions to which these children are exposed, and which may be associated with considerable pain. Although beyond the scope of this chapter, it is noteworthy that children with Down syndrome are at a substantially elevated risk for congenital heart defects, with prevalence rates reported to be as high as 50%–60% of this population (Venugopalan & Agarwal, 2003; Winell & Burke, 2003) compared to only 33% of children without Down syndrome (Venugopalan & Agarwal, 2003). Children with Down syndrome have also displayed high rates of ear, nose, and throat disorders (Mitchell, Call, & Kelly, 2003). Congenital heart defects as well as ear, nose, and throat disorders, and the procedures used to manage them, are potentially quite painful (Hennequin, Morin, et al., 2000). To date, there are virtually no studies documenting the prevalence or incidence of pain among children with Down syndrome who experience these diseases. Given that pain may be a prominent part of the aforementioned conditions, an accurate estimation of pain in vulnerable populations remains an important first step in order to ensure that those most in need receive adequate pain treatment.

Children with Autism

Autism is a severe, pervasive developmental disorder that affects approximately 1 in 400 children, and is characterized by abnormalities in social interaction and communication, and restricted repetitive and stereotyped patterns of behaviors and interests (American Psychiatric Association, 2000). Similar to children with Down syndrome, children with autism have long been thought to be insensitive or indifferent to pain, although we now know that this is not the case (Nader et al., 2004). It has been suggested that the prevailing belief of pain insensitivity among this population may be the result of a sociocommunicative impairment (Craig, Lilley, & Gilbert, 1996). Children with autism often have a delay in or complete absence of language development (Boucher, 2003; Voigt et al., 2000). Moreover, even when speech is present, it tends to lack intonation and inflection, and fails to convey emotions (Peterson, 1986). Deficits in social relatedness are also salient among children with autism, and are closely related to their impairments in communication. These youngsters often do not use the facial expressions or gestures that typically developing children use to communicate their needs or express how they feel (Mash & Wolfe, 1999). Given the pervasive deficits in social relatedness and communication, it is little wonder that the expression of pain may differ among children with autism. Aside from the limited number of studies seeking to either prove or disprove this population's sensitivity to pain (Nader et al., 2004; Tordjman et al., 1999), no studies have documented the prevalence of pain in this group of children, nor have any examined pain in children with other disorders that fall on the autism spectrum (e.g., Asperger syndrome, pervasive developmental disorder not otherwise specified). As noted by Bursch, Ingman, Vitti, Hyman, and Zeltzer (2004), more than 20% of patients at a pediatric pain outpatient clinic at the University of California, Los Angeles, presented with pervasive developmental disorders or autism-like traits, suggesting that pain is indeed a significant problem for a substantial proportion of these youngsters.

Similar to children with Down syndrome, children with autism often have a number of medical conditions that may increase their likelihood of experiencing pain. Epilepsy, a disorder characterized by at least two unprovoked seizures, is highly associated with autism (Muhle, Trentacoste, & Rapin, 2004). Although the prevalence of epilepsy among the general population is estimated to be between 2% and 3%, approximately 30% of children with autism have this disorder, and, by adulthood, the number increases to as many as one third of those with a disorder that falls within the autistic spectrum (Muhle et al., 2004; Munoz-Yunta et al., 2003; Tuchman & Rapin, 2002). Although no study has documented the prevalence of pain associated with epilepsy in children with autism, at least one recent investigation by Breau and associates (2004) reported seizures to be a significant risk factor for recurrent pain among children with cognitive impairment, highlighting that pain may be a problem that is underrecognized in this population.

In addition to epilepsy, a topic of considerable interest in the contemporary scientific literature is the markedly high rate of gastrointestinal diseases in children with autism (Horvath & Perman, 2002; Kuddo & Nelson, 2003). Several studies have noted elevated rates of gastrointestinal symptoms in children with autism relative to their peers without disabilities, many of which are associated with pain (e.g., gastroesophageal reflux, reflux esophagitis) (Horvath & Perman, 2002). Particularly noteworthy is the high prevalence of abdominal pain in children with autism, approaching nearly 40%, relative to only about 16% of age-matched siblings without autism (Horvath & Perman, 2002).

These few examples provide a glimpse into the painful types of comorbid conditions that children with autism may be especially vulnerable to developing. Reports are limited, however, and multicenter epidemiological studies assessing pain among people who fall within the autistic spectrum, including those focusing on subtypes across the autism spectrum, could prove valuable in furthering our understanding of the prevalence of pain as well as the types of pain among these individuals.

Children with Cerebral Palsy

Cerebral palsy (CP) is a group of disorders of the central nervous system manifested by aberrant control of movement or posture. To meet the full criteria for CP, the onset of symptoms must occur early in life, and the symptoms cannot be the result of a recognized progressive disease (Kuban & Leviton, 1994). The motor impairments characteristic of individuals with CP are diverse and may include spasticity (i.e., muscular hypertonicity with increased tendon reflexes), rigidity (i.e., excessive muscle stiffness), dystonia (i.e., disordered tonicity of the muscles), athetosis (i.e., uncontrolled, slow, writhing movements), and ataxia (i.e., a general instability of movement) (Ehde et al., 2003). Having pain associated with these motor impairments is inevitable if one considers, for example, what a person must undergo for the treatment of spasticity. Treatment may include a combination of physiotherapy, orthopedic surgery, neurosurgery, and drug administration (Oberlander & Craig, 2003).

Similar to most others with developmental disabilities, it is difficult to asssess pain in individuals with CP because of their communication difficulties and cognitive impairments (Giusiano, Jimeno, Collignon, & Chau, 1995; Turk et al., 1997). Moreover, the presence of motor impairments poses special challenges to the accurate assessment of pain in CP because pain may be masked by the individual's limited physical response when in pain (e.g., a child with spasticity may be unable to withdraw from a painful stimulus) (Fanurik et al., 1999). Because individuals with CP have potentially severe motor impairments and limited mobility, there is ample reason to suspect that pain may be a serious secondary problem for many of these individuals (Oberlander, O'Donnell, et al., 1999; Schwartz et al., 1999; Turk et al., 1997), thereby underlining the importance of research assessing the types and sources of pain in this population, despite the difficulties in assessment.

Prior to the mid-1990s, very little had been written concerning the nature and scope of pain associated with CP (Ehde et al., 2003). Since then, the few studies that have emerged show that pain is a common part of these individuals' daily lives. The prevalence of pain in children with CP has been reported to be as high as 83% (Hunt et al., 1999), with nearly 50% affected by some form of pain all the time or sometime each day (Hunt et al., 1999), and approximately 11%–23% reported by caregivers to be in *severe* pain constantly or on a daily basis (Houlihan, O'Donnell, Conaway, & Stevenson, 2004; Hunt et al., 1999). In the adult population, approximately 67%–84% report one or more chronic pain problems (Engel, Jensen, Hoffman, & Kartin, 2003; Schwartz et al., 1999; Turk et al., 1997), with about half of those with pain (56%) experiencing pain daily, and a similar number (53%) reporting their pain to be moderate to severe in intensity (Schwartz et al., 1999). Unfortunately, for individuals with CP, there are many potential sources of pain, and the presence of multiple types of pain appears to be the norm (Engel et al., 2003; Hadden & von Baeyer, 2002; Hunt et al., 1999; Nolan, Chalkiadis, Low, Olesch, & Brown, 2000; Oberlander, O'Donnell, et al., 1999). For example, Hadden and von Baeyer (2002) noted several daily living situations to be painful for children with CP. Of the 67% of caregivers reporting their child to have experienced pain in the previous month, assisted stretching (reported to be painful by 93%), assisted sitting (69.8%), assisted walking (53.5%), putting on splints (58.1%), toileting (55.8%), and independent standing (34.9%) were the most painful daily activities reported.

Children with CP may also undergo more invasive and frequent surgical interventions (e.g., placement of gastric feeding devices, release of muscular contractures) in an attempt to maintain or improve their quality of life (Carter et al., 2002; Long & Harp, 1995; Nolan et al., 2000; Oberlander, O'Donnell, et al., 1999), but which may also be additional sources of pain. Indeed, in the study by Hadden and von Baeyer (2002), needle injections (reported by approximately 40% to be painful), blood pressure tests (14%), surgeries (9%), medical examinations (7%), enemas (7%), and dental procedures (5%) were commonly reported by caregivers to be painful for their child with CP. Range-of-motion manipulation therapy and occupational therapy, typical therapeutic regimens for children with CP (Long & Harp, 1995), were also among the most painful health care situations identified by parents (58% and 2%, respectively) (Hadden & von Baeyer, 2002).

In addition to the considerable discomfort associated with carrying out activities of daily living and the acute episodes of procedural pain they frequently encounter, approximately 50% of children with CP experience gastrointestinal pain, often as a result of gastroesophageal reflux (28%), constipation (28%), and abdominal gas (22%), and a similar percentage (i.e., 48%) report musculoskeletal pain, most notably resulting from muscle spasms (25%), dislocated hips (23%), and joint problems (21%) (Carter et al., 2002; Hunt et al., 1999; Long & Harp, 1995). Although prevalence rates were not provided, Long and Harp (1995) identified hip, knee, and foot pain as common in youth with CP, and similarly attributed these pain problems to a number of factors such as congenital dislocation, joint stress related to hypertonic muscles, and overuse. Headaches, seizures, and earaches also appear to be painful for a significant proportion of these youngsters, affecting approximately 21%, 14%, and 10%, respectively (Hunt et al., 1999).

These findings are comparable to the results reported in the adult literature, in which musculoskeletal (e.g., back, hip) deformities, gastrointestinal disturbances, and spasticity are frequently reported and may all be significant sources of pain (Engel et al., 2003; Schwartz et al., 1999; Turk et al., 1997). Indeed, chronic back pain has been reported in 63%–72% of adults with CP, and lower extremity pain may occur in as many as two thirds (Engel et al., 2003; Schwartz et al., 1999). Hip pain is also extremely problematic for a sizable proportion of adults with this condition, reported in approximately 40%–63% (Engel et al., 2003; Hodgkinson et al., 2001; Schwartz et al., 1999). Among nonambulatory adults with CP-related hip pain, pain associated with mobilization, palpation, and weight bearing on their lower limbs is collectively reported by as many as 67% (Hodgkinson et al., 2001). Pain linked to position or postural changes (i.e., staying in the same position for a long period of time or changing posture after staying in a position for too long) has also been reported by nearly 20% of this population, and spontaneous pain (e.g., at night or associated with weather changes) is reported by approximately 14% (Hodgkinson et al., 2001).

Other pain sites that are reported by 40%–55% of adults with CP include the hands and wrists, neck and shoulder area, arms, feet, and ankles (Engel et al., 2003; Schwartz et al., 1999). The prevalence of headaches in this population has been documented to be between 24% and 32%, and abdominal pain between 16% and 22% (Engel et al., 2003; Schwartz et al., 1999; Turk et al., 1997). The process of aging may also bring with it unique sources of pain among adults, including pain associated with disuse or overuse of muscles and limbs affected by chronic disablement (Schwartz et al., 1999; Turk et al., 1997), although more research in this area is needed.

In summary, although limited, the studies on pain in people with CP indicate that chronic pain is a serious secondary problem for a significant number of children and adults with this condition. Together, CP and its management can also present a multitude of sources of acute pain. The lack of research in this area has left many questions unanswered with respect to CP-related pain, gaps deserving attention in future research. To date, the examination of pain in this population has been confined to studies that are cross-sectional in nature, thereby leaving our understanding of the natural course of pain in both youth and adults with CP incomplete. A similar case may be made for children with cognitive impairments but who do not exhibit the motoric dysfunction characteristic of children with CP. Thus, longitudinal research is needed to document the prevalence and diversity of pain conditions among these populations across the life span. Longitudinal research will be instrumental in the development of treatment strategies and for the identification of which patients may be most in need of services and pain treat-

ments (Ehde et al., 2003). In addition, the available studies examining the prevalence of pain in adults with CP have largely been restricted to those with no or
mild cognitive impairments, making generalizations problematic. Despite the difficulties one may encounter when assessing pain among individuals with moderate to severe cognitive impairment secondary to their CP, research remains crucial
given the severe pain many of these individuals must endure on a daily basis.

CONCLUSION

This chapter has provided a comprehensive analysis of what is currently known,
and not known, regarding the prevalence and types of pain manifest across the
spectrum of developmental disabilities, including individuals with cognitive impairment (e.g., mental retardation, Down syndrome), pervasive developmental
disorders, and CP. Until recently, pain has received negligible attention in people
with developmental disabilities, in large part as a result of the inherent difficulties
associated with the assessment of pain in these individuals, as well as the widespread and pernicious belief that they do not experience pain. Pain assessment and
recognition in individuals with cognitive impairment present a special challenge
to both caregivers and health care professionals, which has obvious implications
for obtaining epidemiological data on pain in populations who have cognitive impairment. However, with the increased attention directed toward identifying a
core set of pain behaviors specific to children with developmental disabilities, behavioral measures are beginning to emerge in an attempt to surpass the difficulties or inability of individuals with disabilities to adequately communicate their
experiences through the typical verbal channels. Unfortunately, when communication via nonverbal means is also compromised, as may be the case with CP, several additional challenges to pain assessment emerge because overt behavioral responses to noxious stimuli may be difficult for others to recognize.

Despite these challenges to pain assessment, the research presented in this
chapter suggests that pain is a very real and common experience among populations with disabilities. The emerging empirical literature highlights that children
with developmental disabilities may be at risk for more injuries from different environmental sources than their peers without disabilities. Furthermore, individuals with disabilities may be particularly vulnerable to more frequent, and unique
sources of, acute pain as a result of the vast array of medical procedures to which
they are exposed in order to treat their underlying disorder or the consequences
associated with their condition that develop over time. Chronic pain is also a serious secondary problem for a substantial proportion of children and adults with developmental disabilities, indicating that the pain that they experience continues to
be inadequately managed.

In the face of this knowledge, it is clear that considerable research effort needs
to be directed toward identifying the pain in general, and the specific types of pain
in particular, characteristic of the diverse groups of individuals covered in this
chapter. The vast majority of the research conducted to date is unfortunately ham-
pered by methodological limitations that render firm conclusions regarding the
experience of pain among people with developmental disabilities difficult if not
impossible. With but a few notable exceptions (e.g., Engel et al., 2003; Hennequin,
Morin, et al., 2000; Nader et al., 2004), the diagnoses of children within each of
the studies discussed encompass a broad spectrum of developmental disabilities,

such as Down syndrome, pervasive developmental disorders, CP, and traumatic brain injury. Such heterogeneity is problematic because it is difficult to ascertain which patient groups experience the pain in question. Furthermore, an individual's pain response may differ dramatically depending upon whether the person presents primarily with cognitive impairment, motor dysfunction, or both. However, because of the small sample sizes characteristic of the majority of epidemiological research to date, any within-group differences documented may not be meaningful, and may actually be misleading, calling attention to the need for more large-scale, multicenter investigations. The degree of cognitive impairment has also varied within studies, which is problematic given the recent acknowledgment that the recognition of pain by caregivers and health care professionals may be based on vastly different cues depending on the child's level of intellectual functioning.

In order to provide a more precise understanding of the nature and scope of pain across the full spectrum of developmental disabilities, it remains critical that future research recruit individuals with similar diagnoses and comparable levels of intellectual functioning. It is of equal importance that studies explicitly specify the criteria used to differentiate the different types of pain (i.e., everyday, acute, and chronic pain), because these descriptions are frequently lacking in the available research. Moreover, a standard definition of what constitutes a developmental disability is sorely needed if meaningful comparisons are to be made between studies. Ultimately, making pain differentiation explicit and the use of a standard definition of a developmental disability in research will provide more accurate estimates of the prevalence and incidence of the various types of pain among specific patient populations explored in this chapter.

Although several research questions remain unanswered at the present time, if the increasing number of researchers and clinicians interested in the assessment of pain in people with developmental disabilities is any indication of the fate of epidemiological pain research, it is likely that great strides will be made in our understanding of the experience of pain among unique populations in years to come. Longitudinal and epidemiological research with individuals with cognitive impairment remains crucial so that pain can be adequately managed and, ultimately, the quality of life and mental and physical functioning can be improved.

REFERENCES

American Psychiatric Association. (2000). *Diagnostic and statistical manual of mental disorders, fourth edition, text revision.* Washington, DC: American Psychiatric Press.

Benini, F., Trapanotto, M., Gobber, D., Agosto, C., Carli, G., Drigo, P., et al. (2004). Evaluating pain induced by venipuncture in pediatric patients with developmental delay. *Clinical Journal of Pain, 20,* 156–163.

Biersdorff, K.K. (1991). Pain insensitivity and indifference: Alternative explanations for some medical catastrophes. *Mental Retardation, 29,* 359–361.

Biersdorff, K.K. (1994). Incidence of significantly altered pain experience among individuals with developmental disabilities. *American Journal on Mental Retardation, 98,* 619–631.

Boucher, J. (2003). Language development in autism. *International Journal of Pediatric Otorhinolaryngology, 67,* S159–S163.

Breau, L.M., Camfield, C., McGrath, P.J., Rosmus, C., & Finley, G.A. (2001). Measuring pain accurately in children with cognitive impairments: Refinement of a caregiver scale. *Journal of Pediatrics, 138,* 721–727.

Breau, L.M., Camfield, C.S., McGrath, P.J., & Finley, G.A. (2003). The incidence of pain in children with severe cognitive impairments. *Archives of Pediatrics and Adolescent Medicine, 157,* 1219–1226.

Breau, L.M., Camfield, C.S., McGrath, P.J., & Finley, G.A. (2004). Risk factors for pain in children with severe cognitive impairments. *Developmental Medicine and Child Neurology, 46,* 364–371.

Breau, L.M., MacLaren, J., McGrath, P.J., Camfield, C.S., & Finley, G.A. (2003). Caregivers' beliefs regarding pain in children with cognitive impairment: Relation between pain sensation and reaction increases with severity of impairment. *Clinical Journal of Pain, 19,* 335–344.

Breau, L.M., McGrath, P.J., Camfield, C., Rosmus, C., & Finley, G.A. (2000). Preliminary validation of an observational pain checklist for persons with cognitive impairments and inability to communicate verbally. *Developmental Medicine and Child Neurology, 42,* 609–616.

Bursch, B., Ingman, K., Vitti, L., Hyman, P., & Zeltzer, L.K. (2004). Chronic pain in individuals with previously undiagnosed autistic spectrum disorders. *Journal of Pain, 5,* 290–295.

Carter, B., McArthur, E., & Cunliffe, M. (2002). Dealing with uncertainty: Parental assessment of pain in their children with profound special neeDown syndrome. *Journal of Advanced Nursing, 38,* 449–457.

Chambers, C.T., Reid, G.J., Craig, K.D., McGrath, P.J., & Finley, G.A. (1998). Agreement between child and parent reports of pain. *Clinical Journal of Pain, 14,* 336–342.

Craig, K.D., Lilley, C.M., & Gilbert, C.A. (1996). Social barriers to optimal pain management in infants and children. *Clinical Journal of Pain, 12,* 232–242.

Defrin, R., Pick, C.G., Peretz, C., & Carmeli, E. (2004). A quantitative somatosensory testing of pain threshold in individuals with mental retardation. *Pain, 108,* 58–66.

Doherty, E., Yanni, G., Conroy, R.M., & Bresnihan, B. (1993). A comparison of child and parent ratings of disability and pain in juvenile chronic arthritis. *Journal of Rheumatology, 20,* 1563–1566.

Donovan, J. (1997). Learning disabilities: Pain signals. *Nursing Times, 93*(45), 60–62.

Ehde, D.M., Jensen, M.P., Engel, J.M., Turner, J.A., Hoffman, A.J., & Cardenas, D.D. (2003). Chronic pain secondary to disability: A review. *Clinical Journal of Pain, 19,* 3–17.

Ekman, P., & Friesen, W.V. (1978). *The Facial Action Coding System.* Palo Alto, CA: Consulting Psychologists Press.

Engel, J.M., Jensen, M.P., Hoffman, A.J., & Kartin, D. (2003). Pain in persons with cerebral palsy: Extension and cross validation. *Archives of Physical and Medical Rehabilitation, 84,* 1125–1128.

Fanurik, D., Koh, J.L., Schmitz, M.L., Harrison, R.D., & Conrad, T.M. (1999). Children with cognitive impairment: Parent report of pain and coping. *Developmental and Behavioral Pediatrics, 20,* 228–234.

Fearon, I., McGrath, P.J., & Achat, H. (1996). 'Booboos': The study of everyday pain among young children. *Pain, 68,* 55–62.

Feldt, K.S., Ryden, M.B., & Miles, S. (1998). Treatment of pain in cognitively impaired compared with cognitively intact older patients with hip-fracture. *Journal of the American Geriatrics Society, 46,* 1079–1085.

Fradet, C., McGrath, P.J., Kay, J., Adams, S., & Luke, B. (1990). A prospective survey of reactions to blood tests by children and adolescents. *Pain, 40,* 53–60.

Franck, L.S., Greenberg, C.S., & Stevens, B. (2000). Pain assessment in infants and children. *Pediatric Clinics of North America, 47,* 487–512.

Gibson, S.J., & Chambers, C.T. (2004). Pain over the life span: A developmental perspective. In T. Hadjistavropoulos & K.D. Craig (Eds.), *Pain: Psychological perspectives* (pp. 113–153). Mahwah, NJ: Lawrence Erlbaum Associates.

Gilbert-MacLeod, C.A., Craig, K.D., Rocha, E.M., & Mathias, M.D. (2000). Everyday pain responses in children with and without developmental delays. *Journal of Pediatric Psychology, 25,* 301–308.

Giusiano, B., Jimeno, M.T., Collignon, P., & Chau, Y. (1995). Utilization of neural network in elaboration of an evaluation scale for pain in cerebral palsy. *MethoDown syndrome of Information in Medicine, 34,* 498–502.

Goodenough, B., Kampel, L., Champion, G.D., Laubreaux, L., Nicholas, M.K., Ziegler, J.B., et al. (1997). An investigation of the placebo effect and other factors in the report of pain severity during venipuncture in children. *Pain, 72,* 383–391.

Goodenough, B., Perrot, D.A., Champion, G.D., & Thomas, W. (2000). Painful pricks and prickle pains: Is there a relation between children's ratings of venipuncture pain and parental assessments of usual reaction to other pains? *Clinical Journal of Pain, 16,* 135–143.

Goodman, J.E., & McGrath, P.J. (1991). The epidemiology of pain in children and adolescents: A review. *Pain, 46,* 247–264.

Grossman, H.J. (1983). *Classification in mental retardation.* Washington, DC: American Association on Mental Deficiency.

Hadden, K.L., & von Baeyer, C.L. (2002). Pain in children with cerebral palsy: Common triggers and expressive behaviors. *Pain, 99,* 281–288.

Hadjistavropoulos, T., von Baeyer, C.L., & Craig, K.D. (2001). Pain assessment in persons with limited ability to communicate. In D.C. Turk & R. Melzack (Eds.), *Handbook of pain assessment* (2nd ed., pp. 134–149). New York: Guilford Press.

Hasle, H., Clemmensen, I.H., & Mikkelsen, M. (2000). Risks of leukaemia and solid tumours in individuals with Down's syndrome. *Lancet, 355,* 165–169.

Hennequin, M., Allison, P.J., & Veyrune, J.L. (2000). Prevalence of oral health problems in a group of individuals with Down syndrome in France. *Developmental Medicine and Child Neurology, 42,* 691–698.

Hennequin, M., Faulks, D., & Allison, P.J. (2003). Parents' ability to perceive pain experienced by their child with Down syndrome. *Journal of Orofacial Pain, 17,* 347–353.

Hennequin, M., Faulks, D., Veyrune, J.L., & Bourdiol, P. (1999). Significance of oral health in persons with Down syndrome: A literature review. *Developmental Medicine and Child Neurology, 41,* 275–283.

Hennequin, M., Morin, C., & Feine, J.S. (2000). Pain expression and stimulus localisation in individuals with Down's syndrome. *Lancet, 356,* 1882–1887.

Hill, D.A., Gridley, G., Cnattingius, S., Mellemkjaer, L., Linet, M., Adami, H.O., et al. (2003). Mortality and cancer incidence among individuals with Down syndrome. *Archives of Internal Medicine, 163,* 705–711.

Hodgkinson, I., Jindrich, M.L., Duhaut, P., Vadot, J.P., Metton, G., & Berard, C. (2001). Hip pain in 234 non-ambulatory adolescents and young adults with cerebral palsy: A cross-sectional multicentre study. *Developmental Medicine and Child Neurology, 43,* 806–808.

Horvath, K., & Perman, J.A. (2002). Autistic disorder and gastrointestinal disease. *Current Opinion in Pediatrics, 14,* 583–587.

Houlihan, C.M., O'Donnell, M., Conaway, M., & Stevenson, R.D. (2004). Bodily pain and health-related quality of life in children with cerebral palsy. *Developmental Medicine and Child Neurology, 46,* 305–310.

Hresko, M.T., McCarthy, J.C., & Goldberg, M.J. (1993). Hip disease in adults with Down syndrome. *Journal of Bone and Joint Surgery: British Volume, 75,* 604–607.

Hunt, A., Goldman, A., Seers, K., Crichton, N., & Mastroyannopoulou, K. (1999). *Pain sources and pain cues of children with severe neurological impairment.* Unpublished manuscript.

Hyams, J.S., Burke, G., Davis, P.M., Rzepski, B., & Androlonis, P.A. (1996). Abdominal pain and irritable bowel syndrome in adolescents: A community-based study. *Journal of Pediatrics, 129,* 220–226.

Kaasalainen, S., Middleton, J., Knezacek, S., Hartley, T., Stewart, N.C., & Robinson, L. (1998). Pain and cognitive status in the institutionalized elderly: Perceptions and interventions. *Journal of Gerontological Nursing, 24*(8), 24–31.

Kioschos, M., Shaw, E.D., & Beals, R.K. (1999). Total hip arthroplasty in patients with Down's syndrome. *Journal of Bone and Joint Surgery: British Volume, 81,* 436–439.

Kuban, K.C.K., & Leviton, A. (1994). Cerebral palsy. *New England Journal of Medicine, 330,* 188–195.

Kuddo, T., & Nelson, K.B. (2003). How common are gastrointestinal disorders in children with autism? *Current Opinion in Pediatrics, 15,* 339–343.

LaChapelle, D., Hadjistavropoulos, T., & Craig, K.D. (1999). Pain measurement in persons with intellectual disabilities. *Clinical Journal of Pain, 15,* 13–23.

Leland, N.L., Garrard, J., & Smith, D.K. (1994). Comparison of injuries to children with and without disabilities in a day-care center. *Developmental and Behavioral Pediatrics, 15,* 402–408.

Ljungman, G., Gordh, T., Sorensen, S., & Kreuger, A. (1999). Pain in paediatric oncology: Interviews with children, adolescents, and their parents. *Acta Paediatrica, 88,* 623–630.

Ljungman, G., Gordh, T., Sorensen, S., & Kreuger, A. (2000). Pain variations during cancer treatment in children: A descriptive survey. *Pediatric Hematology and Oncology, 17,* 211–221.

Ljungman, G., & McGrath, P.J. (2003). The prevalence of pain in children with cancer: An epidemiological study in an inpatient setting [Abstract]. In *Pain in childhood: The big questions.* Poster presented at the 6th International Symposium on Pediatric Pain, Sydney, Australia.

Long, T.M., & Harp, K.A. (1995). Pain in children. *Orthopaedic Physical Therapy Clinics of North America, 4,* 503–518.

Malviya, S., Voepel-Lewis, T., Tait, A.R., Merkel, S., Lauer, A., Munro, H., et al. (2001). Pain management in children with and without cognitive impairment following spine fusion surgery. *Paediatric Anaesthesia, 11,* 453–458.

Manne, S.L., Jacobsen, P.B., & Redd, W.H. (1992). Assessment of acute pediatric pain: Do child self-report, parent ratings, and nurse ratings measure the same phenomenon? *Pain, 48,* 45–52.

Mash, E.J., & Wolfe, D.A. (1999). Autism and childhood-onset schizophrenia. In *Abnormal child psychology* (pp. 372–418). Belmont, CA: WaDown syndromeworth.

McGrath, P.A. (1990). *Pain in children: Nature, assessment, and treatment.* New York: Guilford Press.

McGrath, P.J., Rosmus, C., Camfield, C., Campbell, M.A., & Hennigar, A. (1998). Behaviours caregivers use to determine pain in non-verbal, cognitively impaired individuals. *Developmental Medicine and Child Neurology, 40,* 340–343.

Merskey, H. (1986). Classification of chronic pain: Descriptions of chronic pain syndromes and definitions of pain terms. *Pain, Supplement 3,* S1–S8.

Merskey, H. & Bogduk, N. (1994). *Classification of chronic pain: Descriptions of chronic pain syndromes and definitions of pain terms* (2nd ed). Seattle, WA: IASP Press.

Mitchell, R.B., Call, E., & Kelly, J. (2003). Ear, nose and throat disorders in children with Down syndrome. *Laryngoscope, 113,* 259–263.

Muhle, R., Trentacoste, S.V., & Rapin, I. (2004). The genetics of autism. *Pediatrics, 113,* e472–e486.

Munoz-Yunta, J.A., Salvado, B., Ortiz-Alonso, T., Amo, C., Fernandez-Lucas, A., Maestu, F., et al. (2003). Clinical features of epilepsy in autism spectrum disorders. *Revista de Neurologia, 36,* S61–S67.

Nader, R., Oberlander, T.F., Chambers, C.T., & Craig, K.D. (2004). The expression of pain in children with autism. *Clinical Journal of Pain, 20,* 88–97.

Nolan, J., Chalkiadis, G.A., Low, J., Olesch, C.A., & Brown, T.C. (2000). Anaesthesia and pain management in cerebral palsy. *Anaesthesia, 55,* 32–41.

Oberlander, T.F., & Craig, K.D. (2003). Pain in children with developmental disabilities. In N.L. Schechter, C.B. Berde, & M. Yaster (Eds.), *Pain in infants, children, and adolescents* (pp. 599–619). Philadelphia: Lippincott Williams & Wilkins.

Oberlander, T.F., Gilbert, C.A., Chambers, C.T., O'Donnell, M.E., & Craig, K.D. (1999). Biobehavioural responses to acute pain in adolescents with a significant neurologic impairment. *Clinical Journal of Pain, 15,* 201–209.

Oberlander, T.F., O'Donnell, M.E., & Montgomery, C.J. (1999). Pain in children with significant neurological impairment. *Developmental and Behavioral Pediatrics, 20*, 235–243.

Perquin, C.W., Hazebroek-Kampschreur, A.A.J.M., Hunfeld, J.A.M., Bohnen, A.M., van Suijlekom-Smit, L.W.A., Passchier, J., et al. (2000). Pain in children and adolescents: A common experience. *Pain, 87*, 51–58.

Peterson, T.W. (1986). Recent studies in autism: A review of the literature. *Occupational Therapy and Mental Health, 6*, 63–75.

Porter, F.L., Malhotra, K.M., Wolf, C.M., Morris, J.C., Miller, J.P., & Smith, M.C. (1996). Dementia and response to pain in the elderly. *Pain, 68*, 413–421.

Schechter, N.L., Berde C.B., & Yaster, M. (2003). Pain in infants, children, and adolescents: An overview. In N.L. Schechter, C.B. Berde, & M. Yaster (Eds.), *Pain in infants, children, and adolescents* (pp. 3–18). Philadelphia: Lippincott Williams & Wilkins.

Schwartz, L., Engel, J.M., & Jensen, M.P. (1999). Pain in persons with cerebral palsy. *Archives of Physical Medicine and Rehabilitation, 80*, 1243–1246.

Stallard, P., Williams, L., Lenton, S., & Velleman, R. (2001). Pain in cognitively impaired, non-communicating children. *Archives of Disease in Childhood, 85*, 460–462.

Stallard, P., Williams, L., Velleman, R., Lenton, S., & McGrath, P.J. (2002a). Brief report: Behaviors identified by caregivers to detect pain in noncommunicating children. *Journal of Pediatric Psychology, 27*, 209–214.

Stallard, P., Williams, L., Velleman, R., Lenton, S., & McGrath, P.J. (2002b). Intervening factors in caregivers' assessments of pain in non-communicating children. *Developmental Medicine and Child Neurology, 44*, 212–214.

Stanford, E.A., Chambers, C.T., & Craig, K.D. (2005). A normative analysis of the development of pain-related vocabulary in children. *Pain, 114*, 278–284.

St.-Laurent-Gagnon, T., Bernard-Bonnin, A.C., & Villeneuve, E. (1999). Pain evaluation in preschool children and by their parents. *Acta Paediatrica, 88*, 422–427.

Terstegen, C., Koot, H.M., de Boer, J.B., & Tibboel, D. (2003). Measuring pain in children with cognitive impairment: Pain response to surgical procedures. *Pain, 103*, 187–198.

Tordjman, S., Antoine, C., Cohen, D.J., Gauvain-Piquard, A., Carlier, M., Roubertoux, P., et al. (1999). Study of the relationships between self-injurious behavior and pain reactivity in infantile autism. *Encephale, 25*, 122–134.

Torfs, C.P., & Christianson, R.E. (1998). Anomalies in Down syndrome individuals in a large population-based registry. *American Journal of Medical Genetics, 77*, 431–438.

Tuchman, R., & Rapin, I. (2002). Epilepsy in autism. *Lancet Neurology, 1*, 352–358.

Turk, M.A., Geremski, C.A., Rosenbaum, P.F., & Weber, R.J. (1997). The health status of women with cerebral palsy. *Archives of Physical Medicine and Rehabilitation, 78*, S10–S17.

Van Cleve, L., Bossert, E., Beecroft, P., Adlard, K., Alvarez, O., & Savedra, M.C. (2004). The pain experience of children with leukemia during the first year after diagnosis. *Nursing Research, 53*, 1–10.

Venugopalan, P., & Agarwal, A.K. (2003). Spectrum of congenital heart defects associated with Down syndrome in high consanguineous Omani population. *Indian Pediatrics, 40*, 398–403.

Voigt, R.G., Childers, D.O., Dickerson, C.L., Juhn, Y.J., Reynolds, A.M., Rodriguez, D.L., et al. (2000). Early pediatric neurodevelopmental profile of children with autistic spectrum disorders. *Clinical Pediatrics, 39*, 663–668.

von Baeyer, C.L., Baskerville, S., & McGrath, P.J. (1998). Everyday pain in three- to five-year old children in day care. *Pain Research and Management, 3*, 111–116.

Winell, J., & Burke, S.W. (2003). Sports participation of children with Down syndrome. *Orthopedic Clinics of North America, 34*, 439–443.

6

DEVELOPMENTAL ISSUES
IN ACUTE AND CHRONIC PAIN
IN DEVELOPMENTAL DISABILITIES

Lynn M. Breau, Bonnie Stevens, and Ruth Eckstein Grunau

Approximately 7%–10% of infants in North America are born with medical conditions that require hospitalization in the neonatal intensive care unit (NICU) or the pediatric intensive care unit (PICU). Of these, about 10% are at heightened risk for major neurodevelopmental sequelae (sensory, motor, and/or cognitive impairments). Hospitalization in these settings often entails frequent procedures to monitor medical status or to treat life-threatening conditions. Many procedures induce physiological and behavioral changes consistent with pain.

There is growing concern that cumulative repeated procedures may affect infants' development by adding to the effects of, or interacting with, extreme prematurity or, in full-term infants, major complications such as severe asphyxia, hypoxic-ischemic encephalopathy, cerebral infarcts, and cardiac problems that need surgery, or perinatal conditions requiring extracorporeal membrane oxygenation (ECMO). Furthermore, brain development is rapid at this time, increasing the vulnerability of the neurological system to insult. An emerging literature supports this growing concern in infants born extremely preterm, suggesting that pain may have both short-term and long-term effects on physiology and behavior through its impact on the highly plastic developing central nervous system (Anand, 2000; Grunau, 2002; Porter, Grunau, & Anand, 1999).

Little is known about the possible long-term contributions of prolonged pain exposure as well as the effects of analgesics, sedatives, and other medications used over long periods of time in the neonatal period, although interest has grown steadily (Banos, Ruis, & Guardiola, 2004). Neonates have a lower tactile threshold and heightened pain sensitivity (Andrews & Fitzgerald, 1994; Fitzgerald, Millard, & McIntosh, 1989), which may increase the salience of noxious stimuli. In addition, the fact that typical interactions with the environment are not available to infants in the NICU (Whitfield, 2003) could also affect development. Thus, infants in the NICU setting are particularly vulnerable and sensitive, faced with repeated painful experiences and an environment lacking many of the positive aspects of human contact common in a home setting. Given this picture, it is difficult to argue that there is not the potential for possible long-term consequences.

In this chapter, we examine what is known about early pain in the lives of infants who are at heightened risk for minor or major neurodevelopmental sequelae. Because these sequelae may result in sensory, motor, and/or cognitive impairments and the outcomes of their conditions are not always known early in life, we refer to this group of infants as being "at risk for" neurological impairment (NI). Although there is only a very small literature examining this topic specifically in infants at risk for NI, data from studies of animals and human infants, such as those who are born extremely preterm, can provide some insight.

DEFINING INFANTS AT RISK FOR COGNITIVE IMPAIRMENT

As many as 14.9% of the general population of the United States, outside of institutions, has been diagnosed with a developmental disability, namely cognitive, major sensory, or motor impairment, or some combination of these (Larson et al., 2001). Rates of neurological impairments are higher in infants born extremely prematurely, with as many as 25% showing clinically significant intellectual impairments (Horwood, Mogridge, & Darlow, 1998; Ment et al., 2000). However, rates of major impairments also vary by geographical regions and between institutions, depending on multiple environmental factors associated with sociodemographic status, such as the availability and nature of perinatal care (Tommiska et al., 2001).

Clear signs of neurological impairment are not always evident in infancy, and the majority of conclusive diagnoses are not reached until later. In many cases, the etiology of impairments is never identified because major impairments may occur in the absence of neonatal neurological abnormalities (Cioni et al., 2000; Cooke & Abernethy, 1999; Horwood et al., 1998; Saigal, Hoult, Streiner, Stoskopf, & Rosenbaum, 2000). In fact, in some studies, there are no significant associations between outcomes in childhood and neonatal factors, such as days in the NICU (Whitfield, Grunau, & Holsti, 1997), complications at birth (Gutbrod, Wolke, Soehne, Ohrt, & Riegel, 2000), gestational age at birth (Hutton, Pharoah, Cooke, & Stevenson, 1997), birth weight (Huttner et al., 1998), abnormal ultrasound results (Haataja, Mercuri, Cowan, & Dubowitz, 2000), brain lesions detected by magnetic resonance imaging (MRI) (Cioni et al., 2000; Cooke & Abernethy, 1999), or illness severity (Doussard-Roosevelt, McClenny, & Porges, 2001). Thus, there is no simple one-to-one relationship between known perinatal factors and long-term sensory, motor, or cognitive impairments.

To complicate matters further, ongoing factors may add to, or interact with, perinatal factors to increase risk for future impairments. For example, studies variously report that psychosocial factors do affect (Whitfield, 2003), do not affect (Doussard-Roosevelt et al., 2001; Hutton et al., 1997), or selectively affect long-term development (Resnick et al., 1999). Ongoing medical complications may also contribute to long-term disabilities (Ludman, Spitz, & Lansdown, 1993). For example, infants born prematurely are more likely than infants born at term to be rehospitalized during childhood (Teplin, Burchinal, Johnson-Martin, Humphry, & Kraybill, 1991), to experience multiple surgeries (Hack et al., 1993), and to have ongoing medical conditions that are associated with frequent episodes of acute or chronic pain (Houlihan, O'Donnell, Conaway, & Stevenson, 2004). Findings also suggest that maternal infection during pregnancy is implicated in neonatal brain injury (Kirpalani & Asztalos, 2001), and postnatal infection in the NICU is associated with poor neurodevelopment (Stoll et al., 2004). Thus, many complications thought to be induced in the perinatal or neonatal period may be linked to pre- or postnatal infection. In addition, reduced participation in interventions designed to promote development after NICU discharge has also been associated with poorer long-term outcomes (Hill, Brooks-Gunn, & Waldfogel, 2003). In summary, there is no definitive method of quantifying a given infant's risk for NI as a result of some combination of developmental status at birth or events associated with the NICU environment.

Nevertheless, many infants at risk for future NI spend some time in the NICU. Preterm and low-birth-weight infants represent approximately 10% of these children (Joseph et al., 1998), and their numbers are growing, both through increased rates of birth (Craig, Thompson, & Mitchell, 2002) and increased survival of infants born at younger gestational ages and lower birth weights (Horbar et al., 2002; Kaiser, Tilford, Simpson, Salhab, & Rosenfeld, 2004). Each year, approximately 50,000 infants are born in the United States with birth weights less than 1,500 grams (g) (Bernbaum & Batshaw, 1997). These infants are at risk for some degree of intellectual compromise (Mervis, Decoufle, Murphy, & Yeargin-Allsopp, 1995; Resnick et al., 1999). Prematurity (less than 37 weeks' gestation) and extreme prematurity (less than 28 weeks' gestation) also increase risk (Bernbaum & Batshaw, 1997). Illness may contribute additional risk for NI, although its effects appear independent of those of other perinatal factors (Fowlie, Tarnow-Mordi, Gould, & Strang, 1998). A quantitative review by Lorenz, Wooliever, Jetton, and Paneth (1998) highlights the severity of the risk for NI in these groups. In their review of 42 studies including more than 8,000 infants, they found that a diagnosis of mental retardation was the most common major disability among infants of 26 weeks' gestation or less or weighing less than 800 g at birth, or both, with 14% receiving this diagnosis.

Infants born with congenital anomalies are also at heightened risk for developmental disabilities, with some studies estimating as much as 27 times greater risk (Jelliffe-Pawlowski, Shaw, Nelson, & Harris, 2003). This group also accounts for a large number of admissions to the NICU, with studies reporting that they represent from 4.8% to 27% of admissions (Lindower, Atherton, & Kotagal, 1999; Sheth, 1998; Synnes et al., 2004). The proportion of infants admitted to NICUs with identifiable congenital anomalies also appears to have increased (Sheth, Goulden, & Ronen, 1994). Survival rates in this group have also increased, probably as a result of increased medical management of life-threatening conditions (Liu et al., 2001). These infants have longer NICU stays, require more surgeries, and have more medical conditions that require ongoing support after discharge (Lindower et al., 1999). Thus, the frequency of medical care that could result in pain may be even greater for this group than for other infants being cared for in the NICU setting. Although technological advances and the provision of care in the NICU have advanced a great deal, many children who have no clear signs of neurological compromise in the perinatal and neonatal periods develop later impairments in cognitive, motor, or sensory functioning. The literature examining the role of pain early in life is also in its infancy, and investigations of how pain interacts with or adds to risk as a result of specific infant characteristics are needed. Nevertheless, we do know that infants who are extremely premature or of extremely low birth weight have significantly increased risk, regardless of their perinatal or neonatal characteristics. Researchers have begun to examine the role of prolonged and frequent pain in their development (Grunau, 2000, 2002). The following sections examine what is known about pain early in life for these children.

EVIDENCE OF NEUROLOGICAL IMPACT OF EARLY PAIN

Animal Models

Much of the available evidence for long-term effects of neonatal pain on the developing nervous system is based on animal studies. Although we cannot extrapolate directly from the animal neonatal model to human infants, these studies are useful because the central nervous system of rat pups in their first postnatal week provides an approximation to that of premature infants (Marsh, Hatch, & Fitzgerald, 1997). There is increasing evidence that repeated pain may lead to structural and functional reorganization of pain systems in the peripheral and central nervous systems. Recurrent pain in rat pups is related to long-term changes in the receptive fields of dorsal horn neurons (Reynolds, Alvares, Middleton, & Fitzgerald, 1997). Inflammatory agents applied to neonatal rat pups can lead to changes in spinal nociceptive neuronal circuits, causing altered responses to noxious and non-noxious stimuli in adult rats (Ruda, Ling, Hohmann, Peng, & Tachibana, 2000). Because these changes may also be due to ongoing pain long after the neonatal period, and thus may not reflect changes likely in human preterm infants, interest in the type of animal experiments that may best model pain in the NICU has grown considerably. For example, repetitive pinpricks (Anand, Coskun, Thrivikraman, Nemeroff, & Plotsky, 1999) or a small surgical cut (Reynolds et al., 1997) may better reflect the type of pain induced in human infants during medical care than pain caused by long-lasting inflammatory agents (Ruda et al., 2000).

Animal research has also begun to examine the possibility that pain early in life may result in effects through several mechanisms or processes, leading to a complex presentation when these are acting simultaneously (Ren et al., 2004). Ren et al. proposed that early pain may lead to increased pain perception locally, which appears relatively soon after the injury, but early pain at low levels may also lead to global hypalgesia, reflecting increased activity of pain inhibition systems in response to the early pain. The authors also suggested that there may be periods during which these two processes co-occur.

Research with Human Infants

A small literature has examined the potential for immediate neurological damage caused by pain in human neonates that in turn may contribute to long-term impairments. These studies have indicated that procedures that may cause pain can lead to increased (Volpe, 1995) or decreased (Gagnon, Leung, & Macnab, 1999) cerebral blood flow, which can induce wide changes in cerebral blood flow as a result of immature autoregulation. Furthermore, fluctuations in intracranial pressure caused by painful/stressful events may contribute to or exacerbate neurological complications, such as early intraventricular hemorrhage (IVH) and ischemic changes leading to periventricular leukomalacia (PVL) (Anand et al., 1999). Both of these conditions are associated with neurological, psychological, and developmental sequelae (Anand et al., 1999). There is also evidence that rises in intracranial pressure are procedure specific. Bellieni, Burroni, and colleagues (2003) reported that peak intracranial pressure was reduced when blood sampling was conducted through the external jugular vein rather than by heel prick. In contrast, interventions to reduce pain also reduce rises in intracranial pressure. Because complications have been reported in relation to external jugular vein catheterization in newborns (Bitar et al., 2003), heel prick, accompanied by pain-relieving methods such as sensorial saturation, appears to be the best option explored in this study.

In their seminal studies, Fitzgerald and colleagues established that the tactile threshold is significantly lower at lower gestational ages (Fitzgerald, Shaw, & MacIntosh, 1988; Fitzgerald et al., 1989) and may be significantly lowered by repeated tactile stimulation (Andrews & Fitzgerald, 1994), both factors common to infants in the NICU at risk for NI. More recently, these researchers monitored the abdominal skin reflex during the first year of life in healthy infants 30–95 weeks' postconceptional age (PCA) and infants with unilateral hydronephrosis (Andrews, Desai, Dhillon, Wilcox, & Fitzgerald, 2002). There was a significant increase in reflex threshold with increasing PCA in the healthy group. However, this pattern was not found for either the affected or unaffected side of the abdomen for infants with unilateral hydronephrosis. The authors suggested that these results point to referred visceral hypersensitivity in infants.

Pain is also a specific form of stress. Both pain and stress activate the autonomic nervous system and the hypothalamic-pituitary-adrenal (HPA) axis. These hormonal events are one way in which early experience plays a role in neuronal plasticity (Gunnar & Barr, 1998). Research suggests that premature infants exposed to more cumulative pain and stress in the NICU may show changes in HPA axis function over time. For example, greater exposure to cumulative pain since birth (independent of early illness severity and morphine exposure) has been associated with *lower* plasma cortisol responses to stress at 32 weeks' PCA in the NICU among infants born at 22–32 weeks' gestation (Grunau et al., 2005). Conversely, at a corrected age of 8 months, greater cumulative exposure to neonatal pain was associated with *higher* salivary cortisol levels, both basal and in response to visual novelty (Grunau, Weinberg, & Whitfield, 2004). Although the directions of these effects of cumulative pain appear to differ, they both suggest involvement of pain in HPA axis function long after pain has ceased. There is a dearth of information on the developmental trajectory of cortisol production in preterm infants after discharge from the NICU. Understanding of the cumulative impact of stress in the NICU may be advanced by using a more definitive biological marker such as hair cortisol level, which is currently under investigation (Yamada, Stevens, de Silva, Klein, & Koren, 2003).

There is a growing body of evidence, both human data (primarily on preterm infants) and animal data, that neonatal pain has lasting effects on pain systems and biobehavioral arousal regulation. However, the fact that animal and human studies show that pain systems may be altered does not imply that there is damage to the central nervous system leading directly to future impairments. Although it was hoped that improved pharmacological management of pain would improve neurological outcomes for ventilated preterm infants, this has not been forthcoming to date (Anand et al., 2004). Together, animal models and studies of the immediate neurological effects of procedural pain in infancy are providing increasing evidence of some of the complex mechanisms through which possible effects of pain could operate. However, these studies do not clarify the long-term outcomes of these processes. For that information, researchers have focused on clinical studies of infants admitted to the NICU.

THE LONG-TERM EFFECTS OF PAIN ON FULL-TERM INFANTS

The notion that pain may have long-term effects is not unique to infants at risk for NI. Since early studies revealing that unrelieved circumcision pain may affect infants' responses to pain months later during routine immunizations (Taddio, Goldbach, Ipp, Stevens, & Koren, 1995; Taddio, Katz, Ilersich, & Koren, 1997), concern has grown over the potential lasting effects of untreated pain early in life for both preterm and full-term hospitalized and healthy infants.

A 2003 study suggests that effects may last much longer than months (Peters et al., 2003). Peters and colleagues examined whether major surgery and the number of negative hospital experiences affected responses to immunization at 14 and 45 months. The 50 toddlers who had had major surgery with preemptive morphine analgesia did not differ in facial display of pain, heart rate, or cortisol concentrations during immunization from the 50 matched control infants who had not had surgery. However, within the surgical group, decreased heart rate in response to immunization was related to a combined variable reflecting major surgery, Therapeutic Intervention Scoring System (TISS) score, and NICU stay at 14 months. Although these results are not conclusive, and the effect of pain (decreased heart rate in response to subsequent pain) was opposite from that expected, they do suggest that the lasting effects of early pain on subsequent pain response may reach well beyond the first year of life. Further studies are needed to clarify whether the circumstances of early pain, and of later pain situations, may alter the nature of pain impact on later responses.

Few studies have examined the effects of early pain on other aspects of development. However, McCann, Waters, Goumnerova, and Berde (2004) reported on a relationship between brachial plexus birth injury and self-injury. They found that 6.8% of the 133 infants with brachial plexus birth injury who underwent surgery displayed self-injurious behavior, compared with only 1.4% of the 147 infants who did not undergo surgery. Of the 11 children who self-injured, it most often began 8 months after surgery (average age = 17 months) and was directed most often at the affected limb. Three children reported pain verbally prior to the onset of or during the period of self-injury, and three were observed displaying pain behaviors in addition to self-injury. The authors suggested that early pain, related in this case to surgical care of brachial plexus birth injury, may lead to later maladaptive or self-injurious behavior. However, another explanation, especially given that the children reported pain prior to or during the self-injury, is that these children were responding to ongoing pain.

This concern has been raised in studies of older children. For example, Bosch, Van Dyke, Smith, and Poulton (1997) conducted retrospective chart reviews of 25 children with severe cognitive impairments who displayed self-injurious behavior. Seven children had undiagnosed medical conditions that would be expected to cause pain, and treatment of those medical conditions resulted in decreased self-injury for six of the seven. Self-injury has also been reported as a sign of pain by caregivers of children with severe cognitive impairments (McGrath, Rosmus, Camfield, Campbell, & Hennigar, 1998) and is included in some pain assessment tools designed specifically for children with severe impairments (Giusiano, Jimeno, Collignon, & Chau, 1995; Hunt et al., 2004). Self-injury may be also related to the quality and location of pain in children with severe cognitive impairments, and the nature of pain-related self-injury may differ from self-injury caused by other factors (Breau et al., 2003).

Complicating the long-term effects of pain in early life is the fact that many infants who experience pain have chronic medical conditions that may result in continued exposure to both procedural pain (i.e., including surgery) and pain caused by the condition throughout childhood. Thus, one is left with the question of whether a child's early or continued pain experience has a larger role in his or her development. Ludman and colleagues have begun to tackle this question. They followed infants to age 3 years, at which point they examined cognitive functioning (Ludman, Spitz, & Wade, 2001; Ludman et al., 1993). At 6 months of age, the 30 children who had had only one surgery in the neonatal period did not differ significantly from a group of 29 who did not in terms of General Developmental Quotient (GQ) from the Griffiths Mental Development Scales (Griffiths, 1954, 1970). Maternal depression accounted for 21% of the variation in scores for the surgical group, and number of operations contributed to 15% of the variation in GQs. In contrast, at 12 months, the surgical group achieved significantly lower GQs and only length of hospitalization predicted delays in development at this age. A follow-up of these children was conducted at 3 years of age. The surgical group now scored nonsignificantly lower on the Eye Hand and Performance subscales of the Griffiths Mental Development Scales (Griffiths, 1970), the Reynell Developmental Language Scales (Reynell & Huntley, 1985), and the British Picture Vocabulary Scale (Dunn & Dunn, 1982). Only scores on a single test from the Merrill-Palmer Scale of Mental Tests, assessing motor speed, were significantly lower for the surgical group.

Ludman and colleagues also investigated differences within the surgical group, because the ongoing medical experience of the children varied widely. At 3 years, three highly correlated factors—number of surgeries, total time in the hospital, and number of admissions—predicted developmental scores. Conversely, neonatal factors (mechanical ventilation, type of delivery, obstetrical complications, length of original admission) were not significantly related to scores at 3 years of age. However, children within the surgical group who had repeated admissions after the neonatal period, but no persisting medical problem at age 3, showed lower scores on only one language scale in a test battery, compared to the control group and the group who had only one surgery (Ludman et al., 1993). Subsequent modeling indicated that persistent medical conditions and number of surgeries each independently predicted language comprehension and performance on the nonverbal scales of the Griffiths scales. However, whereas the number of surgeries remained a significant predictor of these outcomes when ongoing medical problems were accounted for, the reverse was not true. The authors concluded that language comprehension and nonverbal abilities are most affected by number of surgeries. In a further follow-up study, the same research group found continued impact of surgeries at 11–13 years of age (Ludman et al., 2001). Children who had more surgeries in infancy performed less well in all areas of academic functioning, after controlling for psychosocial factors and ongoing health factors.

The sample size of this study was small, and there was a great deal of variability within groups in terms of medical experiences. However, the results may be extremely important, and further research is warranted to investigate the magnitude and timing of the impact of pain on long-term development. It is likely that effects will depend on the outcome measures and on the complexity of the developmental outcomes that can be tapped at different ages. However, these studies do point to possible negative effects related to surgery in the neonatal period, as well as ongoing medical problems that may themselves cause pain or lead to medical care that could entail pain. The fact that effects of neonatal surgery were found to persist into early adolescence in this very small group suggests that the effects of early medical stress, pain, or both are not necessarily temporary and that, in at least some areas of functioning, they may persist for years in a measurable form. However, an essential caveat is that these clinical studies provide associations between early events and later outcomes, but one must be extremely careful to recognize that causal relationships between early pain and subsequent development cannot be directly inferred. Moreover, some conditions may have comorbidities such that the medical reasons for the multiple surgeries are associated directly with altered development.

To summarize, this handful of studies with full-term infants suggests that surgery in infancy may be associated with subsequent changes in pain-related behavior, maladaptive behavior, and academic performance. Current evidence cannot be interpreted as supporting a causal role for pain, because surgery is a complex event and other surgical factors, such as length of exposure to the pharmacological agents used to induce anesthesia, may affect development (Anand & Soriano, 2004). Nevertheless, these data suggest a possible role for pain in long-term aspects of functioning that requires further investigation.

RESEARCH WITH INFANTS AT RISK FOR NEUROLOGICAL IMPAIRMENT

If pain can have lasting effects on healthy, full-term infants, then it is likely that the effects may be greater for those infants who are already at risk for future sensory, motor, or cognitive impairments, such as infants born extremely prematurely. In addition to the possibility that they already have a compromised neurological system, the combination of other factors, such as longer NICU stays, greater exposure to potentially painful procedures, and preexisting stress related to the NICU environment, suggests that this group may experience more adverse effects as a result of pain.

Exposure to Pain

Advancements in medical care have led to marked improvement in survival rates of extremely preterm infants (Horbar et al., 2002; Kaiser et al., 2004). However, these survivors are exposed to frequent painful procedures as a means of monitoring and treating their often-complex conditions. Several studies highlight how frequent painful events may be. Stevens et al. (1999) found that neonates born at 27–31 weeks' gestation had a mean of 134 painful procedures in their first 2 weeks of life, with the youngest and sickest having more than 300. Johnston, Stremler, Stevens, and Horton (1997) estimated that infants of 28–32 weeks' corrected age can experience 2–10 procedures per day. The frequency of painful procedures also appears to vary with respect to risk for NI. In a large study of 194 infants in two NICUs, Stevens et al. (2003) compared the number of procedures conducted for infants at high, moderate, and low risk for NI. Infants in the high-risk group had experienced severe intrapartum asphyxia or grade 3 or 4 IVH, or had a recognized syndrome or chromosomal anomaly; those in the moderate-risk group had a severe respiratory abnormality; and those in the low-risk group had experienced respiratory distress or sepsis. Although there was no overall difference in the number or type of procedures performed over the first 7 days of NICU admission, infants at high risk for NI did receive significantly more painful procedures than those at moderate or low risk on their first day.

The impact of this repeated and frequent exposure to pain is compounded by inadequate pharmacological pain management. Sabrine and Sinha (2000) surveyed 86 NICUs and found that analgesia was used for less than 10% of many painful procedures (e.g., intravenous cannulations, venipunctures, lumbar punctures) and less than 16% of highly invasive procedures (e.g., chest drain insertions). Similarly, Simons et al. (2003) found that close to 40% of the 171 neonates studied for the first 14 days of their NICU admission received no analgesics. Physicians and nurses in that study rated 26 of the 31 painful procedures as having a pain intensity of 4 on a scale of 10, suggesting that most were perceived to cause at least moderate pain.

Stevens' group also evaluated the analgesics provided specifically for infants at risk for NI (Stevens et al., 2003) and found that analgesic administration varied with respect to risk level. Infants at high risk received 2–3 times fewer bolus opioids than infants at moderate or low risk over the first 2 days of admission, and differences were not related to duration of ventilation. There was also a significant relationship between the number of procedures performed and both analgesic and sedation use for the low- and moderate-risk groups, but no relation in the group of infants at highest risk. Further modeling indicated that, whereas 35% of the variance in analgesic use was explained by number of procedures for those at low risk for NI, and 61% for those at moderate risk, no variance in analgesic use was explained by number of procedures for the infants at high risk for NI.

Clearly, many infants in the NICU experience significant and repeated pain on a daily basis. Pharmacological treatment of pain also appears to be less than optimal, especially for infants at highest risk for NI. To complicate matters further, recent evidence suggests that morphine may have little efficacy in infants undergoing mechanical ventilation (Anand et al., 2004), which calls into question the belief that greater use of opiates to prevent pain would improve developmental outcomes. In fact, these recent major studies of pharmacological management of pain in preterm infants raise many questions about current management and beg for further research investigating the efficacy and safety of other interventions.

Background Stress

The painful events that infants at risk for NI experience in the NICU setting do not occur in isolation. Pain is set against a backdrop of environmental stimulation that may also be uncomfortable, especially for preterm infants who are not developmentally prepared to handle this input. Lighting (Rivkees, Mayes, Jacobs, & Gross, 2004), noise (Bremmer, Byers, & Kiehl, 2003), repeated handling (Gagnon et al., 1999), and mechanical interventions (Quinn, de Boer, Ansari, & Baumer, 1998), as well as isolation from human contact and interaction (Bellieni, Bagnoli, & Buonocore, 2003), have all been shown to stress the neonate.

Observed Pain Effects in the NICU

Increased Pain Response in the Short Term

In addition to any independent effects of environmental or background stress, there is consistent evidence that prior exposure to pain or stress increases pain reactivity in the short term. Porter et al. (1998) investigated the effects of arousal resulting from handling and immobilization on the pain response to a heel stick in healthy, premature and full-term newborn infants. Handled infants, regardless of gestational age, had a higher mean heart rate and greater behavioral arousal and displayed more facial activity in response to the heel stick than did those who were not handled just prior to the painful event. Similarly, previous pain increased response to a subsequent procedure. Grunau, Holsti, Whitfield, and Ling (2000) found that a greater number of painful procedures in the past 24 hours was associated with more facial grimacing in response to endotracheal suctioning in preterm infants weighing 1,000 g or less at birth. Porter, Wolf, and Miller (1999) reported that magnitude of heart rate change and agitated behavior increased with time spent in the NICU for infants born at less than 28 weeks' gestational age.

Studies from Grunau's group have supported the conclusion that prior stress, in the form of pain or other events, does alter subsequent responses to pain. In a study of 44 preterm infants at 32 weeks' gestation, finger splay in response to heel lance was greater in those infants who had experienced more painful procedures since birth (Holsti, Grunau, Oberlander, & Whitfield, 2004). Additional evidence that prior events sensitize preterm infants in the short term, and that the effects of painful stress and other stress may be similar, is provided by two additional studies by this group. In the first, they reported that the response of 54 infants to clustered care (changing diaper, measuring abdominal girth, taking axillary temperature, cleaning mouth with gauze and sterile water) was increased when it was preceded by a heel lance (Holsti, Grunau, Oberlander, & Whitfield, 2005), suggesting sensitization. In a second study, infants received a blood collection on different days either after a rest period or following routine clustered nursing care (Holsti, Grunau, Oberlander, Whitfield, & Weinberg, in press). These infants showed greater response to heel lance, also evidence of sensitization. Only one study has reported lower physiological and behavioral acute pain response in preterm infants who had undergone a painful procedure recently (Johnston et al., 1999). However, the preterm newborns in this study were of younger gestational age at the time of the study, and asleep. In addition, a different measure of pain was used.

Together these studies consistently demonstrate that prior stress, whether or not it includes pain, affects subsequent pain response, with a greater response being most often reported in the short term. Although the magnitude and direction of response appear to be affected by age at the time of observation, as well as contextual factors and the modality of response being observed, all suggest an interaction between common events in the NICU.

Decreased Pain Response

Cumulative repeated pain in the NICU frequently leads to changes in subsequent pain responses, frequently a reduction in response. For example, Johnston and Stevens (1996) compared pain responses of neonates who were born at 28 weeks' gestation and were hospitalized in a NICU for 4 weeks with those of neonates who were born at 32 weeks' gestation. Infants who had experienced more painful procedures displayed a reduced behavioral response to lancing for blood collection, although response was not related to age, Apgar score, birth weight, illness severity, or weight.

Similarly, Grunau, Oberlander, Whitfield, Fitzgerald, and Lee (2001) found that exposure to a greater number of invasive procedures since birth and previous postnatal steroid exposure were both associated with a dampened response to heel lance at 32 weeks' in preterm infants with birth weight of 1,500 g or less. They proposed that there may be a threshold in terms of number of repeated procedures needed to alter subsequent pain response. Infants in their study who had experienced more than 20 procedures responded less vigorously both behaviorally and autonomically during the heel lance than did those who had had fewer than 20 previous procedures. Total amount of morphine up to the day the infant was observed during a painful procedure appeared to contribute to normalized autonomic response to pain but not to behavioral response. Subsequently, Grunau and colleagues (2004) reexamined this question in a new study with infants who had not received any postnatal steroids, confirming dampened pain and stress responses in infants exposed to more cumulative prior pain. Again, the results of studies appear mixed in terms of direction of effect of pain. However, the studies continue to point to effects of pain on behavior long after pain would be expected to have ceased.

Lasting Effects of Pain Beyond the Neonatal Setting

Only two studies have examined the effects of pain experienced in the NICU on subsequent pain response after discharge. Oberlander et al. (2000) unexpectedly found little effect of neonatal pain on response to a finger lance by 24 extremely low-birth-weight (ELBW) infants at 4 months' corrected age, despite exposure to a large number of invasive procedures in the NICU, compared with full-term controls. However, at 8 months, Grunau, Oberlander, and Whitfield (2001) found that facial response following finger lance was initially significantly higher than that in the full-term infants. Moreover, the preterm infants showed significantly less facial and physiological response during recovery, indicating much more rapid dampening following reactivity.

These two studies suggest that the effects of neonatal pain are not necessarily immediate, nor are they consistent over time. Why the effects of pain might vary over time is unclear. Both sample sizes were small, and, therefore, the results may be influenced by the available power. However, the inconsistent results in direction of response are similar to those of studies conducted in the NICU and may reflect situational or developmental factors, or both. Again, this is an area in which future research would be desirable and revealing.

Lasting Effects of Pain Beyond Infancy

Few researchers have investigated the effects of pain for infants at risk for NI beyond infancy. To do so is a challenge because of the numerous interacting factors that may play into long-term development. However, the few studies that currently exist do suggest that pain may have lasting effects well into childhood.

In a study of 195 toddlers at 18 months' corrected age, parent ratings of their child's reactions to everyday bumps and scrapes were compared across four groups: 1) those weighing less than 801 g at birth, 2) those weighing 801–1,000 g at birth, 3) those weighing 1,500–2,499 g at birth, and 4) those weighing more than 2,499 g at birth (Grunau, Whitfield, Petrie, & Fryer, 1994b). Children in the two lower weight groups were rated by parents as significantly less sensitive to pain compared with the larger neonates. Parenting style and home environment were not associated with reported pain sensitivity.

At age 5 years, two studies found increased somatization in former preterm compared to term-born children (Grunau et al., 1994b; Sommerfelt, Troland, Ellersten, & Markested, 1996). In a later study, 36 former preterm neonates (birth weight less than 1,000 g) were compared with former full-term neonates of comparable sociodemographic background (Grunau, Whitfield, Petrie, & Fryer, 1994a). Somatic complaints were greater among the former preterm neonates than among the former full-term group at 4½ years. Within the group of former preterm neonates, those who had scores for somatization that were above the normal range did not have more actual medical problems between the age of 3 and 4½ years, suggesting that the effect was not due to recent medical problems. Subsequently, however, at age 8–10 years, prevalence of somatization did not differ between ELBW children compared with term-born children (Grunau, Whitfield, & Petrie, 1998). However, at age 8–10 years, former extremely low birth weight children (less than 1,001 g) children rated pictures of children in pain situations differently than did term-born peers. Most notably, duration of stay in the NICU was correlated with higher ratings of affective distress in response to pictures of pain events related to recreation and daily living.

Three studies have looked at lasting effects of preterm birth into adolescence. In a study of health status in adolescence, teenagers who were extremely low weight at birth reported more moderate to severe functional limitations, including pain, than did teenagers who were born at term (Saigal et al., 1996). However, in a subsequent report based on the same cohort, these authors indicated that parents of the teens who were ELBW believed that their children had more sensation impairment (speech, hearing, vision) than did parents of control teens, but parents' opinions of the amount of pain their children currently experienced did not differ (Saigal, Rosenbaum, et al., 2000).

Buskila and colleagues (2003) compared the tenderness threshold in adolescents ages 12–18 years who were born prematurely or at full term. They found that the preterm children had more tender points and lower tender thresholds than did those born at full term. In both groups, girls had significantly more tender points and lower tender thresholds. The authors interpreted this finding as evidence for greater somatic sensitivity.

This small group of studies cannot provide definitive evidence that differences between children in mid-childhood or adolescence based on prematurity are necessarily due to pain. Nonetheless, the evidence does fall in line with that from younger children, suggesting effects lasting years beyond infancy. The direction of effects, whether sensitization or dampening, remains unclear.

CURRENT UNDERSTANDING AND NEW DIRECTIONS

Currently there is no direct evidence that uncontrolled neonatal pain contributes directly to the etiology of long-term impairments in infants at risk for NI, such as major cognitive or motor impairment. However, there is increasing evidence that pain, or aspects of events in the NICU setting or early in life that can cause pain, may change subsequent responses to pain, contribute to maladaptive behavior such as self-injury and somatization, or play a role in long-term cognitive outcomes, despite methodological challenges and small sample sizes. Pain in the NICU is a challenging ongoing problem for compassionate care in high-risk neonates.

As is clear from the scarce available data, our understanding of the long-term effects of pain early in life is sketchy at this point. Our knowledge regarding the effects of early pain for those who are vulnerable or have heightened risk for future NI is smaller yet. However, we do have reason to believe that among the many possible factors early in life, especially for those at risk who spend extended periods in the NICU setting, pain likely plays some role in the dynamic mix of factors that can reach far beyond infancy to alter long-term outcomes. It is imperative, therefore, that we not shy away from attempts to unravel this complex situation. If pain can alter long-term development and functioning, through sensory, motor, or cognitive impairments, understanding how this process unfolds will provide insight into possible interventions that can attenuate the negative effects.

As with all aspects of health, pain must be assessed to be managed. Assessment is one aspect of pain for which efforts must be focused to expand our understanding. There can be little movement on ameliorating pain's effects until we can measure it reliably and validly. Although few measures to assess pain in infants were available only 15 years ago, there are now approximately three dozen such measures. Despite this flood of tool development, few tools have been tested with neonates who are at risk for or have demonstrated NI. Moreover, we know little about attitudes of health professionals and parents toward the existence of pain in these babies or how these attitudes influence pain management. Stevens and colleagues are currently embracing these issues in a program of research on pain in infants at risk for NI. They have commenced a program centered on the development of an observational measure of pain specifically for infants at risk, and that will be sensitive to differences in observable pain response in infants with differing levels of risk. This group has collected data from direct observation of these groups of infants during painful events in the NICU, as well as the opinion of clinicians who work with these infants and experts in both hospital and community settings. It is hoped that the melding of information from these diverse sources will provide a tool that is not only sensitive to the nuances of pain response that infants at risk for NI may display, but will also be feasible and acceptable to those who care for this vulnerable group.

Once valid and reliable measures exist, research can begin in earnest to track the long-term outcomes of groups of infants at different levels of risk for NI. Recent research has evolved in complexity to incorporate the many perinatal factors that may interact to alter expected development in infants without risk for NI. Similar studies must be developed for this most needy and vulnerable group. In addition, more work must be completed documenting the expected trajectory of development for specific groups of at-risk infants. Researchers in the field of pediatric pain, however, must combine forces with those who study child development within a broad sociocultural environment.

Finally, but most important for those infants who are currently in NICU settings, we must gain a better understanding of the current practice of pain management in NICU settings. The existing literature suggests that pain is undertreated for neonates in general, and for neonates at risk for NI in particular. This undermanagement may be due in part to underuse of assessment tools, when they are available. However, results from Stevens' group suggest that this may not account for all behavior by professionals. In one study, they found that professionals with experience in a NICU setting, when they were asked to complete questionnaires, expressed the opinion that infants at risk for NI have a reduced pain experience (Breau et al., in press). However, in a second study, in which professionals were asked to rate video clips of infants experiencing a painful procedure, professionals' ratings of pain did not vary when these individuals were presented with information suggesting the infants had low, moderate, or severe risk for future impairments based on current medical information (Breau et al., 2004). The authors suggested that one interpretation of these contradictory results could be that reduced pain management for infants with greater risk for NI (Stevens et al., 2003) may not solely reflect opinions regarding pain expression in this group or the lack of tools for pain assessment. Undermanagement of pain may also reflect opinions or beliefs about the use of pharmacological methods with this group.

Thus, further research aimed at understanding the long-term effects of early pain for those infants at heightened risk for NI should be informed from several directions: studies of pain assessment, pain management, and the complex interactions among these and other perinatal factors that may affect long-term outcomes, against a backdrop of refined knowledge regarding expected development in a very diverse population. No one source of information will suffice.

REFERENCES

Anand, K.J., Hall, R.W., Desai, N., Shephard, B., Bergqvist, L.L., Young, T.E., et al. (2004). Effects of morphine analgesia in ventilated preterm neonates: Primary outcomes from the NEOPAIN randomised trial. *Lancet, 363,* 1673–1682.

Anand, K.J., & Soriano, S.G. (2004). Anesthetic agents and the immature brain: Are these toxic or therapeutic? *Anesthesiology, 101,* 527–530.

Anand, K.J.S. (2000). Effects of perinatal pain and stress. *Progress in Brain Research, 122,* 117–129.

Anand, K.J.S., Coskun, V., Thrivikraman, K.V., Nemeroff, C.B., & Plotsky, P.M. (1999). Long-term behavioral effects of repetitive pain in neonatal rat pups. *Physiology and Behavior, 66,* 627–637.

Andrews, K.A., Desai, D., Dhillon, H.K., Wilcox, D.T., Fitzgerald, M. (2002). Abdominal sensitivity in the first year of life: Comparison of infants with and without prenatally diagnosed unilateral hydronephrosis. *Pain, 100,* 35-46.

Andrews, K., & Fitzgerald, M. (1994). The cutaneous withdrawal reflex in human neonates: Sensitization, receptive fields, and the effects of contralateral stimulation. *Pain, 56,* 95–101.

Banos, J., Ruis, G., & Guardiola, E. (2004). An analysis of articles on neonatal pain from 1965 to 1999. *Pain Research and Management, 6,* 45–50.

Bellieni, C.V., Bagnoli, F., & Buonocore, G. (2003). Alone no more: Pain in premature children. *Ethics in Medicine, 19,* 5–9.

Bellieni, C.V., Burroni, A., Perrone, S., Cordelli, D.M., Nenci, A., Lunghi, A., et al. (2003). Intracranial pressure during procedural pain. *Biology of the Neonate, 84,* 202–205.

Bernbaum, J.C., & Batshaw, M.L. (1997). Born too soon, born too small. In M.L. Batshaw (Ed.), *Children with disabilities* (4th ed., pp. 115–142). Baltimore: Paul H. Brookes Publishing Co.

Bitar, F.F., Obeid, M., Dabbous, I., Hayek, P., Akel, S., & Mroueh, S. (2003). Acute respiratory distress associated with external jugular vein catheterization in the newborn. *Pediatric Pulmonology, 36,* 549–550.

Bosch, J., Van Dyke, D.C., Smith, S.M., & Poulton, S. (1997). Role of medical conditions in the exacerbation of self-injurious behavior: An exploratory study. *Mental Retardation, 35,* 124–130.

Breau, L.M., Camfield, C., Symon, D.N., Bodfish, J.W., McKay, A., Finley, G.A., et al. (2003). Pain and self-injurious behaviour in neurologically impaired children. *Journal of Pediatrics, 142,* 498–503.

Breau, L.M., McGrath, P.J., Stevens, B., Beyene, J., Camfield, C., Finley, G.A., et al. (in press). Healthcare professionals' beliefs regarding the pain of infants at risk for neurological impairment: A survey. *Clinical Journal of Pain.*

Breau, L.M., Stevens, B., McGrath, P.J., Beyene, J., Camfield, C.S., Finley, G.A., et al. (2004). Healthcare professionals' perception of pain experienced by infants at risk for neurological impairment. *BMC Pediatrics, 4*(23).

Bremmer, P., Byers, J.F., & Kiehl, E. (2003). Noise and the premature infant: Physiological effects and practice implications. *Journal of Obstetric, Gynecologic, and Neonatal Nursing, 32,* 447–454.

Buskila, D., Neumann, L., Zmora, E., Feldman, M., Bolotin, A., & Press, J. (2003). Pain sensitivity in prematurely born adolescents. *Archives of Pediatrics and Adolescent Medicine, 157,* 1079–1082.

Cioni, G., Bertuccelli, B., Boldrini, A., Canapicchi, R., Fazzi, B., Guzzetta, A., et al. (2000). Correlation between visual function, neurodevelopmental outcome, and magnetic resonance imaging findings in infants with periventricular leucomalacia. *Archives of Disease in Childhood, Fetal and Neonatal Edition, 82,* F134–F140.

Cooke, R.W. & Abernethy, L.J. (1999). Cranial magnetic resonance imaging and school performance in very low birth weight infants in adolescence. *Archives of Disease in Childhood, Fetal and Neonatal Edition, 81,* F116–F121.

Craig, E.D., Thompson, J.M., & Mitchell, E.A. (2002). Socioeconomic status and preterm birth: New Zealand trends, 1980 to 1999. *Archives of Disease in Childhood, Fetal and Neonatal Edition, 86,* F142–F146.

Doussard-Roosevelt, J.A., McClenny, B.D., & Porges, S.W. (2001). Neonatal cardiac vagal tone and school-age developmental outcome in very low birth weight infants. *Developmental Psychobiology, 38,* 56–66.

Dunn, L.M., & Dunn, L.M. (1982). *British Picture Vocabulary Scale.* Windsor, UK: NFER-Nelson Publishing Company.

Fitzgerald, M., Millard, C., & McIntosh, N. (1989). Cutaneous hypersensitivity following peripheral tissue damage in newborn infants and its reversal with topical anaesthesia. *Pain, 39,* 31–36.

Fitzgerald, M., Shaw, A., & MacIntosh, N. (1988). Postnatal development of the cutaneous flexor reflex: Comparative study of preterm infants and newborn rat pups. *Developmental Medicine and Child Neurology, 30,* 520–526.

Fowlie, P.W., Tarnow-Mordi, W.O., Gould, C.R., & Strang, D. (1998). Predicting outcome in very low birthweight infants using an objective measure of illness severity and cranial ultrasound scanning. *Archives of Disease in Childhood, Fetal and Neonatal Edition, 78,* F175–F178.

Gagnon, R.E., Leung, A., & Macnab, A.J. (1999). Variations in regional cerebral blood volume in neonates associated with nursery care events. *American Journal of Perinatology, 16,* 7–11.

Giusiano, B., Jimeno, M.T., Collignon, P., & Chau, Y. (1995). Utilization of a neural network in the elaboration of an evaluation scale for pain in cerebral palsy. *Methods of Information in Medicine, 34,* 498–502.

Griffiths, R. (1954). *The abilities of babies.* London: University of London Press.

Griffiths, R. (1970). *The abilities of young children.* London: University of London Press.

Grunau, R.E. (2000). Long-term consequences of pain in human neonates. In K.J.S. Anand, B. Stevens, & P.J. McGrath (Eds.), *Pain in neonates* (2nd rev. enlarged ed., pp. 55–76). Amsterdam: Elsevier.

Grunau, R.E. (2002). Early pain in preterm infants: A model of long-term effects. *Clinics in Perinatology, 29,* 373–394.

Grunau, R.E., Holsti, L., Haley, D.W., Oberlander, T.F., Weinberg, J., Solimano, A., et al. (2005). Neonatal procedural pain exposure predicts lower cortisol and behavioral reactivity in preterm infants in the NICU. *Pain, 113,* 293-300.

Grunau, R.E., Holsti, L., Whitfield, M.F., & Ling, E. (2000). Are twitches, startles, and body movements pain indicators in extremely low birth weight infants? *Clinical Journal of Pain, 16,* 37–45.

Grunau, R.E., Oberlander, T.F., & Whitfield, M.F. (2001). Pain reactivity in formerly extremely low birth weight infants at corrected age 8 months compared with term controls. *Infant Behavior & Development, 1,* 41–55.

Grunau, R.E., Oberlander, T.F., Whitfield, M.F., Fitzgerald, C., & Lee, S.K. (2001). Demographic and therapeutic determinants of pain reactivity in very low birth weight neonates at 32 weeks' postconceptional age. *Pediatrics, 107,* 105–112.

Grunau, R.E., Weinberg, J., & Whitfield, M.F. (2004). Neonatal procedural pain and preterm infant cortisol response to novelty at 8 months. *Pediatrics, 114,* e77–e84.

Grunau, R.E., Whitfield, M.F., & Petrie, J. (1998). Children's judgements about pain at age 8–10 years: Do extremely low birthweight (=1000g) children differ from full birthweight peers? *Journal of Child Psychology and Psychiatry and Allied Disciplines, 39,* 587–594.

Grunau, R.V., Whitfield, M.F., Petrie, J.H., & Fryer, E.L. (1994a). Early pain experience, child and family factors, as precursors of somatization: A prospective study of extremely premature and fullterm children. *Pain, 56,* 353–359.

Grunau, R.V.E., Whitfield, M.F., Petrie, J.H., & Fryer, L. (1994b). Pain sensitivity in toddlers of birthweight <1000 grams compared with heavier preterm and full birth weight toddlers. *Pain, 58,* 341–346.

Gunnar, M.R., & Barr, R.G. (1998). Stress, early brain development, and behavior. *Infants and Young Children, 11,* 1–14.

Gutbrod, T., Wolke, D., Soehne, B., Ohrt, B., & Riegel, K. (2000). Effects of gestation and birth weight on the growth and development of very low birthweight small for gestational age infants: A matched group comparison. *Archives of Disease in Childhood, Fetal and Neonatal Edition, 82,* F208–F214.

Haataja, L., Mercuri, E., Cowan, F., & Dubowitz, L. (2000). Cranial ultrasound abnormalities in full term infants in a postnatal ward: Outcome at 12 and 18 months. *Archives of Disease in Childhood, Fetal and Neonatal Edition, 82,* F128–F133.

Hack, M., Weissman, B., Breslau, N., Klein, N., Borawski-Clark, E., & Fanaroff, A.A. (1993). Health of very low birth weight children during their first eight years. *Journal of Pediatrics, 122,* 887–892.

Hill, J.L., Brooks-Gunn, J., & Waldfogel, J. (2003). Sustained effects of high participation in an early intervention for low-birth-weight premature infants. *Developmental Psychology, 39,* 730–744.

Holsti, L., Grunau, R.E., Oberlander, T.F., & Whitfield, M.F. (2004). Specific Newborn Individualized Developmental Care and Assessment Program movements are associated with acute pain in preterm infants in the neonatal intensive care unit. *Pediatrics, 114,* 65–72.

Holsti, L., Grunau, R.E., Oberlander, T.F., & Whitfield, M.F. (2005). Prior pain induces heightened motor responses during clustered care in preterm infants in the NICU. *Early Human Development, 83,* 293–302.

Holsti, L., Grunau, R.E., Oberlander, T.F., Whitfield, M.F., & Weinberg, J. (in press). Body movements, an important additional factor in discriminating pain from stress in preterm infants. *Clinical Journal of Pain, 21,* 491–498.

Horbar, J.D., Badger, G.J., Carpenter, J.H., Fanaroff, A.A., Kilpatrick, S., LaCorte, M., et al. (2002). Trends in mortality and morbidity for very low birth weight infants, 1991–1999. *Pediatrics, 110,* 143–151.

Horwood, L.J., Mogridge, N., & Darlow, B.A. (1998). Cognitive, educational, and behavioural outcomes at 7 to 8 years in a national very low birthweight cohort. *Archives of Disease in Childhood, Fetal and Neonatal Edition, 79,* F12–F20.

Houlihan, C.M., O'Donnell, M., Conaway, M., & Stevenson, R.D. (2004). Bodily pain and health-related quality of life in children with cerebral palsy. *Developmental Medicine and Child Neurology, 46,* 305–310.

Hunt, A., Goldman, A., Seers, K., Crichton, N., Mastroyannopoulou, K., Moffat, V., et al. (2004). Clinical validation of the paediatric pain profile. *Developmental Medicine and Child Neurology, 46,* 9–18.

Huttner, U., Weiss, P.A.M., Maurer, U., Engele, H., Zehetleitner, G., Hausler, M., et al. (1998). Neonatologic complications and long-term sequelae of extremely low birthweight (ELBW) infants: The Graz experience. *Geburtshilfe und Frauenheilkunde, 58,* 475–482.

Hutton, J.L., Pharoah, P.O., Cooke, R.W., & Stevenson, R.C. (1997). Differential effects of preterm birth and small gestational age on cognitive and motor development. *Archives of Disease in Childhood, Fetal and Neonatal Edition, 76,* F75–F81.

Jelliffe-Pawlowski, L.L., Shaw, G.M., Nelson, V., & Harris, J.A. (2003). Risk of mental retardation among children born with birth defects. *Archives of Pediatrics and Adolescent Medicine, 157,* 545–550.

Johnston, C.C., & Stevens, B.J. (1996). Experience in a neonatal intensive care unit (NICU) affects pain response. *Pediatrics, 98,* 1–6.

Johnston, C.C., Stevens, B.J., Franck, L.S., Jack, A., Stremler, R., & Platt, R. (1999). Factors explaining lack of response to heel stick in preterm newborns. *Journal of Obstetric, Gynecologic, and Neonatal Nursing, 28,* 587–594.

Johnston, C.C., Stremler, R.L., Stevens, B.J., & Horton, L.J. (1997). Effectiveness of oral sucrose and simulated rocking on pain response in preterm neonates. *Pain, 72,* 193–199.

Joseph, K.S., Kramer, M.S., Marcoux, S., Ohlsson, A., Wen, S.W., Allen, A., et al. (1998). Determinants of preterm birth rates in Canada from 1981 through 1983 and from 1992 through 1994. *New England Journal of Medicine, 339,* 1434–1439.

Kaiser, J.R., Tilford, J.M., Simpson, P.M., Salhab, W.A., & Rosenfeld, C.R. (2004). Hospital survival of very-low-birth-weight neonates from 1977 to 2000. *Journal of Perinatology, 24,* 343–350.

Kirpalani, H., & Asztalos, E. (2001). Neonatal brain injury. *Current Opinion in Pediatrics, 13,* 227–233.

Larson, S.A., Lakin, K.C., Anderson, L., Kwak, N., Lee, J.H., & Anderson, D. (2001). Prevalence of mental retardation and developmental disabilities: Estimates from the 1994/1995 National Health Interview Survey Disability Supplements. *American Journal on Mental Retardation, 106,* 231–252.

Lindower, J.B., Atherton, H.D., & Kotagal, U.R. (1999). Outcomes and resource utilization for newborns with major congenital malformations: The initial NICU admission. *Journal of Perinatology, 19,* 212–215.

Liu, S., Joseph, K.S., Wen, S.W., Kramer, M.S., Marcoux, S., Ohlsson, A., et al. (2001). Secular trends in congenital anomaly-related fetal and infant mortality in Canada, 1985–1996. *American Journal of Medical Genetics, 104,* 7–13.

Lorenz, J.M., Wooliever, D.E., Jetton, J.R., & Paneth, N. (1998). A quantitative review of mortality and developmental disability in extremely premature newborns. *Archives of Pediatrics and Adolescent Medicine, 152,* 425–435.

Ludman, L., Spitz, L., & Lansdown, R. (1993). Intellectual development at 3 years of age of children who underwent major neonatal surgery. *Journal of Pediatric Surgery, 28,* 130–134.

Ludman, L., Spitz, L., & Wade, A. (2001). Educational attainments in early adolescence of infants who required major neonatal surgery. *Journal of Pediatric Surgery, 36,* 858–862.

Marsh, D.F., Hatch, D.J., & Fitzgerald, M. (1997). Opioid systems and the newborn. *British Journal of Anaesthesia, 79,* 787–795.

McCann, M.E., Waters, P., Goumnerova, L.C., & Berde, C. (2004). Self-mutilation in young children following brachial plexus birth injury. *Pain, 110,* 123–129.

McGrath, P.J., Rosmus, C., Camfield, C., Campbell, M.A., & Hennigar, A.W. (1998). Behaviours caregivers use to determine pain in non-verbal, cognitively impaired individuals. *Developmental Medicine and Child Neurology, 40,* 340–343.

Ment, L.R., Vohr, B., Allan, W., Westerveld, M., Sparrow, S.S., Schneider, K.C., et al. (2000). Outcome of children in the Indomethacin Intraventricular Hemorrhage Prevention Trial. *Pediatrics, 105,* 485–491.

Mervis, C.A., Decoufle, P., Murphy, C.C., & Yeargin-Allsopp, M. (1995). Low-birth-weight and the risk for mental-retardation later in childhood. *Paediatric and Perinatal Epidemiology, 9,* 455–467.

Oberlander, T.F., Grunau, R.E., Whitfield, M.F., Fitzgerald, C., Pitfield, S., & Saul, J.P.

(2000). Biobehavioral pain responses in former extremely low birth weight infants at four months' corrected age. *Pediatrics, 105,* e6.

Peters, J.W., Koot, H.M., de Boer, J.B., Passchier, J., Bueno-de-Mesquita, J.M., de Jong, F.H., et al. (2003). Major surgery within the first 3 months of life and subsequent biobehavioral pain responses to immunization at later age: a case comparison study. *Pediatrics, 111,* 129–135.

Porter, F.L., Grunau, R.E., & Anand, K.J.S. (1999). Long-term effects of pain in infants. *Developmental and Behavioral Pediatrics, 20,* 253–261.

Porter, F.L., Wolf, C.M., & Miller, J.P. (1998). The effect of handling and immobilization on the response to acute pain in newborn infants. *Pediatrics, 102,* 1383–1389.

Porter, F.L., Wolf, C.M., & Miller, J.P. (1999). Procedural pain in newborn infants: The influence of intensity and development. *Pediatrics, 104,* e13.

Quinn, M.W., de Boer, R.C., Ansari, N., & Baumer, J.H. (1998). Stress response and mode of ventilation in preterm infants. *Archives of Disease in Childhood, Fetal and Neonatal Edition, 78,* F195–F198.

Ren, K., Anseloni, V., Zou, S.P., Wade, E.B., Novikova, S.I., Ennis, M., et al. (2004). Characterization of basal and re-inflammation-associated long-term alteration in pain responsivity following short-lasting neonatal local inflammatory insult. *Pain, 110,* 588–596.

Resnick, M.B., Gueorguieva, R.V., Carter, R.L., Ariet, M., Sun, Y.S., Roth, J., et al. (1999). The impact of low birth weight, perinatal conditions, and sociodemographic factors on educational outcome in kindergarten. *Pediatrics, 104,* e741–e7410.

Reynell, J., & Huntley, M. (1985). *Reynell Developmental Language Scales Manual* (2nd rev.). Windsor, UK: NFER-Nelson Publishing Company.

Reynolds, M., Alvares, D., Middleton, J., & Fitzgerald, M. (1997). Neonatally wounded skin induces NGF-independent sensory neurite outgrowth in vitro. *Brain Research: Developmental Brain Research, 102,* 275–283.

Rivkees, S.A., Mayes, L., Jacobs, H., & Gross, I. (2004). Rest-activity patterns of premature infants are regulated by cycled lighting. *Pediatrics, 113,* 833–839.

Ruda, M.A., Ling, Q.D., Hohmann, A.G., Peng, Y.B., & Tachibana, T. (2000). Altered nociceptive neuronal circuits after neonatal peripheral inflammation. *Science, 289,* 628–631.

Sabrine, N. & Sinha, S. (2000). Use of analgesia in 86 neonatal intensive care units. *Lancet, 355,* 932.

Saigal, S., Feeny, D., Rosenbaum, P., Furlong, W., Burrows, E., & Stoskopf, B. (1996). Self-perceived health status and health-related quality of life of extremely low-birth-weight infants at adolescence. *JAMA, 276,* 453–459.

Saigal, S., Hoult, L.A., Streiner, D.L., Stoskopf, B.L., & Rosenbaum, P.L. (2000). School difficulties at adolescence in a regional cohort of children who were extremely low birth weight. *Pediatrics, 105,* 325–331.

Saigal, S., Rosenbaum, P.L., Feeny, D., Burrows, E., Furlong, W., Stoskopf, B.L., et al. (2000). Parental perspectives of the health status and health-related quality of life of teen-aged children who were extremely low birth weight and term controls. *Pediatrics, 105,* 569–574.

Sheth, R.D. (1998). Frequency of neurologic disorders in the neonatal intensive care unit. *Journal of Child Neurology, 13,* 424–428.

Sheth, R.D., Goulden, K.J., & Ronen, G.M. (1994). Aggression in children treated with clobazam for epilepsy. *Clinical Neuropharmacology, 17,* 332–337.

Simons, S.H., van Dijk, M., Anand, K.S., Roofthooft, D., van Lingen, R.A., & Tibboel, D. (2003). Do we still hurt newborn babies? A prospective study of procedural pain and analgesia in neonates. *Archives of Pediatrics and Adolescent Medicine, 157,* 1058–1064.

Sommerfelt, K., Troland, K., Ellersten, B., Markestad, T. (1996). Behavioral problems in low-birthweight preschoolers. *Developmental Medicine and Child Neurology, 38,* 927–40.

Stevens, B., Johnston, C., Franck, L., Petryshen, P., Jack, A., & Foster, G. (1999). The efficacy of developmentally sensitive interventions and sucrose for relieving procedural pain in very low birth weight neonates. *Nursing Research, 48,* 35–43.

Stevens, B., McGrath, P.J., Gibbins, S., Beyenne, J., Breau, L.M., Camfield, C., et al. (2003). Procedural pain in neonates at risk for neurological impairment. *Pain, 105,* 27–35.

Stoll, B.J., Hansen, N.I., Adams-Chapman, I., Fanaroff, A.A., Hintz, S.R., Vohr, B., et al. (2004). Neurodevelopmental and growth impairment among extremely low-birth-weight infants with neonatal infection. *JAMA, 292,* 2357–2365.

Synnes, A.R., Berry, M., Jones, H., Pendray, M., Stewart, S., & Lee, S.K. (2004). Infants with congenital anomalies admitted to neonatal intensive care units. *American Journal of Perinatology, 21,* 199–207.

Taddio, A., Goldbach, M., Ipp, M., Stevens, B., & Koren, G. (1995). Effect of neonatal circumcision on pain responses during vaccination in boys. *Lancet, 345,* 291–292.

Taddio, A., Katz, J., Ilersich, A.L., & Koren, G. (1997). Effect of neonatal circumcision on pain response during subsequent routine vaccination. *Lancet, 349,* 599–603.

Teplin, S.W., Burchinal, M., Johnson-Martin, N., Humphry, R.A., & Kraybill, E.N. (1991). Neurodevelopmental, health, and growth status at age 6 years of children with birth weights less than 1001 grams. *Journal of Pediatrics, 118,* 768–777.

Tommiska, V., Heinonen, K., Ikonen, S., Kero, P., Pokela, M.L., Renlund, M., et al. (2001). A national short-term follow-up study of extremely low birth weight infants born in Finland in 1996–1997. *Pediatrics, 107,* U9–U17.

Volpe, J.J. (1995). *Neurology of the newborn.* Philadelphia: W.B. Saunders.

Whitfield, M.F. (2003). Psychosocial effects of intensive care on infants and families after discharge. *Seminars in Neonatology, 8,* 185–193.

Whitfield, M.F., Grunau, R.V., & Holsti, L. (1997). Extremely premature (< or = 800 g) schoolchildren: Multiple areas of hidden disability. *Archives of Disease in Childhood, Fetal and Neonatal Edition, 77,* F85–F90.

Yamada, J., Stevens, B., de Silva, N., Klein, J., & Koren, G. (2003). Hair cortisol as a biologic marker of chronic stress in neonates: A pilot study. *Pain Research and Management, 8* (Suppl. 8), 59B.

7

PAIN IN INDIVIDUALS WITH CEREBRAL PALSY

Joyce M. Engel and Deborah Kartin

Cerebral palsy (CP) is a developmental disability that affects individuals across the life span. Although CP has been recognized and studied for many years, only relatively recently has the experience of pain in people with CP been explored. This chapter begins by defining CP, discussing the etiology of CP, and providing a descriptive analysis of the characteristics of CP. Next, potential sources of pain and the unique characteristics of pain assessment for this population are discussed. This is followed by a survey of the study of pain in individuals with CP, and then a consideration of intervention strategies for pain intervention used by individuals with CP. Subsequently, implications for clinical practice and future research are presented.

CEREBRAL PALSY DEFINED

Cerebral palsy refers to a group of chronic conditions affecting body movement, muscle coordination, and posture caused by a lesion of the developing brain. It is the most common condition associated with childhood disability (Kuban & Leviton, 1994). CP affects 764,000 youth and adults in the United States (United Cerebral Palsy, 2004). The incidence of CP is approximately 2.5 per 1,000 live births per year in developed countries (Stanley, Blair, & Alberman, 2001). Despite advances in medicine, the frequency of CP has not declined over time because of the survival rate of preterm infants and infants of multiple births with low birth weight (Dzienkowski, Smith, Dillow, & Yucha, 1996). Seventy percent of CP occurs prior to birth (prenatal), 20% occurs during and shortly after the birthing (perinatal), and 10% occurs during the first 2 years of life (postnatal) (United Cerebral Palsy, 2004).

The term *cerebral palsy* is descriptive. There are no diagnostic tests for CP; however, a developmental history is obtained in addition to physical and neurological examinations that may include neuroimaging (magnetic resonance imaging) of the infant or young child (Bax & Brown, 2004). CP is clinically defined as "an umbrella term covering a group of non-progressive, but often changing, motor impairment syndromes secondary to lesions or anomalies of the brain arising in the early stages of its development" (Mutch, Alberman, Hagberg, Kodama, & Perat, 1992). The key features of the definition are that the pathology is non-progressive and the emphasis is on motor disorder. CP is not a disease entity (Bax & Brown, 2004). One important consideration, however, is that although the

Supported by a grant "Management of Chronic Pain in Rehabilitation" POI HD/NS33988, from the National Institutes of Health, National Institute of Child Health and Human Development (National Center for Medical Rehabilitation Research).

pathology of CP is nonprogressive, the expression of CP changes over time. This occurs with the increasing repertoire of developmental abilities that are expected (and may not be achieved) as the child grows. Changes in the expression of CP may also occur as a function of the development of secondary disabilities (Bax & Brown, 2004).

ETIOLOGY OF CP

To understand the causes of CP, it is helpful to identify whether the injury occurred during prenatal, perinatal, or postnatal development. One common prenatal cause is impaired migration of new brain cells to their destination in the developing brain. Major risk factors for this include infection (intrauterine or from the mother's genitourinary tract), toxins, drugs, and radiation exposure. In addition, poor myelination of neurons, hemorrhage in the developing brain, and the presence of multiple fetuses are other possible causes of CP. Perinatally, major risk factors include low birth weight and prematurity. Other causes include increased pressure on the infant brain during delivery (e.g., breech birth), impaired circulation to the fetal brain (e.g., blood clot in the umbilical cord), and poor respiration (asphyxia), which may result in brain cell death. In postnatal development, risk factors include physical trauma (e.g., head injury), infection, seizures, and cerebrovascular disorders (Dzienkowski et al., 1996; United Cerebral Palsy, 2004). CP is believed to result from numerous factors that all result in hypoxic damage to the nerve cells (Bax & Brown, 2004). Determination of the etiology of CP has implications for prognosis, intervention, and ongoing management of associated conditions (e.g., epilepsy) (Ashwal et al., 2004). There is no cure for CP (Bax & Brown, 2004). Treatment therefore strives to maximize function and minimize secondary disability.

DESCRIPTIONS OF CP

The term *cerebral palsy* can be made more specific by adding descriptors characterizing the types of motor impairment and the part(s) of the body in which the motor disability is manifest. Four different classifications of CP are recognized: spastic, dyskinetic, ataxic, and mixed. Spastic is the most common type of CP and is associated with injury to the cerebral cortex. Involuntary sudden movements, hypertonia, persistent primitive reflexes, and exaggerated deep tendon reflexes are typically present and often result in contractures (shortening of soft tissues) and abnormal curvatures of the spine. Spastic-type CP can be further categorized into three subtypes: spastic quadriplegia (all four extremities equally affected), spastic diplegia (affecting the lower extremities more than the upper extremities), and spastic hemiplegia (affecting one side of the body) (Dzienkowski et al., 1996; Miller, 1988). Spasticity is severe in all extremities in youth with spastic quadriplegia. By adulthood, they often develop scoliosis or kyphosis (Bax & Brown, 2004). Seizures and severe cognitive impairment often occur with spastic quadriplegia (Bax & Brown, 2004). The child with diplegic CP may develop fixed contractures at the hip, knee, and ankle joints. Many youth with diplegic CP develop bony undergrowth of both lower limbs.

Dyskinetic-type CP results from injury to basal ganglia and involves impaired voluntary muscle control that results in incomplete movements that appear random. There are three subtypes of dyskinetic-type CP: athetoid (slow, writhing movements), choreoathetoid (rapid, irregular contractions of small muscle groups), and dystonic (prolonged contractions that cause twisting and repetitive movements). Individuals with dyskinetic CP will typically have fluctuating muscle tone, problems with fine motor skills, facial grimacing, and writhing movements of the hands and fingers. The constant increase in muscle tone of the upper extremities may result in rigidity or tremors (Dzienkowski et al., 1996).

People with ataxic-type CP have irregularities of typical muscle coordination that result in a lack of balance and of sense of position in space. Most individuals with ataxic CP are hypotonic from birth. However, the ataxia, although persistent, typically improves over time. This lack of coordination typically results in a staggering gait with shaking of the trunk and head (Dzienkowski et al., 1996; Miller, 1988).

Some people with CP have more than one type. Mixed-type CP is a combination of two or more of the types described previously that results from injury to two or more regions of the central nervous system. Approximately 15%–40% of people with CP have mixed type, with spasticity plus athetoid movements being most common. Individuals with mixed type may demonstrate predominant symptoms of one type with mild symptoms of another (Dzienkowski et al., 1996; Miller, 1988).

The Gross Motor Function Classification System for Cerebral Palsy (GMFCS) (Palisano et al., 1997; Rosenbaum et al., 2002) is used to classify the usual functional performance of children with CP in the contexts of home, school, and community. Distinctions between the five classifications are based largely on functional limitations and the need for assistive technology (including mobility devices) and, to a lesser degree, on quality of movement. In addition to being a descriptive tool, the GMFCS has been demonstrated to be a useful prognostic tool for children with CP (Rosenbaum et al., 2002). The functional abilities of individuals with CP vary greatly, from total physical dependence to mild motor impairments that do not interfere with activities of daily living. Approximately half of the individuals with CP use assistive devices (e.g., wheelchairs) to help with mobility (Ashwal et al., 2004).

Although disturbances in motor abilities and postural control are among the most common impairments associated with CP, the range of associated impairments is broad. These often include visual (e.g., strabismus, myopia) and auditory (e.g., hearing loss) impairments, seizures, gastrointestinal problems, chronic respiratory disease, cognitive impairment, learning disabilities, speech disorders (dysarthria), and behavior problems (Miller, 1988).

According to Murphy, Yeargin-Ausopp, Decoufee, and Drews (1993) approximately 65% of people with CP have cognitive impairment. The severity of cognitive impairment usually correlates with the degree and type of motor impairment. For example, it is known that people with dyskinetic CP of the athetoid type are more likely to have higher cognitive functioning than those with bilateral spastic syndromes (i.e., spastic quadriplegia or spastic diplegia), and youth with spastic-type quadriplegia are often the most severely affected (Miller, 1988). Individuals with CP can have typical intelligence, but accompanying challenges such as perceptual differences, attention-deficit disorder, depression, and emotional instability can interfere with intellectual growth (Dzienkowski et al., 1996).

The etiology of behavioral and emotional disorders associated with CP is complex and can partly be attributed to the brain injury itself, the symptoms of which may include poor attention and obsessive-compulsive traits. Low self-esteem, frustration, and dependency may also coexist with CP. The combination of motor impairment and CP-associated disorders typically results in functional disabilities (Miller, 1988).

CHRONIC PAIN IN INDIVIDUALS WITH CP

Given the wide variability and complexity in the expression of CP, the potential for an individual with CP to experience related pain across the life span is great, and this pain may have multiple sources. There is, however, controversy regarding the relationship of severity of CP to the presence of pain. Some researchers have found that the severity of CP does not directly relate to reports of pain (Landgraf, Abetz, & Ware, 1996), and others have reported an association between the severity of CP and pain, such that the more severe the CP, the more pain is reported (Houlihan, O'Donnell, Conaway, & Stevenson, 2004).

Spasticity, characterized by hyperactive deep tendon reflexes, clonus, and velocity-dependent resistance to movement, and muscle spasm are also potential causes of pain in CP (Chalkiadis, 2001; Roscigno, 2002). Given that spasticity is common in CP, spasticity-related pain is potentially a widespread source of discomfort (Chalkiadis, 2001).

The motor impairments associated with CP extend into adulthood and can contribute to chronic pain (Jensen, Engel, McKearnan, & Hoffman, 2003). Limitations in mobility may predispose the individual with CP to experience pain for various reasons. For example, an individual with CP may experience pain because of limitations in his or her ability to change position and to relieve pressure from body parts (ischemic pain). Pain may also be related to edema of a dependent extremity. Because of limitations in movement and variations in muscle tone (e.g., spasticity, rigidity), individuals with CP may develop contractures that limit range of motion. These limitations may, for example, result in pain during routine activities of daily living and participation in daily life. Furthermore, individuals with CP may experience pain from compensatory overuse of a body part in one area related to decreased mobility in another area. Chronic overuse, resulting from repetitive use of muscles and joints in a manner that is a biomechanical disadvantage, may result in early degenerative joint disease and cause pain in weight-bearing joints. This can occur in both the upper and lower extremities (Gajdosik & Cicirello, 2001; Murphy, Molnar, & Lankasky, 1995). For example, the involvement of the legs may result in overuse and subsequent arthritic changes over time in the wrists, elbows, and shoulders of an individual with diplegic CP who uses crutches for community ambulation.

Similarly, pain may be caused by specific musculoskeletal deformities that also limit range of motion and function. For example, hip dysplasia, subluxation, and dislocation, frequently observed in individuals with CP, are commonly associated with pain (Chalkiadis, 2001; Murphy et al., 1995). Individuals with CP may undergo surgical procedures to correct orthopedic problems (e.g., open reduction of hip dislocation, derotational osteotomy) and muscle imbalances (e.g., heel cord, adductor, or hamstring lengthenings). Surgical and medical procedures may be associated with both acute and chronic pain for the individual with CP (Geiduschek et al., 1994). Furthermore, individuals with CP may experience pain that is a direct function of rehabilitative interventions. For example, pain in individuals with CP has been associated with range-of-motion exercises and stretching, bracing/splinting, and wearing of orthotics, commonly used rehabilitation interventions (Hadden & von Baeyer, 2002; Kibele, 1989; Kibele & Flint,

1990). Poor wheelchair seating may result in postural back pain (K. P. Murphy et al., 1995).

Given the nature of the condition, an individual with CP may require ongoing rehabilitative interventions throughout his or her life span. Repeatedly experiencing these often painful interventions may result in the individual experiencing an increase in psychological stressors (e.g., anxiety, fear, distress) (McGrath, 1990; Turnquist & Engel, 1994). These stressors may negatively impact his or her quality of life, particularly if they are expressed as withdrawal, limited coping abilities, and depression (Engel, Schwartz, Jensen, & Johnson, 2000; Kibele, 1989; Kibele & Flint, 1990).

Spasticity, contractures, overuse syndromes, nerve entrapments, radiculopathies, and myelopathies are common (Roscigno, 2002). Pain may also originate from orthopedic impairments (e.g., hip subluxation, scoliosis, degenerative arthritis) (Bleck, 1987; Hodgkinson et al., 2001). Other common potential contributors to the experience of pain in people with CP include surgical procedures (e.g., soft tissue releases) (Dzienkowski et al., 1996). It is important not to overlook other potential sources of pain in individuals with CP unrelated to the neuromuscular and musculoskeletal systems. Gastrointestinal problems such as gastroesophageal reflux, gastrointestinal motility disturbances, and gastrostomy have been identified as additional sources of pain in people with CP (Del Giudice et al., 1999; Houlihan et al., 2004).

It is essential for clinicians to explicitly evaluate for the presence of pain and potential pain interference in individuals with CP and be open to the myriad of possible causes for the pain. Given the complex nature of CP, combined with other factors, the possibility of misattributing pain in individuals with CP exists. Researchers have highlighted intrinsic and extrinsic challenges of pain evaluation and intervention in individuals with CP (Hadden & von Baeyer, 2002; K.P. Murphy, 1999; Oberlander, O'Donnell, & Montgomery, 1999). For some individuals with CP, intrinsic factors such as the presence of cognitive, sensory-visual, motor, and communication impairments may make the assessment of pain more challenging by obscuring the recognition of pain and complicating the evaluation and intervention processes (Collignon & Giusiano, 2001; Patterson, Jensen, & Engel-Knowles, 2002). For example, a person with CP and dysarthria may require an extended period of time to complete a face-to-face interview, yet, given the person's motor abilities, this strategy may be the most effective way of gaining self-reports about the pain (Schwartz, Engel, & Jensen, 1999). In addition, interpreting and differentiating involuntary muscle activity and facial grimacing, characteristic of some individuals with CP, from pain behaviors may be difficult.

Other factors that are extrinsic to the individual with CP may also come to bear on this process. Extrinsic factors such as limitations in comprehensive services for individuals with CP and in health care providers' experiences in providing services for individuals with CP may contribute to the underidentification and resultant undertreatment of pain. Even when pain complaints have been recognized, reports of pain with varying causes have been initially erroneously attributed to the developmental disability itself rather than identifying the actual underlying cause (Murphy, 1999). In such circumstances, the delay of accurate evaluation may impede appropriate interventions and result in unnecessary pain and suffering. Chapters 10 and 11 provide more in-depth discussions of pain assessment in children and adults with developmental disabilities.

STUDY OF PAIN IN CP

Although CP has long been recognized as a developmental disability, the study of pain in CP is a relatively recent phenomenon (Ehde et al., 2003). Early reports of pain in individuals with CP are first seen as anecdotal findings in studies whose primary focus was other than pain (Ireland & Hoffer, 1985; Tenuta, Shelton, & Miller, 1993). These were followed by studies of the medical and health status of individuals with CP (Murphy et al., 1995; Turk, Geremski, Rosenbaum, & Weber, 1997) and case reports (Murphy, 1999) of the medical problems of individuals with CP that provided further descriptions of the pain experiences associated with CP. Later studies whose specific purpose was to explore the experience of pain in CP were conducted using self-reports of adults (Engel, Kartin, & Jensen, 2002; Schwartz et al., 1999) and youth (Engel, Petrina, Dudgeon, & McKearnan, in press) with CP.

Early descriptive reports linked pain in adults and youth with CP to conditions such as spasticity (Broseta, Garcia-March, Sanchez-Ledesma, Anaya, & Silva, 1990) and spasticity-related deformities of the spine (Cassidy, Craig, Perry, Karlin, & Goldberg, 1994) and other joints (Ireland & Hoffer, 1985). More recently, researchers, using self-report interview methods, proxy reports, and observations, have demonstrated that pain is a common experience in adults (Engel, Jensen, Hoffman, & Kartin, 2003; Schwartz et al., 1999; Turk et al., 1997) and in youth (Engel et al., in press; Hadden & von Baeyer, 2002; Liptak et al., 2001) with CP that may limit activity and participation.

For many individuals with CP, pain is chronic across the life span (Engel et al., 2003; Jensen, Engel, Hoffman, & Schwartz, 2004; Schwartz et al., 1999; Turk et al., 1997). Pain may occur daily and often is of moderate to severe intensity. Pain locations routinely reported in adults with CP are, in descending order of occurrence, the legs/feet, back, neck or shoulder, arms/hands, buttocks/hips, head, chest, and abdomen (Engel et al., 2002). In youth with CP, the hip, knee, and foot are the most frequently identified pain sites (Long & Harp, 1995). It is important to understand, however, that pain is often reported in multiple sites by both adults (Schwartz et al., 1999) and youth (Engel et al., in press) with CP, and that pain lasting more than 3 months is a common experience of individuals with CP (Engel et al., in press; Schwartz et al., 1999).

Fatigue, stress/depression, and overexertion are among the factors identified as exacerbating pain in self-reports by adults with CP, whereas exercise, stretching, and getting adequate rest have been reported to relieve pain (Schwartz et al., 1999). A comparison of the extent to which pain interferes in the daily lives of individuals with CP to that of people with other disabilities such as spinal cord injuries (Turner, Cardenas, Warms, & McClellan, 2001) or amputations (Ehde, Czerniecki, Smith, Jensen, & Robinson, 1998) suggests that individuals with CP experience less pain interference (Schwartz et al., 1999). This somewhat counterintuitive finding needs to be interpreted cautiously. It is possible that the severity of the disability and other factors may have limited independent function in daily activities in the first place. For some, a lower level of activity and participation in activities of daily life may have made pain interference in daily life less relevant.

We have also begun to learn about how individuals with CP cope with chronic pain. Task persistence, increasing activity, diverting attention, reinterpreting pain sensations, praying and hoping, and using coping self-statements are strategies reportedly used by adults with CP to cope with chronic pain (Engel et al., 2000). Guarding and resting have been reportedly used less often, perhaps reflecting limitations in mobility and the use of postural supports (e.g., splints, orthotics, adaptive seating in wheelchairs) limiting opportunity for guarding from pain. Although a preliminary finding, a strong association between catastrophizing and pain interference and depression has been demonstrated in adults. This finding suggests that cognitive behavioral interventions that decrease catastrophizing may benefit some individuals with CP in ameliorating some of the effects of chronic pain (Engel et al., 2000).

PAIN INTERVENTION IN CP

A variety of specific treatment strategies for pain have been reported to be helpful by adults with CP and chronic pain (Engel et al., 2002; Jensen et al., 2004). Both active and passive treatment strategies for pain are used, but use of passive strategies is more common compared to strategies that require active participation. This is evidenced, for example, by the high use of pain medication compared to more active strategies such as biofeedback, counseling, or exercise. What are not understood, however, are the reasons for this discrepancy.

Passive intervention strategies have included pharmacological interventions ranging from non-narcotic analgesics, to prescription medications directed toward spasticity management, to narcotics. Adults with CP reported using and rating many pain treatments as at least moderately helpful on a temporary basis. These included pain medications, biofeedback, and counseling. Furthermore, invasive procedures for pain, such as nerve blocks, tendon releases, spinal cord stimulators, botulinum toxin, and hip and back surgeries, although used less often, were also reported to be at least moderately helpful (Engel et al., 2002).

One concerning finding is that many adults with CP and chronic pain do not directly access health care for assistance with pain management (Engel et al., 2002). In addition, even though many interventions have been reported to be at least moderately helpful in managing pain, many people with CP did not persist with pain treatments found to be helpful. Given the extent to which chronic pain is reported in individuals with CP, this raises concerns about general access to health care and the extent to which pain is addressed in routine health care. Furthermore, it suggests that pain is undertreated in this population.

RECOMMENDATIONS FOR FUTURE CLINICAL PRACTICE AND RESEARCH

Longitudinal studies on the natural course of pain in people with CP are virtually nonexistent and limited to a 2-year study span in adults (Jensen et al., 2004). Longitudinal studies are needed to better understand pain in individuals with CP and will have significant clinical relevance in both the short- and long-term perspective. For example, if pain were found to increase over time to moderate to severe intensity, aggressive pain treatment might be warranted.

There is a paucity of research designed to identify and determine the efficacy of pain interventions for individuals with CP-related pain. It is important to perform empirical studies on pain interventions and to determine their durability. Ideally, future research would also address pain across the life span of groups of people with CP to determine the magnitude, nature, and repertoire of interventions for CP-related pain at different points in an individual's life.

Adherence is an often-overlooked area in health care. Adherence is an important area for concern because many forms of medical, rehabilitative, and psychological treatments for pain depend upon consumer adherence to intervention procedures. Assessment of adherence is critical in determining the degree of adherence required for clinical improvement and in addressing any difficulties with treatment delivery. A unique feature of adherence to interventions for people with severe motor, sensory, and cognitive impairments is that the individual may need to rely on a caregiver for access to the intervention.

Consumer satisfaction with pain interventions for people with CP has not yet been determined. When consumers (e.g., direct recipient of services, caregiver, practitioner) are satisfied with the rendered interventions and results, it is more likely that these interventions will be used on a consistent basis than if consumers find the interventions to be unacceptable (e.g., too time consuming). Intervention modifications may be necessary to meet the needs of those with severe motor, sensory, and cognitive impairments (Engel & Kartin, 2004; Patterson et al., 2002). Consumer satisfaction feedback is also vital for strategic and marketing planning (Engel, 1991).

In addition, social validity also needs to be directly addressed as an important supplement to outcome measures. The acceptability of treatment goals and procedures in addition to the results of intervention programs can be determined by social validation. Wolf (1975) suggested that social validation should address the social significance of treatment goals, the social appropriateness of treatment procedures, and the social importance of treatment results. Social validation is an inexpensive and time-efficient method for practitioners to determine whether consumers share the same perceptions of therapeutic outcomes (Engel & Kartin, 2004).

In order to provide adults and youth with CP appropriate access to health care services for pain, advocacy efforts may be indicated from several perspectives. Raising service providers' awareness about the incidence of pain in people with CP is an important step. Similarly, advocating that the curricula for professional preparation of health care providers include strategies for pain assessment and strategies for developing and implementing appropriate interventions for pain in individuals with CP is critical. Furthermore, the lack of continuity of interventions reported to be helpful in the relief of pain in people with CP raises important questions as to why this is so (Engel et al., 2002). Advocating for resources for further pain research and improved access to pain management for people with CP may result in improved quality of life for adults and youth with CP.

REFERENCES

Ashwal, S., Russman, B.S., Blasco, P.A., Miller, G., Sandler, A., Shevell, M., et al. (2004). Practice parameter: Diagnostic assessment of the child with cerebral palsy. Report of the Quality Standards Subcommittee of the American Academy of Neurology and the Practice Committee of the Child Neurology Society. *Neurology, 62*, 851–863.

Bax, M., & Brown, J. (2004). The spectrum of disorders known as cerebral palsy. In D. Sutton, D. Damiano, & M. Mayston (Eds.), *Management of the motor disorders of children with cerebral palsy* (2nd ed., pp. 9–21). London: MacKeith Press.

Bleck, E.E. (1987). *Orthopedic management in cerebral palsy.* London: MacKeith Press.

Broseta, J., Garcia-March, G., Sanchez-Ledesma, M.J., Anaya, J., & Silva, I. (1990). Chronic intrathecal baclofen administration in severe spasticity. *Stereotactic and Functional Neurosurgery, 54-55*, 147–153.

Cassidy, C., Craig, C.L., Perry, A., Karlin, L.I., & Goldberg, M.J. (1994). A reassessment of spinal stabilization in severe cerebral palsy. *Journal of Pediatric Orthopedics, 14*, 731–739.

Chalkiadis, G.A. (2001). Management of chronic pain in children. *Medical Journal of Australia, 175*, 476–479.

Collignon, P., & Giusiano, B. (2001). Validation of a pain evaluation scale for patients with severe cerebral palsy. *European Journal of Pain, 5*, 433–442.

Del Giudice, E., Staiano, A., Capano, G., Romano, A., Florimonte, L., Miele, E., et al. (1999). Gastrointestinal manifestations in children with cerebral palsy. *Brain Development, 21*, 307–311.

Dzienkowski, R.C., Smith, K.K., Dillow, K.A., & Yucha, C.B. (1996). Cerebral palsy: A comprehensive review. *The Nurse Practitioner, 21*(2), 45–48, 51–44, 57–49; quiz 60–41.

Ehde, D., Jensen, M., Engel, J., Turner, J., Hoffman, A., & Cardenas, D. (2003). Chronic pain secondary to disability: A review. *Clinical Journal of Pain, 19*, 3–17.

Ehde, D.M., Czerniecki, J.M., Smith, D.G., Jensen, M.P., & Robinson, L.R. (1998). Chronic pain following lower limb amputation. *Archives of Physical Medicine and Rehabilitation, 79*, 1172–1173.

Engel, J. (1991). Social validation of relaxation training in pediatric headache control. *Occupational Therapy in Mental Health, 11*(4), 77–90.

Engel, J.M., Jensen, M.P., Hoffman, A.J., & Kartin, D. (2003). Pain in persons with cerebral palsy: Extension and cross validation. *Archives of Physical Medicine and Rehabilitation, 84*, 1125–1128.

Engel, J.M., & Kartin, D. (2004). Pain in youth: A primer for current practice. *Critical Reviews in Physical and Rehabilitation Medicine, 16*, 53–74.

Engel, J.M., Kartin, D., & Jensen, M.P. (2002). Pain treatment in persons with cerebral palsy: Frequency and helpfulness. *American Journal of Physical Medicine and Rehabilitation, 81*, 291–296.

Engel, J.M., Petrina, T., Dudgeon, B., & McKearnan, K.A. (in press). Youths with cerebral palsy and chronic pain: A descriptive study. *Physical and Occupational Therapy in Pediatrics.*

Engel, J.M., Schwartz, L., Jensen, M.P., & Johnson, D.R. (2000). Pain in cerebral palsy: The relation of coping strategies to adjustment. *Pain, 88*, 225–230.

Gajdosik, C.G., & Cicirello, N. (2001). Secondary conditions of the musculoskeletal system in adolescents and adults with cerebral palsy. *Physical and Occupational Therapy in Pediatrics, 21*(4), 49–68.

Geiduschek, J.M., Haberkern, C.M., McLaughlin, J.F., Jacobson, L.E., Hays, R.M., & Roberts, T.S. (1994). Pain management for children following selective dorsal rhizotomy. *Canadian Journal of Anaesthesia, 41*, 492–496.

Hadden, K., & von Baeyer, C. (2002). Pain in children with cerebral palsy: Common triggers and expressive behaviors. *Pain, 99*, 281.

Hodgkinson, I., Jindrich, M.L., Duhaut, P., Vadot, J.P., Metton, G., & Berard, C. (2001). Hip pain in 234 non-ambulatory adolescents and young adults with cerebral palsy: A cross-sectional multicentre study. *Developmental Medicine and Child Neurology, 43*, 806–808.

Houlihan, C.M., O'Donnell, M., Conaway, M., & Stevenson, R.D. (2004). Bodily pain and health-related quality of life in children with cerebral palsy. *Developmental Medicine and Child Neurology, 46*, 305–310.

Ireland, M.L., & Hoffer, M. (1985). Triple arthrodesis for children with spastic cerebral palsy. *Developmental Medicine and Child Neurology, 27*, 623–627.

Jensen, M.P., Engel, J.M., Hoffman, A.J., & Schwartz, L. (2004). Natural history of chronic pain and pain treatment in adults with cerebral palsy. *American Journal of Physical Medicine and Rehabilitation, 83*, 439–445.

Jensen, M.P., Engel, J.M., McKearnan, K.A., & Hoffman, A.J. (2003). Validity of pain intensity assessment in persons with cerebral palsy: A comparison of six scales. *Journal of Pain, 4,* 56–63.

Kibele, A. (1989). Occupational therapy's role in improving the quality of life for persons with cerebral palsy. *American Journal of Occupational Therapy, 43,* 371–377.

Kibele, A., & Flint, S. (1990). The challenge of pediatric pain: The role of occupational therapy in multidisciplinary management. *Occupational Therapy Practice, 1*(3), 39–46.

Kuban, K.C., & Leviton, A. (1994). Cerebral palsy. *New England Journal of Medicine, 330,* 188–195.

Landgraf, J.M., Abetz, L., & Ware, J.E. (1996). *Child Health Questionnaire (CHQ): A user's manual.* Boston: The Health Institute, New England Medical Center.

Liptak, G.S., O'Donnell, M., Conaway, M., Chumlea, W.C., Wolrey, G., Henderson, R.C., et al. (2001). Health status of children with moderate to severe cerebral palsy. *Developmental Medicine and Child Neurology, 43,* 364–370.

Long, T.M., & Harp, K.A. (1995). Pain in children. *Orthopaedic Physical Therapy Clinics of North America, 4,* 503–517.

McGrath, P.J. (1990). *Pain in children: Nature, assessment, and treatment.* New York: Guilford Press.

Miller, G. (1988). Cerebral palsies: An overview. In G. Miller & D. Clark (Eds.), *The cerebral palsies: Causes, consequences, and management* (pp. 1–9). Woburn, MA: Butterworth-Heinemann.

Murphy, C.C., Yeargin-Ausopp, M., Decoufee, P., & Drews, C.D. (1993). Prevalence of cerebral palsy among ten year old children in metropolitan Atlanta, 1985 through 1987. *Journal of Pediatrics, 123,* 513–519.

Murphy, K.P. (1999). Medical problems in adults with cerebral palsy: Case examples. *Assistive Technology, 11,* 97–104.

Murphy, K.P., Molnar, G.E., & Lankasky, K. (1995). Medical and functional status of adults with cerebral palsy. *Developmental Medicine and Child Neurology, 37,* 1075–1084.

Mutch, L., Alberman, E., Hagberg, B., Kodama, K., & Perat, M.V. (1992). Cerebral palsy epidemiology: Where are we now and where are we going? *Developmental Medicine and Child Neurology, 34,* 547–551.

Oberlander, T.F., O'Donnell, M.E., & Montgomery, C.J. (1999). Pain in children with significant neurological impairment. *Journal of Developmental and Behavioral Pediatrics, 20,* 235–243.

Palisano, R., Rosenbaum, P., Walter, S., Russell, D., Wood, E., & Galauppi, B. (1997). Development and reliability of a system to classify gross motor function in children with cerebral palsy. *Developmental Medicine and Child Neurology, 39,* 214–223.

Patterson, D.R., Jensen, M.P., & Engel-Knowles, J. (2002). Pain and its influence on assistive technology use. In M.J. Scherer (Ed.), *Assistive technology: Matching device and consumer for successful rehabilitation* (pp. 59–76). Washington, DC: American Psychological Association.

Roscigno, C.I. (2002). Addressing spasticity-related pain in children with spastic cerebral palsy. *Journal of Neuroscience Nursing, 34,* 123–133.

Rosenbaum, P.L., Walter, S.D., Hanna, S.E., Palisano, R.J., Russell, D.J., Raina, P., et al. (2002). Prognosis for gross motor function in cerebral palsy: Creation of motor development curves. *JAMA, 288,* 1357–1363.

Schwartz, L., Engel, J.M., & Jensen, M.P. (1999). Pain in persons with cerebral palsy. *Archives of Physical Medicine and Rehabiliation, 80,* 1243–1246.

Stanley, F., Blair, E., & Alberman, E. (2001). Birth events and cerebral palsy: Facts were not presented clearly. *British Medical Journal, 322,* 50.

Tenuta, J., Shelton, Y.A., & Miller, F. (1993). Long-term follow-up of triple arthrodesis in patients with cerebral palsy. *Journal of Pediatric Orthopedics, 13,* 713–716.

Turk, M.A., Geremski, C.A., Rosenbaum, P.F., & Weber, R.J. (1997). The health status of women with cerebral palsy. *Archives of Physical Medicine and Rehabilitation, 78*(12 Suppl. 5), 10–17.

Turner, J.A., Cardenas, D.D., Warms, C.A., & McClellan, C.B. (2001). Chronic pain associated with spinal cord injuries: A community survey. *Archives of Physical Medicine and Rehabilitation, 82,* 501–509.

Turnquist, K.M., & Engel, J.M. (1994). Occupational therapists' experience and knowledge of pain in children. *Physical and Occupational Therapy in Pediatrics, 14*(1), 35–51.

United Cerebral Palsy. (2004). *Cerebral palsy: Facts & figures.* Retrieved September 15, 2004, from http://www.ucp.org

Wolf, M.M. (1975). Social validity: The case for subjective measurement or how applied behavior analysis is finding its heart. *Journal of Applied Behavior Analysis, 11,* 203–214.

8

PAIN, HEALTH CONDITIONS, AND PROBLEM BEHAVIOR IN PEOPLE WITH DEVELOPMENTAL DISABILITIES

Craig H. Kennedy and Mark F. O'Reilly

Quite a sizable proportion of individuals with developmental disabilities exhibit some form of behavior problems, which can make care, support, and inclusion difficult (Sigafoos, Arthur, & O'Reilly, 2003). Since the first applications of behavior analysis (roughly equated with the launch of the *Journal of Applied Behavior Analysis* in 1968), practitioners in this discipline have been interested in the assessment and treatment of behavior problems. Best practices in the behavioral assessment and treatment of problem behavior have changed since the 1960s. These changes are a result of many developments, such as public shifts in attitudes toward people with developmental disabilities (e.g., making the use of aversive treatments less acceptable) and the development of more sophisticated assessment and treatment technologies (e.g., analogue functional analysis methods and functional communication training). We are now at an exciting juncture in behavior analysis where we are beginning to meld our operant understanding of the consequences that maintain challenging behavior with other factors such as the general health status of a person and possible neurogenetic predispositions to problem behavior. This new research may allow us to gain a more complete understanding of factors that predispose to, exacerbate, and maintain problem behavior in this population. Such research may also underscore the development of multifaceted approaches that target medical and behavioral issues in the assessment and treatment of problem behavior, which have previously not been considered.

SCOPE OF THE ISSUE: PROBLEM BEHAVIOR AND DEVELOPMENTAL DISABILITIES

Problem behavior is not unique to individuals with developmental disabilities, but it is 2 to 3 times more common in this population than in people without developmental disabilities (e.g., Einfeld & Tongue, 1996). Estimates of the prevalence of problem behavior in this population vary from as low as 2% to as high as 70% (e.g., Chung, Bickerton, Cumella, & Winchester, 1996; Schroeder, Schroeder, Smith, & Dalldorf, 1978). However, such estimates must be viewed with caution because samples are often small and are selected based on convenience (e.g., residents of an institutional setting versus people receiving supported employment).

Probably the most comprehensive research on prevalence of behavior problems among individuals with developmental disabilities has been conducted in the United Kingdom in 1988 and reported in a number of peer-reviewed papers and book chapters (e.g., Qureshi, 1994; Qureshi & Alborz, 1992). In this research, 4,200 individuals with developmental disabilities were screened across seven major health districts in northwest England. Of these, 694 individuals were identified as having some form of problem behavior according to a series of screening procedures, which were comprehensive and reliable. The overall prevalence of problem behavior in this total population survey was 16.5%. The prevalence of problem behavior in each of the seven health districts surveyed ranged from 15% to 17.3%. A follow-up study of two of these major health districts in 1995 revealed prevalence estimates similar to those in the 1988 survey (Emerson et al., 2001a). Overall, the results of this series of prevalence studies indicate that problem behavior occurs in approximately 15%–17% of this population.

Of those identified with problem behaviors in the 1988 survey, 42% engaged in aggression, 30% in destructive behavior, and 27% in self-injury. Approximately 50% of this group displayed one type of problem behavior (e.g., aggression) only, whereas the remaining 50% displayed two or more general types of problem behavior (e.g., aggression and self-injury).

Emerson et al. (2001a) reported the prevalence of specific forms of aggression, destructive behavior, and self-injury based on the 1995 follow-up survey. Some of the most frequent forms of aggression included hitting with the hand, verbal abuse, hitting with an object, scratching, hair pulling, and biting. Some of the most frequent forms of destructive behavior included hitting objects, breaking glass, and throwing objects. Some of the most frequent forms of self-injury included head hitting with the hand, self-biting, head hitting against objects, or self-pinching/scratching.

From this, we can draw a number of conclusions. First, approximately 16% of individuals with developmental disabilities engage in some form of problem behavior. Problem behavior can be classified into the three general categories: aggression, destructive behavior, and self-injury. Instances of problem behavior can vary widely and include a variety of topographies such as striking others, hitting objects, and/or self-hitting for a single individual. Other research has shown that such behaviors tend to occur early in development and, once present, persist well into the adult years (Emerson et al., 2001b; Green, O'Reilly, Itchon, & Sigafoos, 2005).

BEHAVIOR ANALYSIS AND THE ASSESSMENT AND TREATMENT OF PROBLEM BEHAVIOR

Behavior analysis is a natural science approach to the study of the determinants of volitional behavior (Skinner, 1938). It is an active, independent, and productive discipline that has its own peer-reviewed journals, professional organizations, and professional certification board. As a scientific discipline, behavior analysis is concerned with three general issues: 1) the examination and elucidation of the theoretical underpinnings of the science, 2) the experimental analysis of the basic principles that govern behavior, and 3) the application of basic principles of behavior to issues of social importance. The application of these behavioral principles to issues of human importance is usually termed *applied behavior analysis.* Behavior analysis has proven invaluable by demonstrating successful behavior change in diverse areas of application such as community, developmental, organizational, and clinical psychology; behavioral medicine; general and special education; speech and hearing sciences; and social work, to name but a few.

In this section, we provide a historical overview of the use of behavior analysis methodologies to assess and treat problem behavior in this population. In this overview, we discuss earlier trends characterized by the development of treatments to reduce problem behaviors regardless of why they occur. Next, we describe the change in emphasis from simply reducing problem behavior to analyzing the conditions maintaining problem behavior and developing treatments based on assessment results. Finally, we describe recent attempts to incorporate biological variables into the assessment and treatment of problem behavior.

Treatments Designed to Reduce Problem Behavior

Since the inception of behavior analysis, investigators have been interested in using this approach with individuals with developmental disabilities. In fact, many of the early empirical investigations in behavior analysis were directed at treating behavior problems in this population (e.g., Ferster & DeMyer, 1961; Lovaas & Simmons, 1969; Wolf, Risley, & Mees, 1964). Much of the early research evaluated the use of arbitrary consequences that were used to eliminate or reduce problem behavior, including punishment and differential reinforcement. Punishment technologies can involve administering aversive stimuli such as electric shock, spanking, water mist spray, and ammonia when the individual engages in the behavior (e.g., Cunningham & Linscheid, 1976; Dorsey, Iwata, Ong, & McSween, 1980; Tanner & Zeiler, 1975). Such treatments have fallen out of favor for a number of reasons. Aversive treatments may produce emotional side effects such as crying, tantrums, wetting, and general agitation. In addition, these individuals are unable to give informed consent; in fact, this has been the source of much public controversy, with several state legislatures banning the use of such protocols.

Differential reinforcement strategies provide positive or negative reinforcers, or both, to a person for not engaging in problem behavior. Examples of such strategies include differential reinforcement of other behavior (DRO) or differential reinforcement of incompatible behavior (DRI). With DRO, the individual receives a reinforcing stimulus if he or she does not engage in the problem behavior for a predetermined period of time. In DRI, the individual receives a reinforcer for engaging in a behavior that is incompatible (e.g., washing dishes) with the problem behavior (e.g., striking head with fist). One of the major difficulties with these treatment protocols has been the unevenness in terms of the research findings. For example, although a number of studies showed these protocols to be effective (e.g., Allen & Harris, 1966; Tarpley & Schroeder, 1979), other researchers have reported poor results (Corte, Wolf, & Locke, 1971; Young & Wincze, 1974). These discrepancies appear to be due to the variable effectiveness of stimuli assumed to function as positive or negative reinforcers and a lack of knowledge regarding why problem behaviors occur.

Functional Assessment of Problem Behavior

Since the mid-1970s, there has been a shift in emphasis from the immediate focus on treatment protocols to the development of assessment technologies to guide interventions for problem behavior. Much of this work was spurred by the seminal review of problem behavior published by Carr (1977). In this review, Carr set forth a number of hypotheses for why people with developmental disabilities engage in problem behavior. These hypotheses suggested that problem behavior may be maintained by positive reinforcement (e.g., access to attention from others) or by negative reinforcement (e.g., escape from aversive task demands). Carr also suggested that some forms of problem behavior, such as self-injury, might produce automatic reinforcement (i.e., such behaviors reduce or increase sensory stimulation). In other words, Carr (1977) suggested that problem behavior is an operant response that can be controlled by one or more sources of operant reinforcement. Successful treatment may therefore depend on an initial understanding of what reinforcement contingencies are maintaining problem behavior, which can be determined via a functional assessment.

One functional assessment methodology for problem behavior, and one that is a hallmark of research on this topic, is the analogue functional analysis protocol developed by Iwata and colleagues (Iwata, Dorsey, Slifer, Bauman, & Richman, 1982/1994). This methodology involves systematically and repeatedly exposing the person to a series of social reinforcement contingencies or the lack thereof. Each context is designed to identify potential consequences that may be maintaining problem behavior. For example, a person may be ignored unless he or she engages in problem behavior, at which point the therapist attends to the person with statements of concern (e.g., "Don't do that. You will hurt yourself"). High levels of problem behavior in this situation, relative to other situations, indicate that the behavior is maintained by positive reinforcement in the form of attention from others. In another situation, the person with developmental disabilities is engaged in tasks that he or she has difficulty completing. Problem behavior produces brief removal of the task. High levels of problem behavior in this situation relative to others indicate that the behavior is maintained by negative reinforcement in the form of escape from noxious demands. This methodology has proven to be successful in identifying the consequences maintaining problem behavior in people with developmental disabilities (Hanley, Iwata, & McCord, 2003; Iwata, Pace, et al., 1994).

Research on the functions of problem behavior has led to changes in the way we conceptualize treatment and to the development of new treatment protocols. For example, functional assessments are typically a pretreatment requirement today, and treatment selection is no longer an arbitrary decision, but is determined by the results of the prior assessment. An example of a new treatment that is derived from a function-based understanding of problem behavior (i.e., the consequences maintaining problem behavior) is that of functional communication training. Functional communication training involves a two-step process. First, the communicative intent of problem behavior is identified. This involves identifying the consequences that maintain problem behavior by conducting a functional assessment. Second, the person is taught a functionally equivalent behavior that is designed to obtain the same consequence as the problem behavior. Using functional communication training, problem behavior is conceptualized as a form of communication, and the goal of intervention is to replace the problem behavior with a more appropriate communicative response (Carr et al., 1998).

An Emerging Biobehavioral Understanding of Problem Behavior

The analogue functional analysis model of assessment presents a strict response-consequence paradigm for understanding problem behavior. In other words, the problem behavior is identified and the consequences/contingencies maintaining it are isolated. Other variables may influence the variability, topography, and intensity of challenging behavior. For example, a large proportion of individuals with developmental disabilities have a variety of health conditions such as sleep problems, lower gastrointestinal problems, and recurrent infections. Researchers have hypothesized that such health conditions may influence problem behavior (Kennedy & Thompson, 2000). The development of analogue functional analysis techniques has allowed researchers to begin to examine possible interactions between such health issues and the consequences maintaining problem behavior. Such research may herald the beginning of a truly biobehavioral approach to the assessment and treatment of problem behavior for people with developmental disabilities.

For example, the biobehavioral relation between sleep deprivation and operant responding (i.e., problem behavior) has been demonstrated in several peer-reviewed studies (e.g., Kennedy & Meyer, 1996; O'Reilly, 1995). In these studies, the researchers demonstrated, using analogue functional analysis techniques, that aggressive behavior was maintained by negative reinforcement (i.e., escape from task demands) for the individuals involved. What was novel about these assessments is that the researchers also measured sleep duration (i.e., the number of hours slept each night). The analogue functional analyses were conducted over an extended period of time in order to examine the influence of disrupted sleep patterns on operant responding during the analogue assessments. The authors of these studies were able to demonstrate a positive correlation between sleep disturbance and negatively reinforced aggressive behavior. That is, higher levels of negatively reinforced problem behavior occurred following a night of disturbed sleep. This methodology offers a preliminary model by which we can begin to understand the interaction between biological and operant variables in the onset, maintenance, and exacerbation of problem behavior. We explore these issues further as we more closely examine biobehavioral interactions among pain, health conditions, and problem behavior in the following sections.

PAIN, HEALTH CONDITIONS, AND PROBLEM BEHAVIOR

The primary means by which pain influences problem behavior in people with developmental disabilities is through the presence of health conditions (Kennedy & Becker, in press), thus producing a set of biobehavioral interactions. Health conditions include any illness, injury, impairment, or physical condition that negatively affects a person's well-being (World Health Organization, 2000). The presence of a health condition in a person with developmental disabilities can cause discomfort resulting in a greater probability of aggression, destructive behavior, or self-injury. Of particular interest in this discussion is how health conditions can cause discomfort resulting in increased problem behavior.

Although health conditions can be manifested in a variety of forms, research during the past decade indicates that certain conditions are particularly prevalent among individuals with developmental disabilities. Common health conditions occurring in people with developmental disabilities include allergies, constipation, dysmenorrhea, gastroesophageal reflux disease (GERD), otitis media, and sleep problems. These conditions also occur in the general population, but seem to occur more frequently in people with developmental disabilities (Kennedy & Thompson, 2000). This increased prevalence may be due to sequelae of genetic syndromes, physical complications that result from the disability, and/or side effects produced by polypharmacy.

Examples of the increased prevalence of health conditions among people with developmental disabilities are plentiful. GERD, a dysfunction in the lower esophageal sphincter allowing acid to wash up into the esophagus, occurs in approximately 50% of people with profound mental retardation, compared to 10%–20% of the general population (Bohmer et al., 1999). Another gastrointestinal problem, constipation, occurs in 18% of the general population, but its prevalence may be as high as 70% among people with developmental disabilities (Bohmer, Taminiau, Klinkenberg-Knol, & Meuwissen, 2001). Sleep problems, which occur in approximately 15% of the general population, occur in 35%–90% of people with developmental disabilities, depending on the etiology of the disability (Robinson & Richdale, 2004).

A number of experiments have shown how problem behaviors are increased by the presence of a particular health condition. O'Reilly (1997) showed that otitis media—a painful inner-ear infection—can increase rates of self-injury to reduce ambient noise; these behaviors ceased once the child was free of otitis media symptoms. Similar experiments have been conducted for allergies, constipation, dysmenorrhea, GERD, and sleep problems, showing a relation between problem behaviors and health conditions (Kennedy & Becker, in press).

These cumulative findings suggest that health conditions are present at a high rate in people with developmental disabilities for a variety of reasons, and that they can contribute to the occurrence of problem behavior. We next discuss how these health conditions can be manifested, how noxious stimulation results, and how these events coalesce to cause cyclical patterns of problem behavior. After this discussion, we provide specific examples of how health conditions, pain, and problem behavior interrelate and suggest a possible mechanism of action.

Health Condition Patterns

Health conditions influencing problem behaviors can occur in a wide variety of forms and can be manifested in a variety of patterns. One means of conceptualizing the temporal pattern of health conditions is to bifurcate them into acute versus chronic conditions. Acute health conditions typically last less than 3 months and resolve when treated. Chronic health conditions are those that are not cured within 3 months of diagnosis and continue to affect an individual over time. Although this is a frequently used classification system for health conditions, it does little to help identify specific patterns that may be linked to behavioral concerns using functional assessment because the classification system is too broad and nonspecific. In particular, chronic health conditions may show a variety of temporal patterns that require a finer grained analysis.

An alternative way of classifying health conditions affecting behavior problems is to assess their cyclicity or variation in symptomatology over time in relation to behavioral issues. Because health conditions often change in their intensity from day to day, such variation can provide the basis for classifying their patterns in relation to problem behavior (Fisher, Piazza, & Roane, 2002). Such cyclicity can occur at *ultradian* (e.g., GERD), *circadian* (e.g., sleep cycles), or *longer time scales* (e.g., dysmenorrhea). This approach allows for a greater temporal resolution to be identified for the health condition and possible relations to problem behavior.

A number of behavioral patterns are suggestive of the influence of health conditions. In the case of ultradian patterns, variations in the health condition can occur within a calendar day, sometimes occurring multiple times. A prototypical example of this is GERD, which is often not present until after a meal. That is, the person is asymptomatic until something is ingested. Shortly after a meal or snack, GERD symptoms appear that can include heartburn (i.e., substernal burning in the chest) and regurgitation of stomach contents. Such symptoms resolve within hours of consuming the meal or snack. But they are likely to reappear anytime a meal or snack is consumed. This means that GERD symptoms can occur and resolve three or more times a day, producing a very distinctive temporal pattern.

Another example of an ultradian health condition is a contact allergy, which occurs when some substance is introduced into or onto the skin. Contact allergies can result from sources such as cosmetics (e.g., lipstick) or insects (e.g., a bee sting). These allergic reactions involve immunological reactions to the foreign antigen that may include skin swelling and pain. Often allergic reactions resolve within hours once the allergen is removed, although symptoms sometimes persist for several days. Because the health condition will appear each time the foreign antigen is introduced onto or into the skin, such contact allergies are implicated in the occurrence of problem behavior.

A second general temporal pattern that emerges in the assessment of health conditions is circadian. Most animate life on earth follows a 24-hour periodicity relating to the light and dark cycles arising from the earth's rotational pattern. Circadian rhythms provide an organizational framework for life systems, and, not surprisingly, health conditions often emerge along a similar time scale. A prototypical example of health concerns related to a circadian pattern is sleep problems. Although sleep problems can take a variety of forms (e.g., sleep apnea, night awakenings, and total sleep deprivation), they all interfere with circadian rhythmicity. Sleep problems that result in sleep loss can cause a range of negative symptoms, including memory disruption, altered immune system response, and changes in pain perception (Hobson & Pace-Schott, 2002).

A final, and more complex, pattern for health conditions occurs over longer time scales such as days, weeks, months, or seasons. An example of a health condition causing pain over several days is constipation, which is a decrease in defecation or changes in stool composition typically occurring over several days. A person may not defecate for several days, with stool being retained and abdominal discomfort increasing during this time. Once the constipation is resolved naturally or via medication, the discomfort resides. Often this cycle repeats itself over time. Another example of a health condition that manifests itself over longer time scales is dysmenorrhea. This condition is associated with pain in the lower abdomen/pelvis beginning with the onset of menstruation (see Uphold & Graham, 2003, for a distinction between dysmenorrhea and premenstrual syndrome). In this instance, if a woman's menstrual cycle occurs every 4 weeks, then dysmenorrhea symptoms will coincide with the onset of menstruation, producing a cyclical health pattern manifested on a monthly basis. Seasonal allergies are an example of a health condition that occurs over a much longer time scale. In many instances, seasonal allergies manifest themselves as nasal discharge, red/itching eyes, and sneezing that may last days or weeks, depending on how long the allergen is present in the environment. However, these symptoms may only occur during a particular season of the year (e.g., spring).

Clearly, health conditions can be manifested over a variety of time scales and produce cyclical patterns unique to a particular health problem. As is illustrated in the next section, these health condition patterns often coincide with increases in problem behavior. Such cyclical increases in problem behavior seem to be influenced by the discomfort associated with the aforementioned health conditions.

Interactions Among Pain, Health Conditions, and Problem Behavior

The analysis of how pain is produced by health conditions and results in changes in problem behavior is an exercise in studying interaction effects. The onset of a health condition produces some type of noxious stimulus for an individual (often with only that person directly aware of its presence). In some cases, this increased noxious condition leads to an increase in the probability of problem behavior. Most interaction analyses of pain, health, and problem behavior in people with developmental disabilities have been necessarily correlational and have typically been conducted with single individuals or small samples. This means that results need to be interpreted with caution because there is the possibility that extraneous variables not identified in the analysis may be associated with changes in behavior. This also means that systematic replication across individuals is important to establish the integrity of such complex functional relations (see Kennedy, 2005).

Most analyses of pain, health conditions, and problem behavior begin by tracking physical indicators of a disease. An example of this comes from the literature on GERD. Our current understanding of the relationship of GERD and problem behavior suggests that the pain produced by esophageal regurgitation of acidic stomach contents plays a role in increased problem behavior. GERD produces an intense discomfort that coincides with increased stomach acidity and the presence of the bacterium *Helicobacter pylori* (Uphold & Graham, 2003). Hence, we have self-report and physiological data that coincide with regard to GERD symptoms and pain. As described previously, the onset of GERD symptomatology coincides with the ingestion of food and drink, events that for most people occur three or more times per day. Therefore, if GERD is suspected of being involved in the increased occurrence of problem behavior, the pattern of behavior is likely to coincide with meals and snacks. Such a set of events should produce a cyclical pattern of increased problem behaviors following mealtimes that resolves in a few hours in the absence of any pharmacological treatment of the GERD symptoms.

Just such a pattern of GERD symptoms and problem behavior was reported by Kennedy and Thompson (2000). In this case, a man with developmental disabilities engaged in increased self-injury following mealtimes that produced GERD symptoms. That is, self-injury did not occur during most of the man's waking day, but following each meal there was a precipitous increase in self-injury that only decreased approximately 2 hours after mealtime. When his GERD was treated with antacids, this pattern of problem behavior following mealtimes was eliminated. Such a pattern has been reported in multiple instances of problem behavior in people with developmental disabilities (Bohmer et al., 1999), increasing the possibility that the pain produced by GERD may be related to cases of self-injury, destructive behavior, and aggression in people with developmental disabilities.

An important limitation of the existing literature on GERD and problem behavior is the level of refinement at which analyses have been conducted. This research to date has demonstrated a relation between the occurrence of problem behavior and the presence of GERD. Research on the operant functions of problem behavior has demonstrated that such behaviors are often exacerbated or maintained by environmental consequences. The functional analysis methodology described previously in the chapter explains how such behavior-environment relations can be determined. It would now seem opportune to examine the operant function of problem behaviors (via functional analysis methodologies) that are associated with GERD symptoms. Such analyses may allow us an understanding of how GERD symptoms interact with operant behavioral processes.

The literature on sleep deprivation and problem behaviors offers a clearer insight into such possible interactions between behavioral mechanisms of action and health conditions. A number of studies have looked at combining analogue functional analyses with an examination of sleep disturbance. This allows for an experimental analysis of the reinforcers maintaining problem behavior, occurrences of sleep deprivation, and changes in the frequency and functions of problematic responses. An example of this comes from O'Reilly (1995), who analyzed the aggression of a man who had comorbid sleep problems. O'Reilly tracked the sleep patterns of the individual and also conducted daily analogue functional analyses to assess the functions the behavior served. On days when the individual had slept 5 or more hours, problem behaviors were infrequent. When the man slept less than 5 hours, problem behaviors occurred frequently, but only as a means to escape demands. No other operant function was affected by the disrupted sleep. This pattern regarding negatively reinforced problem behavior and sleep problems is well replicated in the research literature (Kennedy & Meyer, 1996; O'Reilly & Lancioni, 2000; Piazza & Fisher, 1991).

To date, the findings on sleep disruption and problem behavior suggest that disrupted sleep increases rates of negatively reinforced behavior, but does not increase rates of positively reinforced behavior (cf. Horner, Day, & Day, 1997). Preclinical research on sleep deprivation and operant behavior suggests a similar pattern in nonhuman behavior. When behavior is placed on an operant schedule of negative reinforcement using laboratory paradigms, rates of responding increase following sleep deprivation even though they are nonadaptive in the sense of not avoiding more stimuli (Kennedy, Meyer, Werts, & Cushing, 2000). However, when positively reinforced responding is exposed to sleep deprivation, rates of responding decrease or are unaffected (Kirby & Kennedy, 2003). This pattern may be explained by research showing that sleep deprivation induces hyperalgesia in laboratory paradigms, increasing the noxiousness of stimuli used in avoidance procedures, but not appetitive tasks (May et al., in press). This pain-inducing effect of sleep deprivation may be responsible for the differential effect on reinforced responding observed in applied and laboratory experiments relating to sleep deprivation.

In the case of sleep deprivation, the lack of sleep may serve as a "motivating operation" (Friman & Oliver, in press) to increase the noxiousness of stimuli. It is possible that some stimuli (e.g., task demands) are noxious enough to function as negative reinforcers in the absence of sleep deprivation (i.e., they maintain aggression, destructive behavior, and/or self-injury), but the lack of sleep exacerbates their reinforcing properties. In other cases, stimuli such as task demands may not function as noxious stimuli until the individual is sleep deprived. The sleep deprivation then establishes these events as stimuli to be avoided and increases problem behavior for the duration of the sleepless period.

Another example of this process can be illustrated with dysmenorrhea. As noted previously, dysmenorrhea occurs at the onset of menses and includes symptoms such as lower abdominal and pelvic pain. An illustration of how this health condition can influence problem behavior is provided by Carr, Smith, Giacin, Whelan, and Pancari (2003). In this study, Carr et al. analyzed the problem behavior of women under demand situations prior to and during menses. The authors found that problem behaviors increased when women displayed symptoms of dysmenorrhea during menses, when compared with other times in their menstrual cycle. In some instances, dysmenorrhea was associated with increases in avoidance behavior above already high baseline levels. In other instances, this health condition established demands as a noxious stimulus to be avoided. The data suggest that the discomfort associated with dysmenorrhea established or exacerbated demands as noxious stimuli, thus increasing rates of problem behavior that functioned to enable the women to avoid demands.

The data from research on sleep deprivation and dysmenorrhea, as well as other health conditions such as allergy symptoms and otitis media, suggest that health conditions producing discomfort as a symptom can increase problem behavior. That is, these health conditions can function as motivating operations to alter the value of reinforcers. This conceptualization of the interrelations among pain, health conditions, and problem behavior suggests that health conditions producing physical discomfort can increase the noxiousness of other stimuli, increasing their value as reinforcers. If problem behaviors are effective in reducing these noxious stimuli, then such behaviors are likely to be reinforced and maintained, particularly when the health condition exacerbates the noxiousness of these stimuli.

The literature reviewed presents an emerging and interesting pattern of results. All of the examples we have reviewed from the extant literature relating to pain, health conditions, and problem behavior involve negative reinforcement. Behaviors that produce escape or avoidance of stimuli seem to increase in probability in the presence of a health condition, but behaviors occasioning the onset of stimuli (i.e., positive reinforcement) have not been found to increase in probability, or actually decrease following sleep loss. This pattern, if it continues to be replicated, suggests a mechanism of action that is specific to a particular type of reinforcer process. That is, the discomfort produced by the health condition may serve as a motivating operation increasing the value of negatively reinforced behavior, but not altering (or perhaps decreasing) the value of positively reinforcing stimuli.

This interaction between the behavioral processes of motivating operations (antecedents to behavior) and negative reinforcers (consequences of behavior) suggests a complex interaction between antecedents and consequences of behavior that is influenced by health conditions. When these conditions combine, the result can be increased levels of aggression, destructive behavior, and/or self-injury that would be hard to explain if the effect of the health condition is not factored into the behavioral equation of how events reinforce problem behavior. Such an observation has important implications for assessment and treatment of problem behavior in people with developmental disabilities.

IMPLICATIONS FOR ASSESSMENT AND INTERVENTION

Problem behaviors such as self-injury, aggression, and property destruction are relatively prevalent among people with developmental disabilities, much of this behavior seems to be learned, and there seems to be a relation between health status and the level/intensity of problem behavior. In our analysis, the presence of various health conditions can act as biobehavioral events, making demands (be they social demands or task demands) more aversive and hence increasing the probability of problem behavior that is maintained by escape from such demands.

The first implication for assessment and intervention is that this process should be coordinated between disciplines with expertise in health and learning. Behavior analysts, with expertise in functional assessment and behavioral intervention plans, should be involved. Previously in the chapter, we describe in detail the core components of an analogue functional analysis. This assessment process is geared to identify the environmental contingencies that are maintaining problem behavior. Results from such an assessment can be used to build a behavioral intervention plan to teach the person with developmental disabilities alternative appropriate behaviors, such as those used to escape from aversive situations. To illustrate, the person could be taught to say, "I need a break," or "I need help," to escape a noxious task or make it less aversive (e.g., cleaning his or her room). This new phrase could be used in place of self-injury that previously produced escape from the aversive task for the person. In addition, the person should also receive regular medical evaluations to ensure a healthy disposition. If problem behavior appears to be cyclical, as described previously, then such information should be made available to medical personnel.

A coordinated effort between health professionals and behavior analysts should be able to isolate the relative impact of medical conditions and reinforcement contingencies on problem behavior (see Kennedy & Becker, in press). We suggest that a functional assessment of problem behavior be conducted when the putative health condition is present, as well as absent. This allows therapists to evaluate the contingencies maintaining the problem behavior and the influence of the health condition on this behavior. Interventions with these individuals will usually be multifaceted, targeting the health conditions, teaching communication skills, and redesigning the environment to make demanding activities more pleasurable for the person.

In some instances, the problem behavior may arise only in the presence of the health condition. In this situation, the person may tolerate demanding situations when he or she is healthy, but when sick the situation may be less tolerable, and problem behavior occurs. Such conditions may be treated primarily through medical means. In the example of GERD, problem behavior occurred following meals only and was successfully treated using antacids. If the health condition cannot be eliminated by medical means, then the environment could be arranged to place fewer demands on the person, and the person can be taught alternative communication strategies to seek help or to escape for brief periods from the demanding situation.

In other instances, problem behavior may have been initially precipitated by a health condition, but it may have evolved to be maintained by social reinforcement contingencies. For example, Carr and McDowell (1980) reported on a 10-year-old boy who began scratching himself in response to a skin allergy. Once started, the behavior was shaped by social reinforcement contingencies and acquired an operant function (i.e., positive reinforcement in the form of access to attention). Such problem behaviors require health assessments and treatment but also repeated functional assessments and interventions to identify the evolving nature of such cases.

In still other situations, problem behavior may be present when the person is healthy but may occur at higher levels or intensities when the person is ill. For example, in the study by O'Reilly (1995), the person engaged in aggression to escape from demanding tasks. However, when he suffered from disrupted sleep, his aggression was more severe during demanding tasks. Carr et al. (2003) showed a relation between dysmenorrhea and problem behavior maintained by escape from demanding situations. For one of the four participants in this study, dysmenorrhea and problem behavior co-occurred. In other words, problem behavior only occurred when the dysmenorrheic symptoms were present. However, for the other three participants, problem behavior occurred during nonmenses times. For these three participants, dysmenorrhea seemed to exacerbate problem behavior. This interactive effect of health conditions on learned behavior requires both health and behavioral assessments to identify the appropriate intervention combination. In the study by Carr et al. (2003), dysmenorrhea symptoms were treated using prescription medication for pain, hot water bottles for backache, periods of rest for fatigue, and use of pads in place of tampons. Behavioral interventions consisted of teaching the participants appropriate ways to seek help in completing and to take breaks from tasks, redesigning the structure and presentation of tasks when participants seemed to be in pain, and offering choices between tasks.

CONCLUSION

Problem behaviors such as aggression, property destruction, and self-injury occur in 16% of persons with developmental disabilities and are often refractory to amelioration. Using functional assessment techniques, researchers have demonstrated that many of these behaviors are maintained by positive or negative reinforcement contingencies, or both. That is, problem behaviors come under the control of social contingencies related to the presentation or removal of salient stimuli in the person's environment. However, to complicate this analytical picture, people with developmental disabilities also have a very high incidence of health conditions. Research findings indicate that the presence of health conditions can initiate or exacerbate problem behaviors. Indeed, it may be that many inconclusive functional assessments are not conclusive because the presence of a health condition (and its associated pain) has not been adequately assessed.

Health conditions appear to increase behaviors that are negatively reinforced but may not influence (or may decrease) behaviors that are positively reinforced. This pattern suggests that the pain associated with a variety of health conditions may act as a motivating operation to establish noxious stimuli as negative reinforcers or to increase their aversiveness, thus increasing rates of problem behaviors maintained by these contingencies. These findings suggest that health assessments and functional behavioral assessments should be conducted concurrently when the temporal pattern of problem behavior suggests that a health condition may be a contributing factor. The resulting interventions may then need to target the health condition to alleviate or eliminate the pain associated with it, as well as social reinforcement contingencies that may be maintaining the problem behavior. Therefore, assessment and intervention should be interdisciplinary and multifaceted in nature.

REFERENCES

Allen, K.E., & Harris, F.R. (1966). Elimination of a child's excessive scratching by training the mother in reinforcement procedures. *Behavior Research and Therapy, 4,* 79–84.

Bohmer, C.J., Niezen-de Boer, M.C., Klinkenberg-Knol, E.C., Deville, W.L., Nadorp, J.H., & Meuwissen, S.G. (1999). The prevalence of gastroesophageal reflux disease in institutionalized intellectually disabled individuals. *American Journal of Gastroenterology, 94,* 804–810.

Bohmer, C.J., Taminiau, J.A., Klinkenberg-Knol, E.C., & Meuwissen, S.G. (2001). The prevalence of constipation in institutionalized people with intellectual disabilities. *Journal of Intellectual Disability Research, 45,* 212–218.

Carr, E.G. (1977). The motivation of self-injurious behavior: A review of some hypotheses. *Psychological Bulletin, 84,* 800–816.

Carr, E.G., Levin, L., McConnachie, G., Carlson, J., Kemp, D., & Smith, C. (1998). *Communication-based intervention for problem behavior: A user's guide for producing positive change.* Baltimore: Paul H. Brookes Publishing Co.

Carr, E.G., & McDowell, J.J. (1980). Social control of self-injurious behavior of organic etiology. *Behavior Therapy, 11,* 402–409.

Carr, E.G., & Smith, C.E. (1995). Biological setting events for self-injury. *Mental Retardation and Developmental Disabilities Research Reviews, 1,* 94–98.

Carr, E.G., Smith, C.E., Giacin, T.A., Whelan, B.M., & Pancari, J. (2003). Menstrual discomfort as a biological setting event for severe problem behavior: Assessment and intervention. *American Journal on Mental Retardation, 108,* 117–133.

Chung, M.C., Bickerton, W., Cumella, S., & Winchester, C. (1996). A preliminary study on the prevalence of challenging behaviors. *Psychological Reports, 79,* 1427–1430.

Corte, H.E., Wolf, M.M., & Locke, B.J. (1971). A comparison of procedures for eliminating self-injurious behavior in retarded adolescents. *Journal of Applied Behavior Analysis, 4,* 201–213.

Cunningham, C.E., & Linscheid, T.R. (1976). Elimination of chronic infant rumination by electric shock. *Behavior Therapy, 7,* 231–234.

Dorsey, M.F., Iwata, B.A., Ong, P., & McSween, T.E. (1980). Treatment of self-injurious behavior using a water mist: Initial response suppression and generalization. *Journal of Applied Behavior Analysis, 13,* 343–353.

Einfeld, S., & Tongue, B. (1996). Population prevalence of psychopathology in children and adolescents with intellectual disability: II. Epidemiological findings. *Journal of Intellectual Disability Research, 40,* 99–109.

Emerson, E., Kiernan, C., Alborz, A., Reeves, D., Mason, H., Swarbrick, R., et al. (2001a). The prevalence of challenging behaviors: A total population study. *Research in Developmental Disabilities, 22,* 77–93.

Emerson, E., Kiernan, C., Alborz, A., Reeves, D., Mason, H., Swarbrick, R., et al. (2001b). Predicting the persistence of severe self-injurious behavior. *Research in Developmental Disabilities, 22,* 67–75.

Ferster, C.B., & DeMyer, M.K. (1961). The development of performances in autistic children in an automatically controlled environment. *Journal of Chronic Diseases, 13,* 312–345.

Fisher, W.W., Piazza, C.C., & Roane, H.S. (2002). Sleep and cyclical variables related to self-injurious and other destructive behaviors. In S.R. Schroeder, M.L. Oster-Granite, & T. Thompson (Eds.), *Self-injurious behavior: Gene-brain-behavior relationships* (pp. 205–222). Washington, DC: American Psychological Association.

Friman, P., & Oliver, R. (in press). Clinical implications of motivating events with special emphasis on establishing operations. In J.K. Luiselli (Ed.), *Antecedent intervention: Recent developments in community-focused behavioral support* (2nd ed.). Baltimore: Paul H. Brookes Publishing Co.

Green, V., O'Reilly, M.F., Itchon, J., & Sigafoos, J. (2005). Persistence of early emerging aberrant behavior in children with developmental disabilities. *Research in Developmental Disabilities, 26,* 47–55.

Hanley, G., Iwata, B.A., & McCord, B. (2003). Functional analysis of problem behavior: A review. *Journal of Applied Behavior Analysis, 36,* 147–185.

Hobson, J.A., & Pace-Schott, E.F. (2002). The cognitive neuroscience of sleep: neuronal systems, consciousness and learning. *Nature Reviews: Neuroscience, 3,* 679–693.

Horner, R.H., Day, H.M., & Day, J.R. (1997). Using neutralizing routines to reduce problem behaviors. *Journal of Applied Behavior Analysis, 30,* 601–614.

Iwata, B., Pace, G., Dorsey, M., Zarcone, J., Vollmer, T., Smith, R., et al. (1994). The functions of self-injurious behavior: An experimental-epidemiological analysis. *Journal of Applied Behavior Analysis, 27,* 215–240.

Iwata, B.A., Dorsey, M.F., Slifer, K.J., Bauman, K.E., & Richman, G.S. (1994). Toward a functional analysis of self-injury. *Journal of Applied Behavior Analysis, 27,* 197–209. (Reprinted from *Analysis and Intervention in Developmental Disabilities, 2,* 3–20, 1982).

Kennedy, C.H. (2005). *Single-case designs for educational research.* Boston: Allyn & Bacon.

Kennedy, C.H., & Becker, A. (in press). Health conditions in antecedent assessment and intervention of problem behavior. In J.K. Luiselli (Ed.), *Antecedent intervention: Recent developments in community-focused behavioral support* (2nd ed.). Baltimore: Paul H. Brookes Publishing Co.

Kennedy, C.H., Caruso, M., & Thompson, T. (2001). Experimental analyses of gene–brain–behavior relations: Some notes on their application. *Journal of Applied Behavior Analysis, 34,* 539–549.

Kennedy, C.H., & Meyer, K.A. (1996). Sleep deprivation, allergy symptoms, and negatively reinforced problem behavior. *Journal of Applied Behavior Analysis, 29,* 133–135.

Kennedy, C.H., Meyer, K.A., Werts, M.G., & Cushing, L.S. (2000). Effects of sleep deprivation on free-operant avoidance. *Journal of the Experimental Analysis of Behavior, 73,* 333–345.

Kennedy, C.H., & Thompson, T. (2000). Health conditions contributing to problem behavior among people with mental retardation and developmental disabilities. In M. Wehmeyer & J. Patten (Eds.), *Mental retardation in the 21st century* (pp. 211–231). Austin, TX: PRO-ED.

Kirby, M., & Kennedy, C.H. (2003). Variable-interval reinforcement schedule value influences responding following REM sleep deprivation. *Journal of the Experimental Analysis of Behavior, 80,* 253–260.

Lovaas, O.I., & Simmons, J.Q. (1969). Manipulation of self-destruction in three retarded children. *Journal of Applied Behavior Analysis, 2,* 67–84.

May, M.E., Harvey, M.T., Valdovinos, M., Kline, R.J., Wiley, R.G., & Kennedy, C.H. (in press). Nociceptor and age-specific effects of REM sleep deprivation induced hyperalgesia. *Behavioural Brain Research.*

Michael, J. (1993). Establishing operations. *The Behavior Analyst, 16,* 191–206.

O'Reilly, M.F. (1995). Functional analysis and treatment of escape-maintained aggression correlated with sleep deprivation. *Journal of Applied Behavior Analysis, 28,* 225–226.

O'Reilly, M.F. (1997). Functional analysis of episodic self-injury correlated with recurrent otitis media. *Journal of Applied Behavior Analysis, 30,* 165–167.

O'Reilly, M.F., & Lancioni, G. (2000). Response covariation of escape-maintained aberrant behavior correlated with sleep deprivation. *Research in Developmental Disabilities, 21,* 125–136.

Piazza, C.C., & Fisher, W. (1991). A faded bedtime with response cost protocol for treatment of multiple sleep problems in children. *Journal of Applied Behavior Analysis, 24,* 129–140.

Qureshi, H. (1994). The size of the problem. In E. Emerson, P. McGill, & J. Mansell (Eds)., *Severe learning disabilities and challenging behaviours* (pp. 17–36). London: Chapman & Hall.

Qureshi, H., & Alborz, A. (1992). Epidemiology of challenging behaviour. *Mental Handicap Research, 5,* 130–145.

Risley, T.R. (1968). The effects and side effects of punishing the autistic behaviors of a deviant child. *Journal of Applied Behavior Analysis, 1,* 21–34.

Robinson, A.M., & Richdale, A.L. (2004). Sleep problems in children with intellectual disability: Parental perceptions, sleep problems, and views of treatment effectiveness. *Child Care, Health and Development, 30,* 139–150.

Schroeder, S.R., Schroeder, C.S., Smith, B., & Dalldorf, J. (1978). Prevalence of self-injurious behaviors in a large state facility for the retarded: A three-year follow-up study. *Journal of Autism and Childhood Schizophrenia, 8,* 261–269.

Sigafoos, J., Arthur, M., & O'Reilly, M.F. (2003). *Challenging behavior and developmental disability.* London: Whurr Publishers.

Skinner, B.F. (1938). *Behavior of organisms: An experimental analysis.* New York: Appleton-Century-Crofts.

Tanner, B.A., & Zeiler, M. (1975). Punishment of self-injurious behavior using aromatic ammonia as the aversive stimulus. *Journal of Applied Behavior Analysis, 8,* 53–57.

Tarpley, H.D., & Schroeder, S.R. (1979). Comparison of DRO and DRI on rate of self-injurious behavior. *American Journal of Mental Deficiency, 84,* 188–194.

Uphold, C.R., & Graham, M.V. (2003). *Clinical guidelines in adult health* (3rd ed.). Gainesville, FL: Barmarrae.

Wolf, M.M., Risley, T.R., & Mees, H. (1964). Application of operant conditioning procedures to the behavior problems of an autistic child. *Behaviour Research and Therapy, 1,* 305–312.

World Health Organization. (2000). *The world health report 2000.* Geneva: Author.

Young, J.A., & Wincze, J.P. (1974). The effects of the reinforcement of compatible and incompatible alternative behaviors on the self-injurious and related behaviors of a profoundly retarded female adult. *Behavior Therapy, 5,* 614–623.

III

ASSESSMENT AND TREATMENT ISSUES

9

USING THE WHO'S INTERNATIONAL CLASSIFICATION OF FUNCTIONING, DISABILITY AND HEALTH

A Framework in the Management of Chronic Pain in Children and Youth with Developmental Disabilities

Maureen E. O'Donnell

P ain is an experience common to all children and youth; those with disabilities are not an exception. Pain can be an acute or chronic experience related to disability or may occur as part of everyday life. Children with disabilities may have additional unique pain experiences, such as pain related to a pressure area in a wheelchair, that complicate their clinical picture. The assessment of pain in this complex clinical scenario can be confusing because the relationships between pain and its causative factors are frequently confounded by the underlying neurological disorder or disease, and teasing apart these factors can be challenging.

Efforts to understand pain in individuals with a disability require an evaluation of the functional impact of the pain, its role in the quality of life, and its compounding interaction with the disability itself. Studies of pain typically focus on describing symptoms, duration, and intensity of pain without accounting for the functional consequences of the pain, even though this is likely to have a major impact on the individual. The measurement of functional disability related to adult pain outcomes has received considerable attention because of issues related to work and cost effects; however, analogous research in pediatric populations has to date been limited. To further our understanding of the functional impact of pain in a child with a developmental disability, this chapter introduces the World Health Organization (WHO) International Classification of Functioning, Disability and Health (ICF). As with other clinical scenarios, an approach to assessment and management of pain in children with disabilities is aided through the use of an organizing framework. The ICF, published in 2001, provides a framework and classification system that the WHO describes as providing "a unified and standard language and framework for the description of health and health-related states. It defines components of health and some health-related components of well-being such as education" (WHO, 2001). This chapter provides background information regarding the ICF, an overview of the model, and a discussion of its use as a conceptual framework to assess and manage pain in children with disabilities.

RATIONALE FOR DEVELOPMENT OF THE ICF

Systematic efforts to characterize functional disability associated with various childhood disabilities have been reported (Butler & Campbell, 2000; Nagi, 1991; WHO, 1980), but work characterizing the deleterious impact of pain on child and family functioning has been limited (Palermo, 2000); to date, there has been no work examining the functional impact of pain in children with disabilities. The WHO has been interested in promoting timely and reliable collection of information about the health of populations. This information is seen as vital to creation of public policy. In working to meet this goal, the WHO (1992) created the International Classification of Diseases and Related Health Problems, now in its 10th revision (ICD-10). Over the years, the ICD system of classification has been valuable in reporting causes of death and details regarding morbidity; however, it does not capture the complex, multifaceted information required to adequately describe the overall health status of the population. Missing was information regarding health outcomes, that is, functioning and disability.

To meet this gap, the WHO developed a classification system that they described as a "classification of the consequences of disease": namely, the International Classification of Impairments, Disabilities and Handicaps (ICIDH) (WHO, 1980). The underlying construct of the ICIDH is presented in Figure 9.1. The ICIDH represented a significant step forward. It advanced a new approach, conceptualizing disability as the consequence of underlying health conditions attributable to disease or injury. It also differentiated these consequences at three distinct planes of the human experience: at the level of the body (impairment), the person (disability), and society (handicap).

This system represented a significant paradigm shift. However, there were concerns that the ICIDH was heavily weighted in a medical model, and there was quick recognition that it required revision. People were very concerned about the negative portrayal of disability and about the linear and unidirectional connections among the elements of the ICIDH model (Rosenbaum & Stewart, 2004).

Over the next 10 years, the WHO, in collaboration with governmental and nongovernmental organizations including groups representing people with disabilities, participated in a revision of the ICIDH. After numerous drafts, the new version, the International Classification of Functioning, Disability and Health (ICF), was endorsed in May of 2001. The WHO urged that it be used in research, surveillance, and reporting of health. The new name reflected the move beyond a "consequences of disease" approach and highlighted functioning as a component of health. The WHO's aims in creating this system of classification were to 1) provide a scientific basis for understanding and studying health and health-related states; 2) establish a common language for describing health and health-related states in order to improve communication among different users, such as health care work-

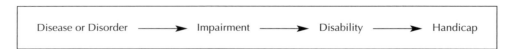

Disease or Disorder ⟶ Impairment ⟶ Disability ⟶ Handicap

Figure 9.1.   The underlying construct of the ICIDH (WHO, 1980; http://who.int). (Please note that WHO does not endorse any products referred to in this publication.)

ers, researchers, and policy makers; 3) permit comparison of data across countries, health care disciplines, services, and time; and 4) provide a systematic coding scheme for health information systems (WHO, 2001).

The ICF belongs to the family of international classifications developed by the WHO. Health conditions (e.g., diseases, disorders, injuries) are classified primarily by the ICD-10, which provides an etiological framework. That is, the ICD-10 describes and classifies a patient's or person's underlying disease condition. Function and disability associated with health conditions or health states are classified by the ICF, making the two classification systems complementary, with the ICF enriching the ICD-10.

The ICF can be used for statistical, research, clinical, social policy, and educational purposes. The approval of this new classification system is a landmark event for medicine and society. With the ICF, patients' functioning, which is described through components of body function and body structures, activity, and participation, became a new central perspective in health care. Patients' functioning is now seen as being associated with, and not merely a consequence of, a health condition. In addition, functioning and health are now seen in relation to health conditions but also in relation to personal and environmental factors (Stucki, Ewert, & Cieza, 2002). This biopsychosocial approach, although not entirely new to rehabilitation and prevention, is now supported by this internationally agreed upon and etiology-neutral framework and a classification on both the individual and population planning level (Cieza et al., 2004) .

CONCEPTUAL FRAMEWORK OF THE ICF

The ICF framework has three major components: 1) "body functions and structures," 2) "activities and participation," and 3) "contextual factors" (made up of "environmental factors" and "personal factors"). Understanding these components and the relationships among them is critical to understanding the ICF. The interactions between the components are shown in Figure 9.2.

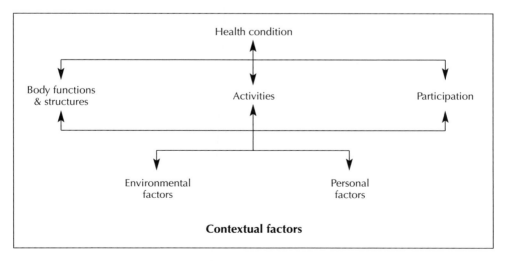

Figure 9.2.   Framework of the ICF (WHO, 2001). (Please note that WHO does not endorse any products referred to in this publication.)

Components of the ICF Framework

Let us consider each of the components in Figure 9.2 as they are defined by the WHO (2001). A *health condition* is an underlying disease or disorder. The health condition usually provides information regarding underlying etiology or pathogenesis. So, for example, Crohn's disease, acquired brain injury, and trisomy 21 might all be examples of health conditions that could cause developmental problems, pain, or both.

Body functions are defined as the physiological functions of body systems (including psychological systems). "Sensation of pain," for example, is considered a specific body function by the ICF. Similarly, muscle tone is an example of body function. *Body structures* are anatomical parts of the body, such as organs, limbs, and their components. "Spinal nerves" is an example of a body structure category within the ICF. Abnormalities of function as well as abnormalities of structure are referred to in the ICF as *impairments,* which are defined as significant deviation or loss of function (e.g., loss of muscle strength, pain, increased tone) or structure (e.g., loss of range of motion of a joint).

Activity is defined by the WHO as the execution of a task by an individual. For the most part, activities can simplistically be thought of as represented by "-ing" verbs, such as reading, communicating with gestures, catching, or driving human-powered transportation, such as a tricycle. *Participation* is defined as involvement in a life situation. This very important component represents social roles, such as the role of being a parent or a sibling, spousal relationships, or taking part in civic or school duties. Difficulties in the activity component are referred to as *activity limitations* (e.g., limitations in walking or buttoning), and problems an individual might experience in the participation component (e.g., restrictions in attending school or scouting and other recreational programs) are called *participation restrictions* by the WHO.

As stated previously, context is a crucially important addition to the ICF. Within the area of contextual factors, *environmental factors* are defined as those factors that make up the physical, social, and attitudinal environment in which people live and conduct their lives. Environmental factors can represent *facilitators* or *barriers.* For example, a curb cut in a sidewalk or an inclusion policy at school are examples of environmental facilitators for children with cerebral palsy who require a wheelchair for transportation. The same curb cut may represent an environmental barrier for a child with visual impairment, who can no longer find the edge of a sidewalk with his or her cane. *Personal factors* are not yet classified well within the ICF system, but the WHO (2001) does provide a brief definition, stating that they "are the particular background of an individual's life and living." These factors include items such as temperament, upbringing, educational experience to date, and character.

Overall, the WHO states that *functioning* is an umbrella term for body functions, body structure, activities, and participation. Functioning denotes the positive aspects of the interaction of an individual (with or without a health condition) with the contextual factors. *Disability* is an umbrella term for impairments of body function or structure, activity limitations, and participation restriction. Disability denotes the negative aspect of the interaction between the individual (with or without a health condition) and his or her contextual factors. It should be noted that, in contrast to the traditional view in which disability resided within the individual person, here disability is a social construct involving interaction of the person, community, and society (Rosenbaum & Stewart, 2004).

Key Differences Between the ICF and Previous Frameworks

What are the key differences between this ICF framework and the impairment, disability, and handicap model of the ICIDH? First, there is interaction between the components and, in contrast to the ICIDH, the relationships between individual components may be bidirectional. This is an acknowledgment of the concept that any aspect of a person's functioning can affect another aspect of functioning. Second, and importantly, contextual factors are added as another component that potentially influences function. This reflects what clinicians have long known: that the functioning of an individual varies, being based not only on the individual's biology, but also on his or her physical, social, and family environment as well as personal factors such as gender and temperament. Third, the language of the ICF is "neutral," meaning it does not have a negative connotation as was the case with the terms "impairment" and "disability" in the ICIDH. Fourth, because of the move to describing the health of all, the system is no longer meant to be used only for those people who have traditionally been thought to have disabilities. In fact, the functioning of every individual, healthy or not, can be described within the ICF framework.

The ICF as a Worldwide Model
for Conceptualizing Relationships Between Components

The ICF provides a very useful conceptual model by which we can consider the many factors and interactions that exist in complex relationships for those with or without an underlying disease. Unlike the ICIDH (see Figure 9.1), in which disease led to impairment, which led to disability, which led to handicap, the ICF (see Figure 9.2) represents bidirectional and complex relationships that are more realistic and like those we see in clinical practice and our own experience. By examining the relationships between the components, and carefully considering each, we may come across strategies for management of health conditions and functional impairments that we had not previously considered. For example, impairments may not lead to activity limitations or participation restrictions if the child's context is changed. Or, activity limitation and participation restrictions may not be linked to an underlying impairment of body function or body structure but rather to an environmental context issue. In addition, this model challenges us to consider the direction of relationships among components. For example, hospitalization of a child—and therefore loss of participation in usual school and home activities—may lead to less opportunity for walking, which could lead to muscle weakness. In this example, there would be links between context and participation limitations that then lead to impairments of body structure—the reverse of the relationships described by the ICIDH, in which the interaction between components was unidirectional. The ICF presents us with a framework that allows us to explore these relationships in the same manner in which others around the globe are exploring these relationships.

The ICF as a Guide to Identify Sources of Influence on Functional States

Bilbao and colleagues (2003) described the ICF as a guide to identify sources of influence on functional states. They stated that the classification system encompasses the different areas of functioning at both the individual and social level as well as incorporating the environmental factors that interact with and have an influence on specific performance in those areas. Arthanat, Nochajski, and Stone (2004) concluded that the ICF has the potential to classify and interpret cognitive impairments on a global level and thereby reflects upon the overall health and functioning of the individual in major life activities.

The ICF as a Communication Instrument

Using a common language about function and using universal codification (by employing the categories and codes that the ICF provides for each of the major components) leads to better understanding and sharing of information. This will lead to improved communication about patient outcomes from treatment and, ultimately, improve services for children and families.

The ICF Beyond the Conceptual

The level of precision offered by the ICF can be enhanced if the categories and coding system are utilized. For each *component* (e.g., the component of "body function") there is a series of *domains*. Example domains of the "body function" component include mental functions, sensory and pain, and voice and speech functions. Similarly, the "activities and participation" component includes domains such as learning and knowledge, mobility, self-care, and interpersonal interactions and relationships. These domains offer more detail to each of the core components.

The ICF then has a series of categories (with codes attached) within each of the domains. Again, the purpose of this detail is to allow precision of definition worldwide. Overall, there are more than 1,400 categories within the ICF system. If the categories are used, especially in conjunction with the coding system for each category, describing a particular clinical and/or life state can be achieved with a great deal of precision.

In the interest of making the 1,400 categories more user friendly in the clinical context, a number of research groups have been working to create what are being called "core sets" for various clinical conditions. For example, two ICF core sets (one brief and one comprehensive) for chronic widespread pain have been developed (Cieza et al., 2004). These sets of categories and codes were developed from a consensus process integrating evidence from preliminary studies including a Delphi exercise, a systematic review, and empirical data collection.

The details of categories and the coding system are beyond the scope of this chapter, which focuses on the framework itself. Readers interested in the names of domains and the categories within each domain are directed to the WHO's publication (2001) which details the categories and codes and their use. The work of Cieza et al. (2004) details the work on the chronic pain core sets to date.

Finally, Australia has been using the ICF as a framework for national data dictionaries (Madden, Choi, & Sykes, 2003). This national effort in data collection may be of interest to some readers who are interested in creating ways to uniformly code function on a provincial, state, or national basis. It remains to be seen how this framework applies to pain and individuals with disabilities.

USES OF THE ICF FOR THE CHILD WITH PAIN AND DISABILITY

The ICF framework is increasingly being used in clinical practice to structure clinical problems (Cieza & Stucki, 2004, Rosenbaum & Stewart, 2004; Steiner et al., 2002; Stucki & Sigi, 2003), particularly in multidisciplinary care and for rehabilitation purposes. The framework will allow those individuals caring for children with pain and their families to use a common approach and a common nomenclature for assessment and treatment of childhood pain in the context of an underlying developmental condition. It is important to note that this approach, however, is equally applicable to all children and adults with or without pain. For the first time in the history of medicine, there is now a universally agreed upon conceptual framework for functioning, disability, and health (Cieza & Stucki, 2004).

Guiding Our Clinical Approach to Assessment and Intervention Planning

Physicians and health professionals can use the ICF framework to identify and document a patient's complaints when taking a patient's history, and to identify and document clinical findings of a clinical examination. This approach may be particularly useful for trainees, who may require structure if they are to have a comprehensive approach to the etiology, impact, and potential treatment of pain that focuses on function and, importantly, participation, as well as the importance of social, physical, and emotional context. The trainee can be directed to consider each of the components (health condition, body structure, body function, activity, participation, and context) in the assessment of pain and in considering what interventions might be helpful for a child and family at the level of each of the components. Many clinics (J. Darrah & R. Adams, personal communication, 2005), even those with experienced clinicians, now keep the figure of the ICF framework (see Figure 9.2) posted in their clinical rooms and team conference rooms. Some have created worksheets rooted in the ICF on which they take their histories, to remind them to consider their assessment and treatment planning in all the ICF domains. This approach has also been described in the literature by Cieza and Stucki (2004), who reported the use of an "ICF Sheet" based on the ICF framework, either on paper or in electronic form, as the most useful way to understand the relationship between selected target problems and impaired body functions, structure, and the psychosocial and environmental factors that exacerbate or help to minimize them (in their case, musculoskeletal/rheumatological problems). They reported that this approach can also improve internal reporting and documentation and can structure multidisciplinary care for the team.

Expanding Our Thinking Beyond "Fixing"

Rosenbaum and Stewart (2004) described what they believe to be the most significant value of the ICF model, its clinical approach. Although they described this with respect to the child with cerebral palsy, their ideas are equally applicable to the child with a developmental condition and pain. They stated that the ICF's importance is in helping us as clinicians to expand our thinking beyond "fixing" primary impairments (e.g., pain or high tone) to a view that places equal value on promoting functional activity and facilitating the child's full participation in all aspects of life. They stated that the ICF enables us to address people's self-determined goals very broadly. Such goals, for example, might include "becoming independently mobile" rather than "walking." This emphasis argues that what people do is more important than the expectation that they do things "normally." Rosenbaum and Stewart suggested that the ICF asks us as clinicians to accept variation and difference rather than use the more traditional approach wherein interventions are based on getting to "normal." Similarly, Yaruss and Quesal (2004) described how using the ICF to address the clinical issue of stuttering allows the clinician to consider the problem and the solution in a broader context.

Looking for Innovative Solutions

The ICF framework, with its interactions, challenges us to consider innovative solutions to a patient's concerns. Historically, clinicians in the rehabilitation and developmental disability setting often have thought of "body structure" solutions to "body structure" concerns. For example, if we were to see a child with cerebral palsy with high tone and pain in the legs, we would often start by examining the lower extremities. We might find contractures and decide that this "body structure" complaint requires a "body structure" solution. However, the ICF facilitates us in taking a broader approach. Instead of prescribing ankle-foot orthoses to provide local stretch, or using botulinum toxin in the gastrocnemius muscle (both of which would be aimed at having a direct effect on body structure), or prescribing pain medication, we might instead consider activity-level and participation-level interventions. Along with the family, we might decide that a recreation program (a participation-level intervention) in which we can ensure that long leg stretches will occur, such as dance or gymnastics, is the solution to the tone and pain issue. This intervention might have a social benefit for the child in addition to achieving a "body structure" goal. The ICF, and the relationships between its components, challenges us to look for such solutions.

Framing Assessment and Outcome Measures

A key function of the ICF classification system for clinicians is its ability to serve as a framework for the use of assessment and outcome measures reflecting the components. With the publication of the ICF taxonomy, reflecting a biopsychosocial approach to disability, an important priority is to examine its promise as a framework for assessment and outcome measures for children (Simeonsson et al., 2003). It is important to note that the ICF itself is not a measure. Rather, it serves as a guide to areas or domains that require measurement. That is, we as clinicians seeing a child with pain and cerebral palsy, for example, can consider the ICF components and the domains within each component that are important to the child and family, and then we must ensure that we are using valid and reliable assessment and outcome measures to tap into those components. Again, the ICF provides a unifying framework for clinical practice, so that the same approach is utilized in countries around the world. Currently, there are limited valid and reliable measures to tap into the participation domain; however, this area is under development.

Counseling and Educating Families

When assisting children and families, one of our tasks is to explain how our therapeutic activities relate to their desired outcomes. An impairment-based approach, focused on body structure and function, suggests to families that by "treating" the body structure we will improve their children's functioning. Although this is implied, it may not always be the case. The ICF model provides an opportunity to talk to parents (and older children) about a different or additional set of goals that focus on function (activity) and social engagement (participation) (Rosenbaum & Stewart, 2004). In this way of thinking, according to Rosenbaum and Stewart, impairment-based interventions may still play an important role in management but the focus widens so that additional perspectives gain currency and can be considered equally valid ways of encouraging children to be functional. This is not meant to diminish the role of interventions aimed at body structures and functions, but rather to expand the horizon and goals of the child and family. This approach, brought forth by the ICF framework, can be used in both outpatient and inpatient settings and by a number of provider disciplines (Kearney & Pryor, 2004; Van Achterberg et al., 2005).

CONCLUSION

The ICF has been developed by the WHO as a framework and mechanism for describing and classifying the health of all people. For the first time in medical history, we have one framework and set of terms that can be used globally. The new common language provided by the ICF enables us in our daily work as clinicians to consider the issues brought forth to us using a biopsychosocial approach that includes interactions of numerous components: body function, body structure, activity, participation, and context. This approach is disease and discipline free, making it particularly useful for multidisciplinary teams but also useful for individual clinicians.

The ICF framework is especially applicable to children with developmental disabilities who have pain. Careful consideration of each of the components with respect to pain, and with respect to the functional goals for the child, makes the framework useful for assessment and for intervention planning. This model enables us to account for multiple compounding and disabling processes, including pain that may occur in a child with a developmental disability. The model illustrates the additive effect of chronic pain on the underlying disability and the role of the context in which the individual lives. Use of this model may enable us to move beyond quantifying the character of pain (frequency, duration, and intensity) and help us to identify the functional consequences of pain, and assess its functional impact in the broader context of the life of an individual with a developmental disability.

As we move forward with the application of this coding and classification system, the ICF may be a useful way of creating common definitions of pain states and its functional consequences. This will allow us to describe clinical issues and the prevalence of conditions across clinical settings and around the world with common data definitions. The clinical and research potential of the ICF for pain in childhood disability is substantial. First steps, however, are to consider it as a guide to frame our clinical approach and to shift our assessments and interventions based on the innovations it produces.

REFERENCES

Arthanat, S., Nochajski, S., & Stone, J. (2004). The International Classification of Functioning, Disability and Health and its application to cognitive disorders. *Disability and Rehabilitation, 26,* 235–245.

Butler, C., & Campbell, S. (2000). Evidence of the effects of intrathecal baclofen for spastic and dystonic cerebral palsy. AACPDM Treatment Outcomes Committee Review Panel. *Developmental Medicine and Child Neurology, 42,* 634–645.

Cieza, A., & Stucki, G. (2004). New approaches to understanding the impact of musculoskeletal conditions. *Clinical Rheumatology, 18,* 141–154.

Cieza, A., Stucki, G., Weigl, M., Kullman, L., Stoll, T., Kamen, L., et al. (2004, July). ICF Core Sets for chronic widespread pain. *Journal of Rehabilitation Medicine, Supplement 44,* 63–68.

Kearney, P., & Pryor, J. (2004). The International Classification of Functioning, Disability and Health (ICF) and nursing. *Journal of Advanced Nursing, 46,* 162–170.

Madden, R., Choi, C., & Sykes, C. (2003). The ICF as a framework for national data: The introduction of ICF into Australian data dictionaries. *Disability and Rehabilitation, 25,* 676–682.

Nagi, S. (1991). Concepts revisited: Implications for prevention. In A. Pope & A. Taylor (Eds.), *Disability in America: Toward a national agenda for prevention* (pp. 309–327). Washington, DC: National Academy Press.

Rosenbaum, P., & Stewart, D. (2004). The World Health Organization International Classification of Functioning, Disability and Health: A model to guide clinical thinking, practice and research in the field of cerebral palsy. *Seminars in Pediatric Neurology, 11,* 5–10.

Simeonsson, R., Leonard, M., Lollar, D., Bjorck-Akesson, E., Hellenweger, J., & Martinuzzi, A. (2003). Applying the International Classification of Functioning, Disability and Health (ICF) to measure childhood disability. *Disability and Rehabilitation, 25,* 602–610.

Steiner, W.A., Ryser, L., Huber, E., Uebelhart, D., Aeschlimann, A., & Stucki, G. (2002). Use of the ICF model as a clinical problem-solving tool in physical therapy and rehabilitation medicine. *Physical Therapy, 82,* 1098–1107.

Stucki, G., & Sigi, T. (2003). Assessment of the impact of disease on the individual. *Best Practice and Research: Clinical Rheumatology, 17,* 451–473.

Stucki, G., Ewert, T., & Cieza, A. (2002). Value and application of the ICF in rehabilitation medicine. *Disability Rehabiliation, 24,* 932–938.

Van Achterberg, T., Hlleman, G., Heijnen-Kaales, Y., Van der Brug, Y., Roodbol, G., Stallinga, H., et al. (2005). Using a multidisciplinary classification in nursing: The International Classification of Functioning, Disability and Health. *Journal of Advanced Nursing, 49,* 432–441.

World Health Organization. (1992). *ICD-10: International statistical classification of diseases and related health problems* (10th ed.). Geneva: Author.

World Health Organization. (1980). *ICIDH: International classification of impairments, disabilities and handicaps: A manual of classification relating to the consequences of disease.* Geneva: Author.

World Health Organization. (2001). *International classification of functioning, disability and health.* Geneva: Author.

Yaruss, J., & Quesal, R. (2004). Stuttering and the International Classification of Functioning, Disability and Health (ICF): An update. *Journal of Communication Disorders, 37,* 35–52.

10

ASSESSING PEDIATRIC PAIN AND DEVELOPMENTAL DISABILITIES

Lynn M. Breau, Patrick J. McGrath, and Marc Zabalia

Most research specifically addressing the pain of children with cognitive impairments has emerged since the 1990s. This group has been included in few studies of pain in children in the general population because most of these studies incorporate some aspect of self-report, which is not always available from this group, or because it is assumed that their pain experience or response will differ from that of typically developing children. They are also typically excluded from studies of specific painful conditions because they often have several medical conditions that may complicate assessment or management of pain or both. Children with cognitive impairments form a heterogeneous group. Those with mild intellectual impairments may have no visible physical impairments and can communicate verbally. In contrast, those with the most severe intellectual impairments frequently have severe physical limitations and may neither speak nor understand spoken language to any practical extent. Children with cognitive impairments are more likely to be blind or deaf, and many display autistic behaviors. This has led some to believe that their pain behavior is erratic and cannot be used to reliably judge their pain. However, this also means that pain assessment tools developed for typically developing children may not be suitable for this group.

The exclusion of this group from most research into pediatric pain has serious implications; they are particularly susceptible to pain resulting from their physical disabilities or medical problems associated with those disabilities (Ehde et al., 2003; Konstantareas & Homatidis, 1987; Nordin & Gillberg, 1996), from treatments for those problems (Hadden & von Baeyer, 2002), or from reduced detection or management of typical health problems (Allison & Lawrence, 2004; Hennequin, Faulks, & Roux, 2000). They may also be at greater risk for accidental injury (Leland, Garrard, & Smith, 1994), especially among those who are mobile (Breau, Camfield, McGrath, & Finley, 2004). Their injuries may also be more severe and may result in more long-term care needs than those of typically developing children (Braden, Swanson, & Di Scala, 2003).

Children with cognitive impairments may also have pain for a longer period because of difficulties in detecting their pain, and, in some groups, this can have fatal effects (Jancar & Speller, 1994). The complexity of their multiple medical conditions may also make it more difficult to manage pain well, even when it is detected. In summary, there is mounting evidence that pain presents a greater problem for children with cognitive impairments than for typically developing children, and this is occurring within a population that is growing as advancements in medical technology have increased survival rates and life span (Lorenz, Wooliever, Jetton, & Paneth, 1998).

A study aimed at documenting the nature and incidence of the children's pain suggests that the pain experienced by this group is not trivial (Breau, Camfield, McGrath, & Finley, 2003). These authors reported that pain resulting from minor accidental injuries had an average rating of 4 on a 0–10 scale of pain intensity completed by caregivers, and more common types of pain, resulting from chronic conditions such as gastrointestinal disorders, musculoskeletal problems, or illnesses, was rated on average at 6.1 of 10. Given that a score of 30 of 100 is considered clinically significant (equivalent to 3 of 10 in this study), and a level at which many parents give medication (Finley, McGrath, Forward, McNeill, & Fitzgerald, 1996), it is obvious that children with cognitive impairments are frequently suffering from clinically significant pain.

Despite increasing evidence that pain is a significant problem for this group, and the emergence of measures to assess their pain, there remains controversy over whether their pain experience differs from that of typically developing children, with some suggesting that problems in pain assessment are due to the fact that individuals with cognitive impairments do not display pain behavior because they are insensitive to pain (pain insensitivity) or may not interpret what they feel as negative (pain indifference) (Biersdorff, 1991, 1994; Lu, 1981). However, studies using validated measures suggest that children with cognitive impairments may show more pain behavior (Nader, Oberlander, Chambers, & Craig, 2004). In addition, adults with cognitive impairments may have more difficulty with localizing pain specifically (Hennequin, Morin, & Feine, 2000) and may respond to pain more slowly (Defrin, Pick, Peretz, & Carmeli, 2004), but their sensitivity to pain (Defrin et al., 2004) and reaction to pain (Porter et al., 1996) may be greater.

PAIN ASSESSMENT

Against this backdrop of difficulties with pain detection and management, and questions about the actual experience of pain in individuals with cognitive impairments, a small literature has slowly laid the groundwork for better pain assessment in this vulnerable group of children. The following sections describe the emergence of this literature about pain assessment in children with children with developmental disabilities and associated cognitive impairments.

First Reports of Observable Pain Response

In 1965, Reynell published the first study that documented the pain response of children with cognitive impairments as part of a study following children with cerebral palsy after surgery. No relationship was found between children's pain-related behavior and their level of intellectual functioning. This was the first evidence that children with multiple disabilities do display a pain response that can be observed and quantified. A series of papers describing case reports followed over the next two decades (Collignon, Giusiano, Porsmoguer, Jimeno, & Combe, 1995; Collignon, Porsmoguer, Behar, Combe, & Perrin, 1992; Mette & Abittan, 1988). Most often they described distinct behaviors that led professionals to investigate the possibility of pain.

Finding Common Pain Behaviors

Only in 1995, 30 years after Reynell's original study (Reynell, 1965), did the next study appear that attempted to quantify observable pain behavior in individuals with cognitive impairment (Giusiano, Jimeno, Collignon, & Chau, 1995). This group developed a list of behaviors based on observations during a physical examination of 100 residents, ages 2–33 years, in a long-term care facility. All were nonverbal, and 70% were described as having a "chronic vegetative state." This groundbreaking study provided the first evidence of common pain behaviors in this population. One difficulty with the results, however, was that the items generated were based on change from "usual" behavior, making the tool difficult to use for people not familiar with an individual.

The same year, Hunt and Burne (1995) reported on parents' perceptions of the pain behaviors of 120 people ages 1–25 years with static or progressive encephalopathies. The most common signs of pain included postural and physiological changes, crying, and facial expression. The majority of parents also reported that their child's mood changed with pain.

The following year, Fanurik, Koh, Harrison, and Conrad (1996) reported a study of 66 children with cognitive impairments. In this study, 41% of children had severe cognitive impairments, but 48% did have verbal skills. Parents' descriptions of their child's reaction to a previous needle stick included verbalization, localization of the painful area, cry, behavioral or emotional changes, facial expression, body movement, and self-abusive behavior. Unfortunately, the retrospective nature of the study limits conclusions.

This group later interviewed a set of parents regarding their children's pain experience, expression, and treatment (Fanurik, Koh, Schmitz, Harrison, & Conrad, 1999). Parents' descriptions of how their child displays pain varied with the level of their child's cognitive impairment. For example, 57% of parents of children with mild or moderate impairments said that their child made direct verbal statements about pain, but only 7% of parents of children with severe to profound cognitive impairments reported this. Many parents also thought that their child's pain was underestimated or undertreated by health care professionals (Fanurik, Koh, Schmitz, Harrison, & Conrad, 1999). Twenty-nine percent believed their child's pain was treated differently because of the child's cognitive impairments.

Investigating Physiological Pain Response

Another avenue investigated has been the possibility that there may be physiological responses to pain that could be used to detect pain, especially in children with cognitive impairments who have very limited or no verbal ability. In one study, response to pain in eight adolescents with spastic quadriplegia (Oberlander, Gilbert, Chambers, O'Donnell, & Craig, 1999) was evaluated as they received both a mock and a real injection in random order. No significant increase in heart rate was found during the injection, nor did facial action increase. Although these results suggest that physiological measures may not be sensitive to pain for children with altered neurological systems, the sample size was small, making it possible that there was insufficient statistical power.

Research with adults with similar impairments also suggests that Oberlander et al.'s (1999) results may reflect not pain insensitivity but, rather, a lack of physiological reactivity to pain. One study found relatively lower heart rate and blood pressure response to a cold pressor test as well as a hand-grip test in individuals with cognitive impairments than in typically developing controls (Fernhall & Otterstetter, 2003). The authors suggested that this reflects a general decreased sympathetic modulation in this population. A similar attenuation of autonomic response to pain was found by another group when they investigated the pain response of adults with Alzheimer's disease (Rainero, Vighetti, Bergamasco, Pinessi, & Benedetti, 2000). In a subsequent study, they found that pain sensation was unrelated to brain electrical activity or cognitive status, whereas heart rate increase in response to pain was related to delta and theta frequencies of brain activity (Benedetti et al., 2004). They concluded that pain sensation is not altered by cognitive status, whereas autonomic status is. Porter et al. (1996) reported a similar blunting of heart rate increase in response to venipuncture in a sample of older adults with Alzheimer's disease. Again, in their sample, behavioral response to pain was not diminished.

In summary, the bulk of research to date suggests that physiological response to pain in individuals with cognitive impairments may be reduced or qualitatively different relative to that in other groups. However, this appears to reflect differences in the mounting of response to pain, rather than a decrease in pain sensation. This idea that there may be a disconnect between pain sensation and pain response in some individuals with cognitive impairments is supported by adults in which the threshold for heat pain was increased relative to controls if a measure that depended on response time was used. In contrast, when a measure of threshold that was independent of response time was used, those individuals with cognitive impairments displayed reduced conduction velocity and reaction time, but lower pain thresholds (Defrin et al., 2004).

Thus, at this time, physiological responses to pain do not appear promising as a method of clinical pain assessment. It appears that those individuals with cognitive impairments may have altered responses to many external stimuli, and that this reflects differences in physiological response but not pain perception. Given the heterogeneity of this population, it may be some time before we have an indication of whether reliable physiological responses can be used to detect or measure pain.

Research of Pain Assessment Tools
Designed for Typically Developing Children

Measures of Facial Reaction to Pain

Facial expression has also been explored as a key to pain assessment in children with cognitive impairments. Research suggests that typically developing children display a facial response to pain (Breau, McGrath, et al., 2001). Oberlander et al. (1999) were the first to explore this possibility, in their previously described study of adolescents. However, they found no increase in facial activity in response to pain using the Child Facial Coding System (Chambers, Cassidy, McGrath, Gilbert, & Craig, 1996). This may reflect their methodology. They chose to analyze only facial action occurrence, through summing the occurrence of all actions over each period of time examined. Research suggests that the intensity of facial action carries important information regarding pain, and inclusion of this parameter may have altered the results (Breau, McGrath, et al., 2001).

Other studies have found facial responses to pain in groups with cognitive impairments. Porter et al. (1996) reported that the older adults with Alzheimer's disease in their study displayed a greater, but less easily classified, facial response to pain than did those without cognitive impairments. Similarly Nader et al. (2004) found increased facial activity in children with autism relative to controls, when they were observed during venipuncture. Mercer and Glenn (2004) also studied facial response in infants with and without developmental delays. They found that facial response was not diminished, but was more diffuse in the infants with impairments.

Overall, this small literature suggests that facial activity may have merit as a method of pain assessment for children with cognitive impairments. However, there is clearly a great deal of work to be done in this area before clinical use is feasible. Those children with impairments may not show the same pattern of facial response as typically developing children, necessitating the development of new coding schemes for deciding which pattern does reflect pain. Most current systems are also time consuming and coded from film, making bedside application impractical at this time.

Multidimensional Pain Assessment Tools

Several studies have examined the validity of multidimensional pain tools designed for typically developing children when used with those who have cognitive impairments. Voepel-Lewis, Merkel, Tait, Trzcinka, and Malviya (2002) investigated the validity of nurses' scores for 79 children on the Face, Legs, Activity, Cry, Consolability (FLACC) scale for postoperative pain in children with cognitive impairments. Parents also provided estimates of their child's pain using a visual analogue scale (VAS) of pain ranging from 0 to 10. Correlations between FLACC scores and parent VAS ratings ranged from .52 to .65, although parent ratings appeared to be higher. FLACC scores decreased significantly with administration of analgesia. However, children with mild pain who were not administered analgesics were omitted from these analyses. Thus, caution must be taken in interpreting this finding because it can only speak to reductions in scores for children with moderate to severe pain. Likewise, the authors reported that agreement between observers was not as good for moderate pain as for mild or severe pain. This suggests that observers were able to use the scale to distinguish very low versus very high pain, but may have had more difficulty when pain was at neither extreme.

Soetenga, Pellino, and Frank (1999) used the University of Wisconsin Children's Hospital Pain Scale and the Wong-Baker Faces Scale (Wong & Baker, 1988) with 74 children admitted to the hospital, 15 of whom were older than age 3 but nonverbal (Soetenga, 1999). The University of Wisconsin Children's Hospital Pain Scale contains four subscales: Vocal, Facial, Behavior, and Body Movement. The correlation between the two scales was .53 for parents and .89 for nurses. Scores were significantly lower after analgesic administration, and interrater reliability was excellent. Unfortunately, the authors did not report subgroup analyses for the nonverbal children in the sample, so it is difficult to conclude whether the psychometrics presented would be similar had the scores for the subgroup been examined separately.

Solodiuk and Curley (2003) suggested the use of an individualized VAS for children with severe cognitive impairments. A caregiver is asked to provide descriptors for the 0 and 10 anchors and for points between. The authors reported that this method has worked well clinically but have not yet reported data on the validity or reliability of this adaptation of a tool commonly used by typically developing children.

Overall, there is not convincing evidence that the tools described here are satisfactory for children with cognitive impairments. Although further research may provide additional evidence to support their use clinically, they are not recommended at this time.

The Emergence of Multidimensional Pain Tools Specifically Constructed for Children with Cognitive Impairments

Since the first attempt by Giusiano et al. (1995) to determine a common set of pain behaviors in individuals with severe cognitive impairments living in residential facilities, several groups have developed multidimensional pain assessment tools specifically for children with cognitive impairments. Although there is some overlap between these tools, each also has its unique characteristics, and some have focused on broader populations (e.g., children and adults), while others have primarily looked at a specific subgroup (e.g., individuals living in residential facilities) or situation (e.g., postoperative pain). Table 10.1 depicts the items contained in three of these tools, which gives a sense of the similarities.

Echelle Douleur Enfant San Salvadour

Since their first study published in English (Giusiano et al., 1995), Collignon and Giusiano and their group have continued their development of the Echelle Douleur Enfant San Salvadour (DESS). In a second study published in English, they reported refinement of the scale (Collignon & Giusiano, 2001). After reducing the number of items to 10, they reported that a score of 2 indicates attention should be paid to the child, because pain is possible, and a score of 6 on their scale indicates definite pain that requires treatment. Two problems exist with the items of this scale. First, there is overlap between items. For example, the addition of crying or jerking to some behaviors (e.g., protection of painful areas) increases scores for that item. However, because crying and jerking are also included as specific scorable items, this means that scores for the items are not independent, undermining assumptions for statistical analyses. Second, an item that involves the individual seeking a comfortable position also includes the possibility that the nurse placed the person in that position. Thus, the judgment of the nurse becomes incorporated in behavior ratings. Unfortunately, the DESS is also designed so that items are rated in relation to the individual's typical behavior. This may be possible, or even preferred, in situations in which an adult familiar with the individual is assessing pain, such as in the home setting or in large, long-term residential centers. However, this format is not appropriate in other situations, such as in emergency situations or in the hospital, where staff may frequently change. Using change from typical behavior also means that scores cannot be used across situations (e.g., home versus school/hospital) because children's usual behavior may differ across these settings. Finally, validation of the DESS was conducted in French. Caution should be taken in using the DESS cutoff values if one is using an English version of the scale until systematic translation and validation in English are completed, because cultural and language differences can affect both pain behavior and our perception of pain behavior.

Table 10.1. Items from three observational tools that provide clinical cut-off scores for pain

NCCPC-R	PPP	DESS
Moaning, whining, whimpering (fairly soft)	Cries/moans/groans/screams or whimpers	Moaning or inaudible cries (cries with manipulation or spontaneously, in an irregular or continuous way)
Crying (cries with or without tears)		
Screaming/yelling (very loud)		Crying (moderately loud)
A specific sound or word for pain (for example: a word, cry, or type of laugh)		
Eating less, not interested in food	Is reluctant to eat/difficult to feed	
Increase in sleep	Has disturbed sleep	
Decrease in sleep		
Not cooperating, cranky, irritable, unhappy	1. Is cheerful (reverse scored) 2. Is hard to console or comfort	Ability to communicate with the nurse (by searching, expressions or babbles, spontaneously or when being solicited)
Less interaction with others, withdrawn	1. Is sociable or responsive (reverse scored) 2. Appears withdrawn or depressed	Spontaneous interest for the surroundings (negatively rated)
Seeking comfort or physical closeness		
Being difficult to distract, not able to satisfy or pacify		
A furrowed brow	Frowns/has furrowed brow/ looks worried	
A change in eyes, including squinching of eyes, opening eyes wide, frowning eyes	1. Grimaces/screws up face/ screws up eyes 2. Looks frightened (with eyes wide open)	Painful expression (face shows pain; a paradoxical laugh can correspond to a painful rictus)
Turning down of mouth, not smiling		
Lips puckering up, tight, pouting or quivering		
Clenching or grinding teeth, chewing or thrusting tongue out	Grinds teeth or makes mouthing movements	
Not moving, less active, quiet		
Jumping around, agitated, fidgety	1. Is restless/agitated or distressed 2. Has involuntary or stereotypical movements/ is jumpy/startles or has seizures	Increase in spontaneous movement (voluntary motricity or not, coordinated or not, choreoathetotic movements of limbs or head)
Floppy		
Stiff, spastic, tense, rigid	Tenses/stiffens or spasms	Aggravation of tonic troubles (increase in stiffness, tremulations, hypertonic spasms)
Gesturing to or touching part of the body that hurts	Tends to touch or rub particular areas	
Protecting, favoring or guarding part of the body that hurts	Resists being moved	Protection of painful areas (protects the area supposed painful with his/her hand in order to avoid contact)

(continued)

Table 10.1. *(continued)*

NCCPC-R	PPP	DESS
Flinching or moving the body part away, being sensitive to touch	Pulls away or flinches when touched	Coordinated defensive reaction or equivalent on examination of an area supposed painful (grazing, touching, or mobilization induces a coordinated bodily reaction or equivalent that we can interpret as a defensive reaction)
Moving the body in specific way to show pain (e.g., head back, arms down, curls up)	1. Flexes inward or draws legs up towards chest 2. Twists and turns/tosses head/writhes or arches back	Spontaneous analgesic position (search for an unusual position that calms or placed in analgesic position by nurse)
Shivering Change in color, pallor Sweating, perspiring Tears Sharp intake of breath, gasping Breath holding		
	Self harms, (e.g., biting self or banging head)	

The Non-Communicating Children's Pain Checklist

McGrath and his group initiated a program to develop an observational pain tool specifically for children with severe impairments in the mid-1990s (Breau, McGrath, Camfield, Rosmus, & Finley, 2000). Items were generated through semistructured interviews with the primary caregivers of 20 individuals ages 6–29 years (McGrath, Rosmus, Camfield, Campbell, & Hennigar, 1998). Thirty-one behaviors were extracted and grouped into seven subscales (Vocal, Eating/Sleeping, Social/Personality, Facial Expression, Activity, Body & Limbs, and Physiological). Although specific behaviors varied among individuals, all individuals displayed some behavior from each subscale.

In a subsequent study, this new pain measure, the Non-Communicating Children's Pain Checklist (NCCPC), was validated in a home setting (Breau et al., 2000). One item was dropped because of low endorsement, leaving 30 items that were rated as present or absent. Thirty-three caregivers indicated whether each item was present for four observations, two in which pain was present, one in which the individual with cognitive impairments was distressed but had no pain, and one calm period. An important aspect of this study was that the pain events observed by the caregivers were heterogeneous, including both acute pain, such as bee stings, minor burns, falls, and intravenous line insertions, and longer term pain, such as severe burns, throat/urinary tract/sinus infections, and postoperative pain. The results indicated that scores were consistent over the two pain events, despite the differing causes of pain in most cases. Scores during calm were also significantly lower, suggesting that the tool was sensitive to pain.

In a second study, information was collected from caregivers about their children's typical pain behavior in order to predict behavior during a subsequent pain event (Breau, Camfield, McGrath, Rosmus, & Finley, 2001). A core set of NCCPC items that were reported as "typical" by caregivers had significant odds of appearing during subsequent pain episodes. The seven items were "not co-operating, cranky, irritable, unhappy"; "seeking comfort"; "change in eyes"; "less active"; "gestures to part that hurts"; tears"; and "sharp intake of breath." A multiple correlation (R) of .70 indicated that the seven items also played a significant role in predicting pain intensity, and a nonsignificant R of .31 indicated that they played a significant role in predicting distress, suggested that the items were specific to pain. A replication, in which 63 new caregivers' ratings of these seven items were used to predict the presence of pain, provided additional evidence that these behaviors are particularly consistent. The presence of the seven NCCPC items during the subsequent episode correctly identified the presence of pain in 69% of cases and its absence in 95% of cases.

A third study of the NCCPC investigated its use for postoperative pain (Breau, Finley, McGrath, & Camfield, 2002). Items from the Eating/Sleeping subscale were excluded and more detailed responses from observers were added, such that they now provided ratings to indicate whether each item was observed "not at all," just a little," "fairly often," or "very often" during 10-minute pre- and postoperative observations of 24 children. Caregivers' and researchers' total scores were significantly higher after surgery. The correlation between caregiver and researcher NCCPC–Postoperative Version (NCCPC-PV) scores was .72, indicating good interrater reliability. A score of 11 was found to be best for detecting moderate to severe pain. The equivalent 100-mm VAS ratings for children with mild pain were 12.0 (SD = 11) and for moderate to severe pain, 53.5 (SD = 17).

The NCCPC-R was also reexamined in a home setting with a larger sample than in the early studies. This 30-item version also incorporated the rating system developed for the postoperative version (not at all, just a little, fairly often, very often). Seventy-one caregivers completed the NCCPC–Revised (NCCPC-R) for 2-hour observations of their child at home. Scores for children who experienced pain during the observations were compared to scores for children who did not have pain. Pain in this group was due to a wide variety of causes, including falls, self-injury, gastroesophageal reflux, constipation, and surgery. Fifty-two caregivers also completed the NCCPC-R for a second episode of pain to assess consistency in scores across pain episodes. Scores during pain for the two pain episodes differed significantly from scores when pain was absent. A total score of 7 had very good sensitivity (84%) and good specificity (65%–77%) for detecting any pain. The results also indicated that total NCCPC-R scores were consistent across the two episodes of pain, as were the number of items children displayed. The number of items displayed was consistent with that reported in the first study (Breau et al., 2000), indicating good consistency across samples. Because of concerns that children display pain erratically, further analyses of children's individual consistency in scores was conducted. These indicated that 93% of the 55 children who were observed during two episodes of pain had scores during their second observed episode of pain that fell within the 95% confidence intervals of the scores they received for their first episode of pain (Breau, McGrath, et al, 2002).

The NCCPC and NCCPC-R were specifically designed for children who had very limited verbal abilities because of their cognitive impairments. However, Hadden and von Baeyer (2002) have also used the NCCPC-R with children with cerebral palsy and varying levels of verbal abilities. Parents identified items from the checklist that occurred when their child had pain. The reported presence of 24 items from the NCCPC-R did not vary with the children's communication ability. However, caregivers of children who could not communicate verbally reported a greater frequency of several items, including "decreased sleep"; "jumping around, agitated, fidgety"; "stiff, spastic, tense, rigid"; and "lips pucker up tight, pout, quiver." In contrast, caregivers of children who could communicate verbally reported a greater frequency of the items "gestures to or touches part of the body that hurts" and "protects or favors part of body that hurts." Thus, it appears that the children displayed different patterns of items, but achieved similar total scores, when parents used the tool retrospectively.

In another study, Hadden and Von Baeyer (2001) investigated the scores of 129 children with cerebral palsy, with a wide range of verbal abilities, during home physiotherapy exercises that were expected to cause pain. Although children's facial expression did not change significantly during active stretching, scores on the NCCPC-PV were significantly higher. Thus, there is some evidence that the various NCCPC versions may be valid for higher functioning children with physical impairments. However, further research is needed to examine possible differences in sensitivity and specificity for higher functioning groups before clinical use with these groups is recommended.

Breau, Camfield, Symons, et al. (2003) also examined whether the NCCPC-R is valid for children who display self-injurious behavior. This is a concern because there is a greater belief that these children may be insensitive to pain (Gillberg, Terenius, & Lonnerholm, 1985; Sandman, Barron, Chicz-DeMet, & DeMet, 1990) or may display pain differently. There were no significant differences in NCCPC-R total scores for observed episodes of pain in 101 children with ($n = 44$) and without ($n = 57$) self-injury. In fact, children who self-injured received nonsignificantly higher total NCCPC-R scores and higher scores on the Vocal and Social/Personality subscales. The results also suggested that children who had chronic pain might show a different pattern of self-injury, suggesting that self-injurious behavior might be a reaction to pain in some children, rather than evidence of insensitivity to pain.

Nader et al. (2004) also used the NCCPC-R in their study of venipuncture pain in children with autism. In this case, parents were asked to complete the NCCPC-R retrospectively for a past pain event. Unexpectedly, scores for the past event were negatively correlated with facial response to pain during the venipuncture, as well as ratings of distress using the Observational Scale of Behavioral Distress (Jay, Ozolins, Elliott, & Caldwell, 1983). Nader et al. suggested that this finding may reflect the inappropriateness of the two measures of venipuncture pain, or the fact that children with autism may display very different behaviors in strange or new situations. Given the mixed results described previously regarding the facial display of pain in several samples of children with cognitive impairments, the former explanation may be valid. However, it is also possible that the children reacted atypically during this event, especially since they were restrained through bundling with a blanket by adults with whom they were not familiar. This may have resulted in a great deal of distress, distracting them from the actual pain caused by venipuncture. Thus, it may be that the behaviors observed were more specific to distress than pain.

At this time, eight studies have included one of the NCCPC versions, with five studies specifically examining the psychometrics of the two tools for everyday pain and for postoperative or acute pain (NCCPC-R and NCCPC-PV, respectively).

The data supporting the validity and reliability of the tools look promising, and cutoff scores have been developed, making the two useful clinically. One problem with the validation of the NCCPC-R is that it was conducted with 2-hour observations, which are impractical in a hospital setting. We have recommended that caregivers use the NCCPC-PV and 10-minute observations if observation periods of 2 hours are not feasible. As with all pain assessment tools, however, repeated evidence is required with different samples and in different situations to provide cumulative support for clinical use. Currently, evaluations of several translations of the NCCPC-R and NCCPC-PV are underway (French, Swedish, and German), and these will provide additional information regarding the situations and populations for which these tools are valid. Research examining the validity of the NCCPC-R and NCCPC-PV with subgroups of children, such as those with Batten disease, are also planned.

The Pain Indicator for Communicatively Impaired Children

Stallard et al. (2002) developed the Pain Indicator for Communicatively Impaired Children (PICIC). Numerical (0–5) pain ratings of their children made by 49 caregivers were predicted using ratings provided by parents of six different pain cues, rated as occurring "not at all," "a little," "often," or "all the time," as well as individual pain cues identified by caregivers. Five of the six cues proposed by Stallard's group achieved 67% sensitivity, three of the cues were associated with ratings of pain severity on a 1–5 scale, and 20 additional pain cues were identified by caregivers.

Unfortunately, cutoff scores have not yet been developed for this scale, and interrater reliability was not assessed in the study. The authors also did not provide information about the time frame of the observations upon which the parents based their ratings. However, the scale is short, making it quick to use. Further studies should provide additional information regarding its psychometric properties.

The Paediatric Pain Profile

The Paediatric Pain Profile was developed through interviews with 21 caregivers of children with cognitive impairments (Hunt, Mastroyannopoulou, Goldman, & Seers, 2003). From an original pool of 56 items, a set of 20 was selected for the final version. Items are rated as occurring "not at all," "a little," "quite a lot," or "a great deal." The scale was then examined in a subsequent study (Hunt et al., 2004). When asked retrospectively, parents' ratings of their child on the scale were significantly higher with respect to a typical pain the child had than when the child was "at their best," and they correlated with parents' VAS pain ratings for that typical pain. Simultaneous ratings by 54 parents and another observer familiar with the child in the home indicated that interrater reliability was good (.73). Forty-one parents also provided ratings for their child prior to and after administration of a short-acting analgesic in the home. Scores were significantly lower after analgesics were given. Finally, scores were examined in 30 children having gastrointestinal or orthopedic surgery. However, scores did not decline from the first to the fifth postoperative day.

This set of studies provides some preliminary evidence of the validity and reliability of the Paediatric Pain Profile. Although the interrater reliability appears good, it was based on ratings from two adults familiar with the child. Further research is needed to determine if the Paediatric Pain Profile displays similar reliability and validity when used by professionals who do not know the children being rated well. Similarly, although a cutoff score is provided, it was developed through averaging the pain ratings of two observers familiar with the child, something that would not be available in most clinical settings. Furthermore, 96 pairs of ratings were used to develop the cutoff scores, but it appears that only 54 of these were conducted simultaneously, and the time frame of the observations is unclear. The scale should be simple to complete, making clinical use feasible. However, the unclear time frame for observations is a problem in terms of determining the length of time upon which observations should be based. In addition, several items are reverse scored, adding somewhat to the task of computing scores. One positive attribute of the scale is that the developers have generated a package that caregivers can complete, documenting their child's baseline behavior and behavior during common pains. This might be particularly helpful in cases in which children have multiple conditions that cause chronic or recurrent pain.

Other Scales in Development

Whereas the PICIC and the Paediatric Pain Profile have focused primarily on pain outside the hospital setting, another group has developed a pain assessment tool for postoperative pain. Terstegen, Koot, de Boer, and Tibboel (2003) generated 209 potential items through interviews with parents and professionals who work with children with cognitive impairments; through observations of children during events expected to be painful, such as physiotherapy, vaccinations, and dental treatment; and through review of the literature. This pool of items was reduced to 23 that appeared to be sensitive to pain in 52 children who had surgery. They also found that 13 items achieved higher ratings during pain caused by a procedure than during pain after surgery, suggesting a possible difference in pain display depending on whether pain is short/acute or longer lasting. Few additional psychometrics of the scale are presented, so this tool is not yet appropriate for clinical use. However, it shows promise for differentiating pain types.

Summary

In all, five English-language tools have been developed specifically for children with cognitive impairments in the space of only a few years. Each has been developed by a different group, and through slightly different methods. Interestingly, there is a great deal of overlap in the items included in each. For example, all items of the PICIC (Stallard et al., 2002) are included in the NCCPC-R and NCCPC-PV (Breau, McGrath, et al., 2002; Breau, Finley, et al., 2002), the Paediatric Pain Profile (Hunt et al., 2004), and the tool in development by Terstegen et al. (2003). Twelve items from the NCCPC-R and NCCPC-PV are also included in Terstegen et al.'s new tool, and all but 2 of the 20 items of the Paediatric Pain Profile assess behaviors included in the NCCPC versions. It is also notable that three of the four tools incorporate between 20 and 30 items. This supports the notion that children with cognitive impairments, especially those with severe impairments and limited verbal ability, may exhibit a core group of pain signs across situations.

At this time, the NCCPC-R and NCCPC-PV have accumulated the most support for their psychometric properties, and these scales are used clinically to supplement clinical judgment. Several large-scale studies of English, French, and Swedish versions of the tools are also underway, aimed at providing new information about their use and possibly refinements to make them more feasible in clinical practice. For example, in several studies, assessments are being made using observations of only 5 minutes to determine if reducing the observation period will affect the sensitivity of these tools to pain. It is also hoped that more cutoff scores can be developed with these larger groups so that scores can be equated with points on a VAS of pain intensity.

That fact that so many groups have begun development of scales in such a short period of time highlights a growing recognition of the difficulties that clinicians and parents encounter in judging pain in children with cognitive impairments. Almost all of the children involved in these studies had moderate to severe cognitive impairments, with little or no ability to communicate their pain verbally. However, many children have milder impairments and may be able to provide some indication of their pain. The literature investigating the reliability of their self-report, however, consists of only a few studies.

Self-Report of Pain

Fanurik, Koh, Harrison, Conrad, and Tomerlin (1998) were the first group to investigate the self-report abilities of children with cognitive impairments. Their study included 47 children with varying levels of cognitive impairments and 111 children without impairments scheduled for surgery. Children's ability to use a 0–5 numerical rating scale of pain was assessed through several tasks. Children's ability to understand the concepts of magnitude and order were tested using tasks in which they were required to order wooden blocks by size and to arrange numerals in order. Children were then asked to match cards depicting faces at different levels of pain with cards depicting pain intensity (1, 3, and 5).

Only 10 (21%) of the children with cognitive impairments could complete all three tasks, and all had mild to borderline impairments. An additional 23 (44%) of the children could complete some part of the tasks, and none of these children completed the final task of assigning numerals to faces depicting pain intensity. In contrast, all children without impairments who were above age 8 completed all tasks, and 18% of children without impairments who were between ages 4 and 7 were able to complete all tasks, with 32% of this age group completing at least some tasks.

An interesting secondary analysis in this study examined nurses' ability to predict which children were capable of using a numerical rating scale. Only 47% of children with cognitive impairments who were deemed capable by nurses did demonstrate the ability. In most cases, nurses tended to overestimate the abilities of children with mild to moderate impairment. Nurses also overestimated the skills of 33% of children without impairments.

Benini et al. (2004) described a study of the self-report skills of 16 children ages 7–18 years with mild to moderate cognitive impairments. In this novel study, children were administered a 1-hour training session on use of the pain tools that were then used prior to receiving a venipuncture. Children then completed original and adapted versions of a 10-cm VAS of pain, the Eland Color Scale (Eland, 1985), which depicts a picture of a body that the child uses to indicate pain location, and the Faces Scale (Wong & Baker, 1988). There were no differences in children's ability to use the scales based on level of impairment (mild, moderate) or diagnosis (tetraplegia, Down syndrome). The authors reported that more children completed the modified scales (numbers of faces in Faces Scale reduced; body parts enlarged on Eland Color Scale; set of 5 cubes replaced 10-cm VAS). Unfortunately, relationships between parent ratings of pain and each instrument were not provided, but there was a moderate consistency between the VAS ratings provided by parents and a researcher and those provided by children.

Only one other study has examined the self-report skills of children with cognitive impairments. Zabalia et al. (2005) investigated the ability of 14 children with mild to moderate cognitive impairments ages 8–18 years to use a 100-mm VAS of Pain and the Faces Pain Scale–Revised (Hicks, von Baeyer, Spafford, van Korlaar, & Goodenough, 2001) to rate the pain of vignettes and the pain they believed they would feel were they to experience the events in the vignettes. The vignettes depicted individuals in pain as a result of a burn from a hot casserole, falling from a bicycle, falling from roller skates, and a vaccination. After ratings were provided, the children were also asked to describe the quality of the pain each event would cause.

The children's pain ratings for both the vignettes and the pain they would feel in those situations did vary by the cause of pain, suggesting that they did distinguish between the pain events. The children also provided up to nine words to describe the quality of the pain for the events, a number that is similar to that reported by typically developing children of a similar mental age, and the words were appropriate for the pain depicted (e.g., "burning," "pinching"). One weakness of the study is that the children did not rate their own pain for an actual experienced event. However, the results do indicate that the children had some skill in rating pain and, most important, that they could describe pain quality.

In summary, there is only a small body of research evaluating the ability of children with cognitive impairments to provide self-report of pain. This indicates that children with mild impairments may be able to use some self-report tools to provide a firsthand rating of the intensity of their pain. The research also suggests that children with mild to moderate impairments can distinguish between different types of pain and may be able to provide descriptions of the quality of their pain that could be useful for diagnosing the cause of pain. Clinicians should investigate each child's abilities to use self-report tools, because it appears that they may overestimate children's skills. Using simple analogue tasks may be feasible in some situations. Clinicians should also request estimates from parents or caregivers in addition to child self-report, or use observational pain tools, until further evidence is available to show that children can provide reliable self-report in clinical situations that may be more distressing (and, possibly, more painful), or until the psychometric properties of modified tools, such as those described by Benini et al. (2004), have been evaluated more fully.

The Role of the Observer in Pain Assessment

Parents have identified pain as one area of concern for their children who cannot communicate verbally (Stephenson & Dowrick, 2000). They have also expressed concern that some professionals may discount their reports that their child has pain (Hunt et al., 2003) and that their child's pain is treated differently than that of typically developing children (Fanurik, Koh, Schmitz, Harrison, & Conrad, 1999).

In interview studies, parents also reported that familiarity with their child is required to assess the child's pain (Carter, McArthur, & Cunliffe, 2002; Hunt et al., 2003). No scientist or clinician would argue the fact that each child is unique. However, parents may be basing this assumption on past experience in which professionals failed in attempts to discern pain because of lack of training, lack of literature to provide guidance, and lack of structured tools to use. However, our knowledge of the process of developing structured tools and of gathering evidence for their validity has grown. In addition, variation in individuals' pain behavior does not preclude the use of measures that have been empirically and scientifically tested for clinical use. We must keep sight of our primary goal, which is not to generate a precise picture of the child's pain experience, but rather to have sufficiently accurate information upon which to base treatment decisions. For most professionals, a tool that can distinguish between no pain and mild, moderate, or severe pain is sufficient for everyday practice.

Research also suggests that, when provided with information in a structured way, or when using a validated tool, observers who are unfamiliar with children with cognitive impairments may provide very reliable judgments. For example, the good interrater reliability between parents and a researcher reported by Breau, Finley, et al. (2002) suggests that use of a structured tool may facilitate agreement between parents and an unfamiliar observer. Two studies by Stevens' group also suggest that structured information and tools may also help to minimize preexisting beliefs on the part of observers that could impact judgments of pain in children with cognitive impairments. In one study, professionals who completed a questionnaire asking about the pain of infants at risk for cognitive impairments indicated a belief that greater impairment led to a reduced pain experience (Breau et al., in press). In contrast, when presented with the task of assessing from videotape the pain of infants at varying levels of risk for neurological impairment, using 0–10 VAS pain ratings, the pain ratings of a similar group of professionals did not vary with descriptions of the infants' level of risk for neurological impairment (Breau, Stevens, et al., 2004). Similarly, when presented with vignettes, pain ratings by professionals in a study by Fanurik, Koh, Schmitz, Harrison, Roberson, et al. (1999) also did not differ with the described level of cognitive impairment of the children.

To date, we do not know if biases or preexisting beliefs affect adults' judgments of pain in children with cognitive impairments. A belief that individuals with cognitive impairments have a reduced pain experience has been reported for caregivers (Breau, MacLaren, McGrath, Camfield, & Finley, 2003) and professionals (Breau, Stevens, et al., 2004). However, it is not clear whether these operate through effects on pain assessment or management, or whether professionals are able to set these aside in clinical situations. This is an important area for future research if optimal care is to be provided for this very vulnerable group.

Clearly, assessment is only the first step in the process of alleviating a child's pain. Whereas the literature regarding pain assessment for this vulnerable group is small, that regarding pain treatment is almost nonexistent. The next section of this chapter describes issues regarding treatment of acute and chronic pain in children with cognitive impairments and highlights the difficulties clinicians face in their efforts to manage what can be very complex pain problems.

TREATMENT OF PAIN

There has been very little research on treatment of pain in infants or children with cognitive impairments. Almost all studies of treatments of pain have excluded these children. This is in spite of the fact that they are more likely to have painful conditions and more likely to undergo painful procedures than other children

(Breau, Camfield, McGrath, et al., 2003; Stallard, Williams, Lenton, & Velleman, 2001).

There are two major strategies for determining what treatment to use for pain in children with cognitive impairment. The first and the preferred method should be to diagnose the cause of the pain and treat this underlying cause. The second approach is to symptomatically treat the pain without knowing its cause.

Acute Pain

For procedure pain and for postoperative pain, the diagnosis is usually obvious. Lacking any evidence, we should assume that, in general, treatments that are effective in typically developing children will be effective in children with cognitive impairments. However, a study of infants at risk for neurological impairment in a neonatal intensive care unit suggests that this may not always be the case. In their study of 194 infants, Stevens et al. (2003) reported that infants with greater risk for neurological impairment received fewer analgesics for procedure-related pain on the first day of life. They also found that analgesic administration was related to the number of procedures performed for most infants but not for those at highest risk for future impairments.

Many treatments found effective for typically developing children could easily be implemented with children with cognitive impairments. For example, the use of EMLA, a eutectic mixture of lidocaine and prilocaine, is likely to be effective in reducing pain from needles in children (Halperin, McGrath, Smith, & Houston, 2000). Similarly, distraction is effective in reducing pain from short procedures (Cohen, Blount, & Panopoulos, 1997).

However, treatment may not always be straightforward. There may be more problems in implementing treatment in the child with cognitive impairments than in other children. In the case of EMLA, for example, some children with cognitive impairment will not tolerate the presence of the EMLA patch for an hour before the needle is used. Some children with cognitive impairments may be so distressed by the medical situation that they are difficult to distract. Adults who are unfamiliar with a child may also find it difficult to determine a child's developmental level, in order to decide upon an activity that could be distracting. Modeling, shaping, and other behavioral techniques may be helpful in reducing children's distress and optimizing cooperation. Souders, Freeman, DePaul, and Levy (2002) provided an excellent description of techniques used for children with autism spectrum disorders, based on experiences during a large trial that entailed venipuncture (Levy et al., 2003). Many of these techniques may be effective with other children with cognitive impairments.

Postoperative pain management for children with limited cognitive abilities also generally follows the strategies that are useful in other children, with a few exceptions. The selection, dosages, and schedules of drugs used should be no different from those used with other children. Specific challenges may arise. Children with airway problems may need to be monitored even more carefully than a child without any respiratory difficulties. Several case studies have reported specific instances of anesthesia management in children with particular syndromes that involve cognitive impairments (Adhami & Cancio-Babu, 2003; Courreges, Nieuviarts, & Lecoutre, 2003; Critchley, Gin, & Stuart, 1995; Iacobucci, Galeone, & De Francisci, 2003; Shenkman, Krichevski, Elpeleg, Joseph, & Kadari, 1997). Children with cognitive impairment are unlikely to be able to use patient-controlled analgesia. However, successful use has been reported for typically developing children over 5 years of age (Birmingham et al., 2003; McDonald & Cooper, 2001). Thus, with older children with cognitive impairments who have mental abilities greater than a typically developing 5-year-old, patient-controlled analgesia may be possible.

There is evidence that children with cognitive impairments do not receive the same care as children without cognitive impairments postoperatively. In one of the few studies of postoperative pain management in children with cognitive impairment, Malviya et al. (2001) compared the pain assessment and management practices in 42 children (19 with cognitive impairment and 23 without impairment) undergoing spinal fusion. They found that children with cognitive impairment received smaller total opioid doses.

Koh et al. (2004) prospectively examined 152 children with cognitive impairment of different severities and 138 children without cognitive impairments. They found that children with cognitive impairment undergoing surgery received less opioid in the perioperative period than did children without cognitive impairment. However, in the postoperative period, both groups of children were given similar amounts and types of analgesics. Koh et al. (2004) suggested that anesthesiologists believe that children with cognitive impairment are more sensitive to the side effects of opioids than other children. Unfortunately, there is no research investigating this phenomenon.

In summary, there is a dearth of data on acute pain in infants and children with cognitive impairment that can guide their care, and they may receive fewer analgesics than children without cognitive impairment. The use of nonpharmacological treatments has been most neglected and, yet, might offer many options for treating children's acute pain when their complex conditions raise concerns about analgesic administration.

Chronic and Recurrent Pain

Diagnosis of the Etiology of Pain

Clinicians are well aware of the methods of diagnosis, and diagnosis of pain in children with cognitive impairment is fundamentally no different than diagnosis of pain in other children. However, it is important to emphasize issues that are particularly important with this population. These issues arise because children with severe cognitive impairment cannot verbally communicate and because many of these children often suffer significant comorbidities, especially speech defects, epilepsy, and cerebral palsy (Arvio & Sillanpaa, 2003).

The first step in diagnosis is to take a thorough history of the pain problem and the child. In this population, the history must be taken almost exclusively from the adults in the child's world. Continuity of care may be even more important in these children than in other children because knowledge of the child's typical problems and usual behavior may help in diagnosis. Nevertheless, each problem that every child presents with deserves a careful and detailed analysis. It is also important to keep in mind the child's abilities and estimated developmental level, because children with cognitive impairments may display pain behavior that more closely resembles that of mental-age peers than chronological-age peers, and caregivers may not always be aware that these behaviors may reflect pain.

A problem arises if the accompanying adult is not well acquainted with the history of the child's current problem. This may be the case if the child lives in a residential facility, such as a group home. In these situations, it is important to obtain supplementary information from caregivers who know the child, which can be done by telephone. Encouraging the child's caregivers to keep written reports of any problems will help.

The importance of a thorough physical examination cannot be overemphasized with this group of children. Children must be undressed, taken out of their chairs, and thoroughly examined. Because children cannot verbally localize pain for the clinician, it is imperative to examine the entire child. Children with cognitive impairment may be fearful of examination, and it is often necessary to proceed gently and slowly with the physical examination to avoid causing distress.

Children with significant cognitive impairments are at higher risk for several conditions that do not present as frequently in children with typical cognitive functioning. Clinicians should have an increased index of suspicion for these problems. In a two-round Delphi poll, we surveyed an international panel of clinicians with experience with pain in children with significant cognitive disability (Choo, McGrath, Finley, Camfield, & Breau, 2001). We found good concordance among these clinicians that gastrointestinal problems were a major source of pain. They also agreed that children with cognitive impairment frequently suffer musculoskeletal pain, pain as the result of infection, headache, pain from skin problems, neuropathic pain, dental pain, and pain from self-injury. Other research by our group indicates that children's characteristics may also heighten their risk for specific types of pain (Breau, Camfield, et al., 2004).

Although recommendations for use of a directed history and behavioral changes for diagnosis of particular health problems have been presented by Bosch (2002), and Tracy and Wallace (2001) outlined the ways in which developmental delays may impact the presentation of physical conditions, there has not been a systematic mapping of the painful conditions from which children with cognitive impairment suffer. This type of mapping would be of considerable value to the clinician. We are currently using the tacit wisdom of expert clinicians who deal with these children to develop clinical algorithms to help in the diagnosis of different causes of pain. This web-based program will work from symptoms to suggest possible diagnoses that may be relevant, or it will give symptoms for a chosen diagnosis. In addition, an algorithm will indicate predisposing factors and treatment options.

For example, a clinician might indicate that his or her patient appears to be in pain, has a cough and fatigue, and is floppy and irritable. A list of diagnoses that these symptoms could be associated with is produced. In this case, four symptoms match pneumonia and two symptoms match gastroesophageal reflux, osteomyelitis, septic arthritis, and inflammatory arthritis. The clinician can then review the other symptoms listed for each possible diagnosis and use these to narrow down the final diagnosis. Different tests are suggested as possibilities. The program is still under development and testing. It will not diagnose problems but can provide prompts for clinicians who may not be thinking of a possibility.

Treating Pain Without Knowing Its Cause

Pain clinicians treating adults or children with pain often cannot find the cause of the pain. This is also true with children with cognitive impairment. In these situations, the treatment will be symptomatic. General principles of good clinical care are used. Interventions are chosen on the basis of an analysis of what is known.

If there is evidence of inflammation, a drug with analgesic and anti-inflammatory properties will be used. If the pain has some characteristics of neuropathic pain, one of the drugs commonly used for that type of pain is used. If pain seems to occur when the child is sitting for a lengthy period of time, alterations may be made to the number of hours he or she is sitting. Both the intended actions and the side effects of each intervention (whether a drug or a behavioral intervention) have to be considered.

Optimally, one treatment is given at a time, and the effect of that treatment is observed over a few days. If the pain is alleviated, the treatment may be withdrawn for a short period of time to see if the pain begins to reoccur. This simple reversal design can be a clear indication that the treatment is what is helping the pain.

Research on all types of pain management in children with cognitive impairments is seriously lacking. Only scattered studies are available. Without any specific research, the pain management approaches shown to be effective with other children should be tried. However, it is likely that outcomes could be significantly improved if research were able to detail specific strategies that were optimal for children with cognitive impairment.

CONCLUSION

As our knowledge in pain assessment and management for children with cognitive impairments grows, it is vital that we use the information we currently have at hand in caring for children now. There is a history of undertreatment of pain in vulnerable groups, with children with cognitive impairments representing only one of these. It can be easy for us to assume differences in pain sensation when no evidence exists, because of our preexisting beliefs about pain, about the relation between pain and intellectual functioning, and about the pain tolerance of those who may express pain differently from us.

Undoubtedly, pain is a subjective experience. It may vary as a result of many factors, such as age, gender, and culture, and sensitivity, and tolerance to pain can be subject to the psychoemotional context. The suffering associated with pain is also subjective. It is the very subjectivity of pain and suffering that raises obstacles for us. Empathy is fundamental to evaluating the pain of another, and this requires identification with the person suffering pain when we have no objective source of information. However, it is difficult to identify with those who we see as "different," leaving us feeling helpless and inadequate to the task. Thus, we may develop mechanisms to deal with our frustrations when working with those who we view as "impaired." This can include minimizing their experience, or its impact on their lives. These attitudes are as likely to influence pain management as they are other aspects of care for these groups.

A child with cognitive impairments can elicit our pity and charity. Conversely, humans still display a general tendency to "blame the victim" in our efforts to make sense of suffering. These two feelings can lead to an ambivalence that can also interfere with good pain management, and may be one reason that recognition of pain may be delayed for this group. This highlights the fact that the effectiveness of any tool is dependent upon the hand that holds it.

In all, there is little doubt that objective assessment is the best guarantee that treatment will be administered and will be effective. Objective tools can help to minimize our biases, to detect patterns in pain, and to adapt treatment on an ongoing basis. They also make it possible to communicate reliable information among all involved in the care of a child and help professionals to become proficient in pain assessment and management strategies. Objective assessment also allows us to collect information across children to improve our understanding of specific pain problems.

The insistence that children with cognitive impairments are idiosyncratic underlies not only resistance to the use of structured pain assessment, but also arguments that pain treatments will not be effective for them. When benefits outweigh potential harm, we have little evidence that treatments that are effective for specific pain problems in typically developing children will not be so in those with cognitive impairments.

Our challenge at this juncture is to achieve balance. We must accept and be sensitive to the uniqueness of each child and his or her personal experience of pain, while pressing on in our efforts to validate objective pain assessment tools that will aid in consistent high-quality diagnosis, to gather evidence regarding the effectiveness of pain management strategies for these very complex children, and to promote the use of scientifically tested methods in all aspects of pain care.

REFERENCES

Adhami, E.J., & Cancio-Babu, C.V. (2003). Anaesthesia in a child with Sotos syndrome. *Paediatric Anaesthesia, 13,* 835–840.

Allison, P.J., & Lawrence, H.P. (2004). A paired comparison of dental care in Canadians with Down syndrome and their siblings without Down syndrome. *Community Dentistry and Oral Epidemiology, 32,* 99–106.

Arvio, M., & Sillanpaa, M. (2003). Prevalence, aetiology and comorbidity of severe and profound intellectual disability in Finland. *Journal of Intellectual Disability Research, 47,* 108–112.

Benedetti, F., Arduino, C., Vighetti, S., Asteggiano, G., Tarenzi, L., & Rainero, I. (2004). Pain reactivity in Alzheimer patients with different degrees of cognitive impairment and brain electrical activity deterioration. *Pain, 111,* 22–29.

Benini, F., Trapanotto, M., Gobber, D., Agosto, C., Carli, G., Drigo, P., et al. (2004). Evaluating pain induced by venipuncture in pediatric patients with developmental delay. *Clinical Journal of Pain, 20,* 156–163.

Biersdorff, K.K. (1991). Pain insensitivity and indifference: Alternative explanations for some medical catastrophes. *Mental Retardation, 29,* 359–362.

Biersdorff, K.K. (1994). Incidence of significantly altered pain experience among individuals with developmental disabilities. *American Journal on Mental Retardation, 98,* 619–631.

Birmingham, P.K., Wheeler, M., Suresh, S., Dsida, R.M., Rae, B.R., Obrecht, J., et al. (2003). Patient-controlled epidural analgesia in children: Can they do it? *Anesthesia and Analgesia, 96,* 686–691.

Bosch, J.J. (2002). Use of directed history and behavioral indicators in the assessment of the child with a developmental disability. *Journal of Pediatric Health Care, 16,* 170–179.

Braden, K., Swanson, S., & Di Scala, C. (2003). Injuries to children who had preinjury cognitive impairment: A 10-year retrospective review. *Archives of Pediatrics and Adolescent Medicine, 157,* 336–340.

Breau, L.M., Camfield, C., Symons, F.J., Bodfish, J.W., McKay, A., Finley, G.A., et al. (2003). Pain and self-injurious behaviour in neurologically impaired children. *Journal of Pediatrics, 142,* 498–503.

Breau, L.M., Camfield, C.S., McGrath, P.J., & Finley, G.A. (2003). The incidence of pain in children with severe cognitive impairments. *Archives of Pediatrics and Adolescent Medicine, 157,* 1226.

Breau, L.M., Camfield, C.S., McGrath, P.J., & Finley, G.A. (2004). Risk factors for pain in children with severe cognitive impairments. *Developmental Medicine and Child Neurology, 46,* 364–371.

Breau, L.M., Camfield, C.S., McGrath, P.J., Rosmus, C., & Finley, G.A. (2001). Measuring pain accurately in children with cognitive impairments: Refinement of a caregiver scale. *Journal of Pediatrics, 138,* 721–727.

Breau, L.M., Finley, G.A., McGrath, P.J., & Camfield, C.S. (2002). Validation of the Non-Communicating Children's Pain Checklist–Postoperative Version. *Anesthesiology, 96,* 528–535.

Breau, L.M., MacLaren, J., McGrath, P.J., Camfield, C.S., & Finley, G.A. (2003). Caregivers' beliefs regarding pain in children with cognitive impairment: Relation between pain sensation and reaction increases with severity of impairment. *Clinical Journal of Pain, 19,* 335–344.

Breau, L.M., McGrath, P.J., Camfield, C., & Finley, G.A. (2002). Psychometric properties of the Non-communicating Children's Pain Checklist–Revised. *Pain, 99,* 349–357.

Breau, L.M., McGrath, P.J., Camfield, C., Rosmus, C., & Finley, G.A. (2000). Preliminary validation of an observational pain checklist for persons with cognitive impairments and inability to communicate verbally. *Developmental Medicine and Child Neurology, 42,* 609–616.

Breau, L.M., McGrath, P.J., Craig, K.D., Santor, D., Cassidy, K.L., & Reid, G.J. (2001). Facial expression of children receiving immunizations: A principal components analysis of the Child Facial Coding System. *Clinical Journal of Pain, 17,* 178–186.

Breau, L.M., McGrath, P.J., Stevens, B., Beyene, J., Camfield, C., Finley, G.A., et al. (in press). Healthcare professionals' beliefs regarding the pain of infants at risk for neurological impairment: A survey. *Clinical Journal of Pain.*

Breau, L.M., Stevens, B., McGrath, P.J., Beyene, J., Camfield, C.S., Finley, G.A., et al. (2004). Healthcare professionals' perception of pain experienced by infants at risk for neurological impairment. *BMC Pediatrics, 4*(23).

Carter, B., McArthur, E., & Cunliffe, M. (2002). Dealing with uncertainty: Parental assessment of pain in their children with profound special needs. *Journal of Advanced Nursing, 38,* 449–457.

Chambers, C.T., Cassidy, K.L., McGrath, P.J., Gilbert, C.A., & Craig, K.D. (1996). *Child Facial Coding System: A manual.* Halifax, Nova Scotia/Vancouver: Dalhousie University and University of British Columbia.

Choo, S.A., McGrath, P.J., Finley, G.A., Camfield, C., & Breau, L.M. (2001). *Causes of pain in non-verbal cognitively impaired children—a Delphi study.* Unpublished manuscript.

Cohen, L.L., Blount, R.L., & Panopoulos, G. (1997). Nurse coaching and cartoon distraction: An effective and practical intervention to reduce child, parent, and nurse distress during immunizations. *Journal of Pediatric Psychology, 22,* 355–370.

Collignon, P., & Giusiano, B. (2001). Validation of a pain evaluation scale for patients with severe cerebral palsy. *European Journal of Pain, 5,* 433–442.

Collignon, P., Giusiano, B., Porsmoguer, E., Jimeno, M.E., & Combe, J.C. (1995). Difficultés du diagnostic de la douleur chez l'enfant polyhandicapé. *Annals of Pediatrics, 42,* 123–126.

Collignon, P., Porsmoguer, E., Behar, M., Combe, J.C., & Perrin, C. (1992). L'automutilation: Expression de la douleur chez le sujet déficient mental profond. In *La douleur de l'enfant quelles réponses?* (pp. 15–21). Paris: UNESCO.

Courreges, P., Nieuviarts, R., & Lecoutre, D. (2003). Anaesthetic management for Edward's syndrome. *Paediatric Anaesthesia, 13,* 267–269.

Critchley, L.A., Gin, T., & Stuart, J.C. (1995). Anaesthesia in an infant with Rubinstein-Taybi syndrome. *Anaesthesia, 50,* 37–38.

Defrin, R., Pick, C.G., Peretz, C., & Carmeli, E. (2004). A quantitative somatosensory testing of pain threshold in individuals with mental retardation. *Pain, 108,* 58–66.

Ehde, D.M., Jensen, M.P., Engel, J.M., Turner, J.A., Hoffman, A.J., & Cardenas, D.D. (2003). Chronic pain secondary to disability: A review. *Clinical Journal of Pain, 19,* 3–17.

Eland, J.M. (1985). The child who is hurting. *Seminars in Oncology Nursing, 1,* 116–122.

Fanurik, D., Koh, J.L., Harrison, D., & Conrad, T.M. (1996). Children with cognitive impairment: Parent report of pain and coping [Abstract]. Proceedings of the 8th World Congress on Pain (Progress in Pain Research and Management, p. 299). Seattle: IASP Press.

Fanurik, D., Koh, J.L., Harrison, R.D., Conrad, T.M., & Tomerlin, C. (1998). Pain assessment in children with cognitive impairment: An exploration of self-report skills. *Clinical Nursing Research, 7,* 103–124.

Fanurik, D., Koh, J.L., Schmitz, M.L., Harrison, R.D., & Conrad, T.M. (1999). Children with cognitive impairment: Parent report of pain and coping. *Journal of Developmental and Behavioral Pediatrics, 20,* 228–234.

Fanurik, D., Koh, J.L., Schmitz, M.L., Harrison, R.D., Roberson, P.K., & Killebrew, P. (1999). Pain assessment and treatment in children with cognitive impairment: A survey of nurses' and physicians' beliefs. *Clinical Journal of Pain, 15,* 304–312.

Fernhall, B., & Otterstetter, M. (2003). Attenuated responses to sympathoexcitation in individuals with Down syndrome. *Journal of Applied Physiology, 94,* 2158–2165.

Finley, G.A., McGrath, P.J., Forward, S.P., McNeill, G., & Fitzgerald, P. (1996). Parents' management of children's pain following 'minor' surgery. *Pain, 64,* 83–87.

Gillberg, C., Terenius, L., & Lonnerholm, G. (1985). Endorphin activity in childhood psychosis: Spinal fluid levels in 24 cases. *Archives of General Psychiatry, 42,* 780–783.

Giusiano, B., Jimeno, M.T., Collignon, P., & Chau, Y. (1995). Utilization of a neural network in the elaboration of an evaluation scale for pain in cerebral palsy. *Methods of Information in Medicine, 34,* 498–502.

Hadden, K.L., & von Baeyer, C.L. (2001). Measuring pain in children with cerebral palsy during home stretching exercises: Facial actions and global ratings. In

Hadden, K. L., & von Baeyer, C.L. (2002). Pain in children with cerebral palsy: Common triggers and expressive behaviors. *Pain, 99,* 281–288.

Halperin, S.A., McGrath, P., Smith, B., & Houston, T. (2000). Lidocaine-prilocaine patch decreases the pain associated with the subcutaneous administration of measles-mumps-rubella vaccine but does not adversely affect the antibody response. *Journal of Pediatrics, 136,* 789–794.

Hennequin, M., Faulks, D., & Roux, D. (2000). Accuracy of estimation of dental treatment need in special care patients. *Journal of Dentistry, 28,* 131–136.

Hennequin, M., Morin, C., & Feine, J.S. (2000). Pain expression and stimulus localisation in individuals with Down's syndrome. *Lancet, 356,* 1882–1887.

Hicks, C.L., von Baeyer, C.L., Spafford, P.A., van Korlaar, I., & Goodenough, B. (2001). The Faces Pain Scale–Revised: Toward a common metric in pediatric pain measurement. *Pain, 93,* 173–183.

Hunt, A., & Burne, R. (1995). Medical and nursing problems of children with neurodegenerative disease. *Palliative Medicine, 9,* 19–26.

Hunt, A., Goldman, A., Seers, K., Crichton, N., Mastroyannopoulou, K., Moffat, V., et al. (2004). Clinical validation of the Paediatric Pain Profile. *Developmental Medicine and Child Neurology, 46,* 9–18.

Hunt, A., Mastroyannopoulou, K., Goldman, A., & Seers, K. (2003). Not knowing—the problem of pain in children with severe neurological impairment. *International Journal of Nursing Studies, 40,* 171–183.

Iacobucci, T., Galeone, M., & De Francisci, G. (2003). Anaesthetic management of a child with Pallister-Killian syndrome. *Paediatric Anaesthesia, 13,* 457–459.

Jancar, J., & Speller, C.J. (1994). Fatal intestinal obstruction in the mentally handicapped. *Journal of Intellectual Disability Research, 38,* 413–422.

Jay, S.M., Ozolins, M., Elliott, C.H., & Caldwell, S. (1983). Assessment of children's distress during painful medical procedures. *Health Psychology, 2,* 133–147.

Konstantareas, M.M., & Homatidis, S. (1987). Ear infections in autistic and normal children. *Journal of Autism and Developmental Disorders, 17,* 585–594.

Leland, N.L., Garrard, J., & Smith, D.K. (1994). Comparison of injuries to children with and without disabilities in a day-care center. *Journal of Developmental and Behavioral Pediatrics, 15,* 402–408.

Levy, S.E., Souders, M.C., Wray, J., Jawad, A.F., Gallagher, P.R., Coplan, J., et al. (2003). Children with autistic spectrum disorders. I: Comparison of placebo and single dose of human synthetic secretin. *Archives of Disease in Childhood, 88,* 731–736.

Lorenz, J.M., Wooliever, D.E., Jetton, J.R., & Paneth, N. (1998). A quantitative review of mortality and developmental disability in extremely premature newborns. *Archives of Pediatrics and Adolescent Medicine, 152,* 425–435.

Lu, D.P. (1981). Clinical investigation of relative indifference to pain among adolescent mental retardates. *ASDC Journal of Dentistry for Children, 48,* 285–288.

Malviya, S., Voepel-Lewis, T., Tait, A.R., Merkel, S., Lauer, A., Munro, H., et al. (2001). Pain management in children with and without cognitive impairment following spine fusion surgery. *Paediatric Anaesthesia, 11,* 453–458.

McDonald, A.J., & Cooper, M.G. (2001). Patient-controlled analgesia: An appropriate method of pain control in children. *Paediatric Drugs, 3,* 273–284.

McGrath, P.J., Rosmus, C., Camfield, C., Campbell, M.A., & Hennigar, A.W. (1998). Behaviours caregivers use to determine pain in non-verbal, cognitively impaired individuals. *Developmental Medicine and Child Neurology, 40,* 340–343.

Mercer, K., & Glenn, S. (2004). The expression of pain in infants with developmental delays. *Child Care, Health and Development, 30,* 353–360.

Mette, F., & Abittan, J. (1988). Essais d'évaluation de la douleur chez le polyhandicapé. *Annales Kinésithérapie, 15,* 101–104.

Nader, R., Oberlander, T.F., Chambers, C.T., & Craig, K.D. (2004). Expression of pain in children with autism. *Clinical Journal of Pain, 20,* 88–97.

Nordin, V., & Gillberg, C. (1996). Autism spectrum disorders in children with physical or mental disability or both. I: Clinical and epidemiological aspects. *Developmental Medicine and Child Neurology, 38,* 297–313.

Oberlander, T.F., Gilbert, C.A., Chambers, C.T., O'Donnell, M.E., & Craig, K.D. (1999). Biobehavioral responses to acute pain in adolescents with a significant neurologic impairment. *Clinical Journal of Pain, 15,* 201–209.

Porter, F.L., Malhotra, K.M., Wolf, C.M., Morris, J.C., Miller, J.P., & Smith, M.C. (1996). Dementia and response to pain in the elderly. *Pain, 68,* 413–421.

Rainero, I., Vighetti, S., Bergamasco, B., Pinessi, L., & Benedetti, F. (2000). Autonomic responses and pain perception in Alzheimer's disease. *European Journal of Pain, 4,* 267–274.

Reynell, J.K. (1965). Post-operative disturbances observed in children with cerebral palsy. *Developmental Medicine and Child Neurology, 7,* 360–376.

Sandman, C.A., Barron, J., Chicz-DeMet, A., & DeMet, E.M. (1990). Plasma B-endorphin levels in patients with self-injurious behavior and stereotypy. *American Journal on Mental Retardation, 95,* 84-92.

Shenkman, Z., Krichevski, I., Elpeleg, O.N., Joseph, A., & Kadari, A. (1997). Anaesthetic management of a patient with Leigh's syndrome. *Canadian Journal of Anaesthesia, 44,* 1091–1095.

Soetenga, D., Pellino, T.A., & Frank, J. (1999). Assessment of the validity and reliability of the University of Wisconsin Children's Hospital Pain Scale for preverbal and nonverbal children. *Pediatric Nursing, 25,* 670–676.

Solodiuk, J., & Curley, M.A. (2003). Pain assessment in nonverbal children with severe cognitive impairments: the Individualized Numeric Rating Scale (INRS). *Journal of Pediatric Nursing, 18,* 295–299.

Souders, M.C., Freeman, K.G., DePaul, D., & Levy, S.E. (2002). Caring for children and adolescents with autism who require challenging procedures. *Pediatric Nursing, 28,* 555–562.

Stallard, P., Williams, L., Lenton, S., & Velleman, R. (2001). Pain in cognitively impaired, non-communicating children. *Archives of Disease in Childhood, 85,* 460–462.

Stallard, P., Williams, L., Velleman, R., Lenton, S., McGrath, P.J., & Taylor, G. (2002). The development and evaluation of the Pain Indicator for Communicatively Impaired Children (PICIC). *Pain, 1-2,* 149.

Stephenson, J.R., & Dowrick, M. (2000). Parent priorities in communication intervention for young students with severe disabilities. *Education and Training in Mental Retardation and Developmental Disabilities, 35,* 25–35.

Stevens, B., McGrath, P.J., Gibbins, S., Beyenne, J., Breau, L.M., Camfield, C., et al. (2003). Procedural pain in neonates at risk for neurological impairment. *Pain, 105,* 27–35.

Terstegen, C., Koot, H.M., de Boer, J.B., & Tibboel, D. (2003). Measuring pain in children with cognitive impairment: Pain response to surgical procedures. *Pain, 103,* 187–198.

Tracy, J.M., & Wallace, R. (2001). Presentations of physical illness in people with developmental disability: The example of gastro-oesophageal reflux. *Medical Journal of Australia, 175,* 109–111.

Voepel-Lewis, T., Merkel, S., Tait, A.R., Trzcinka, A., & Malviya, S. (2002). The reliability and validity of the Face, Legs, Activity, Cry, Consolability observational tool as a measure of pain in children with cognitive impairment. *Anesthesia and Analgesia, 95,* 1224–1229.

Wong, D.L., & Baker, C.M. (1988). Pain in children: comparison of assessment scales. *Pediatric Nursing, 14,* 9–17.

11

ISSUES IN PAIN ASSESSMENT FOR ADULTS WITH SEVERE TO PROFOUND MENTAL RETARDATION

From Research to Practice

James W. Bodfish, Vicki N. Harper,
Jennifer M. Deacon, Joseph R. Deacon, and Frank J. Symons

Although people with severe to profound mental retardation may experience a tremendously painful medical condition or procedure, they are frequently unable to express their pain through conventional means. In fact, it is one of the paradoxes of life for people with severe to profound mental retardation that while their neurodevelopmental disorders place them at a significantly *greater* risk for pain-related medical conditions and procedures, their level of cognitive impairment often precludes the conventional communication of their pain to others. To further complicate matters, individuals with this degree of cognitive and physical impairment typically rely on others to meet their needs. If a person needs relief for his or her pain but cannot express it to those who care for him or her, the consequence can be untreated pain and a concomitant significantly reduced quality of life.

The paradox of pain in people with mental retardation has remained a largely unexamined issue to date. This chapter begins to address this issue with respect to adults with severe to profound levels of mental retardation. First, we examine the issue conceptually: What is the nature of severe to profound mental retardation, and how can it affect pain experience, pain sensitivity, pain expression, and the recognition of pain by others in clinical settings? Next, we address this issue empirically: How have pain sensation and pain expression been measured and studied in individuals with severe to profound mental retardation? Finally, we address the applied aspects of this issue: How can the findings of these studies be translated to guide the routine care of people with mental retardation? In this last section, we examine results from clinical service settings for adults with mental retardation where pain assessment and pain management services have been in place.

Because the first step in clinical pain management is identifying pain, we focus on issues surrounding the identification and measurement of pain in clini-

This work was supported by a grant from the Foundation of Hope and by Public Health Service Grant HD35682 (National Institute of Child Health and Human Development).

The impetus and direction for this work were derived from the Millcroft Inn Symposium on Pain in Significant Neurological Impairment, sponsored by the Mayday Foundation (Alton, Ontario; January 2000). Copies of the Pain and Discomfort Scale and Pain Examination Procedure are available from the first author.

The authors thank Dawn Parker, Jamie Clary, Nancy Poteet, and Bill Heeth for their assistance with the studies conducted to develop the PADS.

cal settings. In line with this, much of the material in this chapter covers empirically derived and psychometrically sound (i.e., reliable, valid) methods for the clinical identification and measurement of pain that have been developed for use in routine service settings for people with severe to profound mental retardation, including a specific clinical assessment instrument for adults with severe to profound mental retardation. Issues in the treatment of pain are not covered in this chapter, however, because other chapters focus specifically on this, and there is very little empirical work to draw on specific to treating pain for individuals with severe cognitive impairment.

CONCEPTUALIZING PAIN EXPERIENCE

How do people view individuals with disabilities with respect to pain? The International Association for the Study of Pain (IASP) has defined pain as "an unpleasant sensory and emotional experience associated with actual or potential tissue damage, or described in terms of such damage" (Merskey & Bogduk, 1994). The definition proposed by the IASP suggests that pain is a subjective experience, with the understanding of the word's meaning learned through early life experiences with injury. This definition emphasizes the role of self-report as the primary means for relating pain or gaining assistance to deal with pain. Thus, based on this IASP definition, self-report of pain has come to be considered the "gold standard" for relating pain. Consequently, the vast majority of pain assessment tools rely heavily on language and cognitive skills. This is problematic when considering people with developmental disabilities, who have limited cognitive and language skills.

There exists a large body of research on the identification, assessment, and treatment of pain among people without disabilities. Consequently, identification and management of pain in the general population has become a routine practice in most medical settings. However, very little systematic work has been done in the area of recognition of pain and discomfort among people with cognitive or communication deficits or both. This is not because people with disabilities do not experience the procedures or the conditions that are known to produce pain. In fact, many individuals within this population experience painful medical conditions (Oberlander, Gilbert, Chambers, O'Donnell, & Craig, 1999). They also may be more frequently subjected to a variety of potentially painful medical procedures. However, the emphasis on effective communication of the subjective pain experience can create a barrier to the identification of pain among people with cognitive and communicative limitations. Individuals who do not or cannot report the information required by the typical pain assessment procedures may be in danger of misdiagnosis and undertreatment when ill or injured (Biersdorff, 1991; Hadjistavropoulos et al., 1998; Kovach, Weissman, Griffie, Matson, & Muchka, 1999). Indeed, it has been reported that health care professionals fail to note the presence of pain when verbal reports are absent (Jancar & Speller, 1994). Thus, the dependence on self-report pain assessment tools places people with limited cognitive and communication skills at risk for substandard health care.

The absence of self-report behaviors not only is a barrier to the assessment of pain among some populations but also may lead to the belief that these individuals have a reduced sensitivity to pain. How well caregivers respond to the pain management needs of those they serve seems related to their understanding and beliefs about the sensitivity of these individuals to pain (Schechter & Allen, 1986; Vortherms, Ryan, & Ward, 1992). The results of previous studies have demonstrated clearly that both the recognition and management of pain in patients are influenced strongly by the beliefs and attitudes of their health care workers (Vortherms et al., 1992; Watt-Watson, 1987). This effect is likely to be even stronger in the case of the care and treatment of people with severe developmental disabilities given that such individuals are often totally reliant on others both to recognize their needs and to respond to them. History has shown that this was indeed the case for "preverbal" clinical populations such as typically developing neonates and infants who underwent known pain-related medical procedures (Schechter, 1989). Historically, prevailing false beliefs about infants' insensitivity to pain led to widespread undertreatment of pain in pediatric clinical settings (Gadish & Gonzalez, 1988; Oberlander, O'Donnell, & Montgomery, 1999; Schechter, 1989).

Unfortunately, little is known about the beliefs of direct care providers and health care clinicians with respect to the pain experience in people with mental retardation. Early reports of fatalities among adults with severe to profound mental retardation with presumably preventable medical conditions (e.g., intestinal obstructions) initially thought to be due to pain insensitivity in this population are more likely to be related to the fact that care providers can fail to notice such conditions when conventional means of pain reporting are lacking (Jancar & Speller, 1994; Roy & Simon, 1987). In these instances, it is possible that care providers tend to believe that because pain is a subjective experience, it is identified best through patient self-report, and thus the absence of self-report also suggests the absence of the awareness or sensitivity of pain. In a study of clinicians' knowledge of pain in children, Turnquist and Engel (1995) found that clinicians were more likely to believe that pain was associated with a particular condition commonly known to be painful in adults (e.g., arthritis, acquired immunodeficiency syndrome, cancer) than with a nonspecific condition such cerebral palsy or mental retardation. Oberlander and O'Donnell (2001) surveyed clinicians who had extensive experience in working with children with severe neurological impairments (including mental retardation). They found that, although most experienced clinicians believed that such patients were sensitive to pain and that they could recognize the presence of pain in this group, even experienced workers were often uncertain about whether the source of pain could be isolated, whether expressions of distress could be equated with pain per se, and whether they could distinguish accurately between pain and other affective states in this group.

With respect to adults with mental retardation, Symons, Hinze, Sutton, and Bodfish (1999) used a standardized questionnaire (the Pain & Discomfort in Developmental Disabilities Questionnaire [P3DQ]) to examine beliefs about pain experience among 98 clinicians (nurses, medical doctors, occupational therapists, and physical therapists) who cared for adults with mental retardation in inpatient residential settings. Whereas only one third of clinicians surveyed believed that people with *mild or moderate* levels of disability experienced pain differently from people without disabilities, two thirds of those surveyed believed that people with *severe to profound* levels of disability experienced pain differently from people without disabilities (Figure 11.1). Furthermore, although the majority of clinicians surveyed indicated that orofacial signs were most indicative of pain and discomfort in individuals with severe disabilities, overall there was considerable disagreement among the clinicians surveyed as to what domains of functioning could be used to most accurately signal the presence of pain in people with severe to profound levels of disability (e.g., verbalizations, vocalizations, changes in functioning level, body movements, orofacial expression).

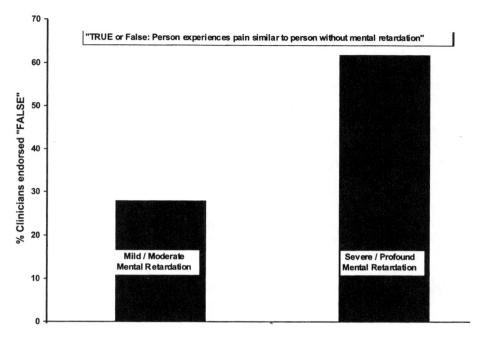

Figure 11.1.   Beliefs of clinicians who work with adults with mental retardation about whether adults with mild to moderate mental retardation and adults with severe to profound mental retardation experience pain in the same way that adults without disabilities experience pain. Results are based on responses for a total sample of 98 clinicians (nurses, physicians, occupational therapists, and physical therapists) on the Pain and Discomfort in Developmental Disabilities Questionnaire (P3DQ).

Symons et al. also examined 1 year of daily medical chart entries for five adults with profound mental retardation and multiple comorbid potential pain sources (e.g., cerebral palsy [CP]/contractures, feeding tubes, gastrointestinal disorders) to identify the behaviors that direct care providers used to signal the need for a referral to a physician for pain-related issues. Figure 11.2 displays the mismatch that was found between clinicians' beliefs about the best signs of pain in this population and the actual signs used by direct care providers to initiate a pain treatment referral in this population. Whereas direct care providers tended to initiate referrals to physicians most often on the basis of a change in activities of daily living performance (e.g., eating, sleeping, response to self-care) and least often based on changes in body movements or orofacial expression, the opposite pattern was found for clinicians' beliefs about what signs are most important for the identification of pain.

Variations in beliefs and practices concerning pain in this population may be due to the potential for common conceptualizations of "mental retardation" (e.g., neurological damage, cognitive deficits, language deficits) and "pain" (e.g., a subjective experience, communicated through introspection by verbal self-report) to lead to assumptions of relative pain insensitivity or lack of pain expression even in the face of recognized sources of pain (e.g., medical procedures, medical conditions) that are frequent facts of life for people with mental retardation. Given the potential for common conceptualizations of these phenomena to lead to the "pain insensitivity + diminished pain expression" assumption, researchers in this area have examined whether this assumption is accurate for individuals with mental retardation. In other words, the pain insensitivity issue is an empirical issue—one

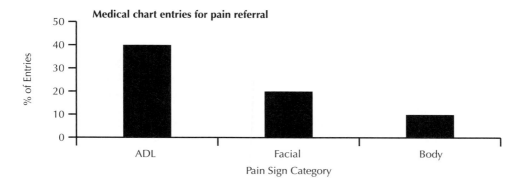

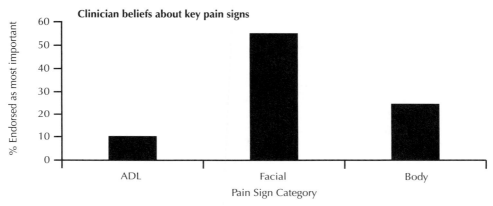

Figure 11.2. A comparison of clinicians' beliefs about specific pain signs that can be used to identify pain in people with severe to profound mental retardation to the pain signs that were logged in medical charts by direct care health workers (e.g., nurses, nurses' aides) to initiate referrals to physicians for suspected pain in patients with severe to profound mental retardation. Data for clinicians' beliefs were taken from P3DQ responses from a sample of 98 clinicians. Data on medical chart entries were taken from a 1-year retrospective longitudinal chart review for five adults with severe to profound mental retardation and comorbid gastrointestinal or musculoskeletal conditions.

that can be examined through clinical research with this population. Are people with severe disabilities insensitive to pain? If not, then, in the absence of the ability to verbalize pain experiences, how do these individuals reliably signal the experience of pain? Research on presumed pain insensitivity in people with mental retardation has been guided by previous research with other clinical populations such as typically developing infants, about whom clinicians and care providers have in the past held similar beliefs regarding the importance of verbal self-reports of pain and the presumed absence of pain in the absence of such self-reports.

EMPIRICAL STUDIES OF PAIN SENSITIVITY AND PAIN EXPRESSION

Are people with mental retardation insensitive to pain? How do they express pain if they feel it? These are difficult questions that focus on essentially subjective experiences in people who generally lack the ability to tell us about them in a conventional manner. Similar questions have been posed and addressed in the area of pediatrics concerning preverbal neonates and infants. A previous bias in pediatrics held that neonates and infants had only limited sensitivity to pain. This bias was presumably related in part to the absence of verbal self-reports of pain in neonates and infants. That is, a general reliance on verbal self-reports of pain as the gold standard of pain assessment led practitioners to believe that, in the absence of such reports, pain either could not be identified or likely was not present. This bias has been diminished as a result of research demonstrating that neonates and infants reliably display nonverbal signs of pain and thus can be shown to be sensitive to pain and to have pain experiences in association with known pain sources. Behaviors that even preterm infants have been noted to display in response to painful stimuli include a variety of facial actions, withdrawal, and cry. These nonverbal pain signs have been validated through association with objective physiological signs of pain and distress (Craig, 1992; Grunau, Oberlander, Holsti, & Whitfield, 1998; Johnston & Strada, 1986). Several standardized pain rating scales incorporating these nonverbal behaviors have been developed and are now part of standard clinical practice for use with neonates and infants.

Researchers have used the techniques for measuring nonverbal pain signs in infants as methods for identifying specific indices or signs of pain in people with mental retardation. In a seminal study in this area, LaChapelle, Hadjistavropoulos, and Craig (1998) used the Facial Action Coding System (Ekman & Friesen, 1978) to measure the facial reactions of 40 adults with mental retardation (47% with moderate to profound levels of retardation) to routine intramuscular injection under blinded rating conditions. The intensity of objectively coded facial activity showed significant increases from baseline to injection, indicating a significant degree of pain sensitivity and nonverbal (facial action) pain expression in this group. Furthermore, the authors found no correlation between either the frequency or the intensity of facial activity in response to injection and degree of cognitive disability (as measured by IQ), indicating that degree of cognitive disability does not appear to moderate the ability to express pain nonverbally in the way that it likely moderates the verbal expressions of pain. This study provides evidence that not only refutes the commonly assumed pain insensitivity notion for people with mental retardation but also provides support for the utility of nonverbal behavioral signs as measures of pain in this population.

Once the shift has been made from a focus on whether a person is sensitive to pain to whether a person is currently expressing pain, consideration of the variety of potential forms of pain expression becomes important. Pain can be considered to be an emotional state, and, like other emotional states, pain can be expressed both *verbally* and *nonverbally*. Although most pain assessment procedures have relied heavily on verbal indices of pain (e.g., verbal self-report), the assessment of pain can be expanded to include a focus on nonverbal signs or behaviors that are reliably associated with pain states. This is consistent with two notions. First, assessment procedures should capitalize on an individual's available communication repertoire (Anand & Craig, 1996). Second, behavioral expressions of pain are merely a nonverbal form of self-report. Such an addition to the material available for the assessment of pain can be used to facilitate the development of tools for individuals with limited cognitive or communication abilities or both. Previous research has shown that a relatively distinct pattern of facial actions can be observed in relation to the experience of pain (Grunau et al., 1998; Prkachin, 1992). Furthermore, in addition to specific facial actions, a wide range of other nonverbal behaviors that have received similar research support as nonverbal indices of pain are viewed as potential external reflections of the internal pain state. Thus, a variety of nonverbal behaviors can be used to index the expression of pain among people whose disability constrains their ability to express pain verbally.

In a systematic series of seminal studies, McGrath, Breau, Stallard, and colleagues established the range of nonverbal behaviors that can be associated with pain experiences in children and adolescents with a variety of neurological impairments, including mental retardation (Breau, Finley, McGrath, & Camfield, 2002; Breau, McGrath, Camfield, & Finley, 2002; Breau, McGrath, Camfield, Rosmus, & Finley, 2000; McGrath, Rosmus, Camfield, Campbell, & Hennigar, 1998; Stallard, Williams, Velleman, Lenton, & McGrath, 2002; Stallard, Williams, Velleman, Lenton, McGrath, & Taylor, 2002). In these studies, 31 separate observable nonverbal behaviors were found to be associated with the full variety of pain sources that can occur in people with mental retardation of all levels of disability. These nonverbal behaviors were grouped into seven subcategories: Vocal Behaviors (e.g., moaning, crying), Eating/Sleeping Behaviors (e.g., eats less, increased sleep), Social Personality Behaviors (e.g., fewer interactions, difficult to distract), Facial Expressions (e.g., grimace), Activity (e.g., fidgety), Body and Limbs (e.g., floppy, protects/favors part of body), and Physiological (e.g., shivering, sweating, gasping). Across these studies, these nonverbal behaviors 1) have been identified by caregivers (e.g., parents) as occurring in association with well-defined pain-related events (e.g., gastrostomy tube insertions, gastrointestinal illness); 2) could be used to distinguish pain from nonspecific distress (e.g., unwanted self-care, feared noises); 3) could be used to identify the presence of acute pain that occurs as a result of medical procedures; and 4) could be used to identify both a set of common pain signs that tends to be elicited by painful experiences in this population and also individualized sets of specific pain profiles that tend to recur within individuals over time in response to painful experiences.

Because the nonverbal pain signs identified by the McGrath et al. studies were developed based on relatively small samples ($n = 20-72$ participants) of children and adolescents, only a percentage of whom had severe to profound mental retardation, Bodfish, Harper, Deacon, and Symons (2001) sought to establish the validity of these items for the assessment of potential pain signs in adults with severe to profound mental retardation. In this study, the 31 nonverbal behaviors identified in the original McGrath study (McGrath et al., 1998) were used to screen a sample of 304 adults (mean age = 36.1 years) with severe to profound levels of mental retardation who resided in an inpatient residential setting. A "specific pain condition" subset of 81 cases was identified through medical chart diagnoses of known pain conditions (e.g., gastrointestinal disorder, musculoskeletal disorder) that required ongoing medical treatment and that had persisted for a minimum of 6 months. Care providers for all participants (nurses and nurses' aides) who were familiar with the participants (i.e., had a minimum of 6 months of daily interaction with the participant) were asked to endorse all of the behaviors listed that the participant in question had displayed during a presumed pain-related experience. A subset of 4 of the 31 items was excluded from analyses because endorsement had occurred at least monthly in less than 20% of all cases. Sixteen of the remaining items (including items from all seven of the nonverbal behavior domains identified in the McGrath et al. studies) were found both to occur frequently in at least 20% of cases and to distinguish specific pain condition cases from the remainder of the sample (Table 11.1). These results validate the findings of the McGrath et al. studies, and also indicate that a variety of nonverbal behaviors can be used to identify potential pain experiences in adults with severe to profound mental retardation.

Table 11.1. The frequency of occurrence of the 31 nonverbal pain signs from the Non-Communicating Children's Pain Checklist (NCCPC) in a sample of adults with severe to profound levels of mental retardation ($N = 304$).

NCCPC Item	Never	> Monthly	Monthly	Weekly	Daily	> Hourly	Hourly
Vocal							
Moaning, whining, whimpering (fairly soft)*	39.0%	13.0%	9.0%	13.0%	20.0%	2.7%	3.3%
Crying (moderately loud)*	45.0%	16.0%	12.3%	17.0%	9.0%	0.3%	0.3%
Screaming/yelling (very loud)*	30.9%	13.5%	11.5%	18.2%	21.2%	3.4%	1.4%
A specific sound or vocalization for pain "word," cry, type of "laugh"	33.0%	17.3%	15.0%	17.3%	15.0%	1.0%	1.3%
Eating/Sleeping							
Eats less, not interested in food	36.2%	21.9%	13.8%	20.6%	7.5%	0.0%	0.0%
Increase in sleep	41.9%	27.1%	11.3%	13.0%	6.7%	0.0%	0.0%
Decrease in sleep	45.2%	30.0%	12.4%	9.9%	2.5%	0.0%	0.0%
Social/Personality							
Not cooperating, cranky, irritable*	13.3%	19.5%	17.6%	27.2%	18.6%	1.7%	2.3%
Less interaction, withdrawn*	25.2%	23.5%	10.4%	20.1%	17.5%	2.4%	1.0%
Seeks comfort or physical closeness	28.3%	16.0%	7.7%	16.0%	28.3%	2.0%	1.7%
Difficult to distract, not able to pacify*	25.9%	22.9%	13.6%	19.9%	13.9%	2.3%	1.7%
Facial Expression of Pain (Cringe, Grimace)							
Cringe/grimace*	30.2%	21.1%	15.1%	18.8%	13.1%	0.3%	1.3%
Furrowed brow*	41.5%	19.3%	14.3%	15.3%	8.3%	0.3%	1.0%
Change in eyes, including eyes closed tight, eyes opened wide, eyes as if frowning*	33.9%	16.1%	11.7%	22.2%	13.8%	0.0%	2.4%
Turn down of mouth, not smiling	27.0%	22.3%	13.0%	19.0%	17.3%	0.3%	1.0%
Lips pucker up tight, pout or quiver*	53.2%	14.3%	8.9%	12.3%	9.9%	0.3%	1.0%
Clenches/grinds teeth, thrusts tongue*	52.0%	15.2%	5.4%	8.5%	15.5%	1.7%	1.7%

Activity							
Not moving, less active, quiet	29.6%	27.9%	7.4%	16.2%	13.8%	2.7%	2.4%
Jumping around, agitated, fidgety	38.1%	15.7%	9.4%	15.4%	13.4%	4.0%	4.0%
Body and Limbs							
Floppy	68.9%	9.0%	3.7%	5.0%	11.4%	1.0%	1.0%
Stiff, spastic, tense, rigid	41.7%	11.3%	7.3%	9.7%	21.0%	3.3%	5.7%
Gestures/touches part of body that hurts	63.6%	11.5%	12.1%	7.4%	4.0%	0.7%	0.7%
Protects/guards part of body that hurts*	58.6%	18.9%	12.2%	6.4%	2.4%	0.3%	1.0%
Flinches or moves body part away, sensitive to touch*	45.7%	21.7%	14.7%	8.3%	5.7%	1.3%	2.7%
Moves body to show pain (e.g., head back, arms down, curls up)	58.4%	18.8%	10.7%	6.4%	5.0%	0.7%	0.0%
Physiological							
Shivering	73.6%	13.0%	3.7%	3.3%	6.4%	0.0%	0.0%
Change in color, pallor	60.4%	22.2%	10.4%	3.4%	3.7%	0.0%	0.0%
Sweating, perspiring	57.4%	19.8%	10.4%	6.0%	5.4%	0.3%	0.7%
Tears*	56.5%	18.9%	11.9%	10.3%	2.3%	0.0%	0.0%
Sharp intake of breath, gasping*	73.1%	10.6%	4.9%	4.3%	6.6%	0.3%	0.0%
Breath-holding*	87.9%	4.0%	2.3%	2.0%	3.3%	0.3%	0.0%

*These items discriminated the subset of cases with a specific pain condition (gastrointestinal disorder and/or muscle-skeletal disorder) ($n = 81$) from the remainder of the cases ($p < .05$).

Development of Pain Assessment Tools for Children with Mental Retardation

Researchers have used the array of nonverbal behaviors that have been found to be potential pain signals to construct empirically derived and psychometrically sound clinical assessment scales for the routine measurement of pain in people with mental retardation. Giusiano, Jimeno, Collignon, and Chau (1995), McGrath et al. (1998), and Hunt et al. (2004) have developed separate pain assessments tools for use with children with mental retardation, each focusing on specific sets of observable nonverbal behaviors that can be used to signal pain. Bodfish et al. (2001) have extended this work to develop an empirically derived clinical assessment scale and pain examination procedure for people with severe to profound mental retardation.

Giusiano et al. (1995) and Collignon and Giusiano (2001) developed an observational scale for assessing pain in children with CP based on behaviors considered to be associated with pain by a group of physicians (Evaluation Scale for Pain in Cerebral Palsy). The items included on the scale were various facial expressions, cry behaviors, movement and posture changes, and change in social behaviors. The behaviors identified were those induced by a specific, brief invasive procedure and typically observed in a physical examination type of setting. This type of pain experience may be considered more reflective of acute pain than chronic, long-term pain. Further research is needed to establish the reliability and validity of this scale, its applicability in populations other than children with CP, and its validity for pain other than acute pain, as well as the practicality of this scale in routine clinical settings.

McGrath et al. (1998) generated items for the original version of the Non-Communicating Children's Pain Checklist (NCCPC) from interviews with 20 parents of children with CP. Subsequently, Breau et al. (2000) examined the reliability and validity of the NCCPC as a pain assessment instrument by having parents of 54 children with mental retardation prospectively assess whether the items from the NCCPC were present or absent in four situations: acute pain, long-term pain, a nonpainful but distressing situation, and when the child was calm. On average, NCCPC items were more than four times more likely to be reported by parents during pain states. Furthermore, although the total number of NCCPC items did not differentiate pain states from distress states, scores for the Eating/Sleeping and the Body & Limbs subscales did discriminate pain from distress states. Evaluation of the psychometric properties of the checklist was also conducted, and the checklist was found to have acceptable levels of internal consistency and test-retest reliability. To examine the validity of the scale as a measure of postoperative pain, Breau, Finley, et al. (2002) evaluated a postoperative version of the NCCPC (NCCPC-PV) that added a 4-point ordinal scale for rating the frequency of occurrence of each of the NCCPC items. A sample of 24 children with mental retardation was rated both before and after surgery by parents, research assistants, and nurses; total scores for the NCCPC-PV were significantly higher postoperatively and did not differ significantly by observer. Furthermore, acceptable levels of internal consistency, interrater reliability, and sensitivity/specificity were found for the NCCPC-PV. Thus, the NCCPC is a rigorously developed and psychometrically sound clinical rating scale that can measure validly the variety of pain sources routinely encountered by children with mental retardation (procedural pain, acute pain, long-term pain).

Hunt and colleagues (2004) developed the Paediatric Pain Profile (PPP) as a clinical rating scale of nonverbal pain behaviors that can be used with children with severe to profound mental retardation. Interviews combined with question-naires from parents of 121 children with severe to profound levels of mental re-tardation were used to develop a list of 56 cues taken to be indicative of pain in this group. Subsequent item analysis and psychometric testing were used to refine this list of potential nonverbal behavioral cues into a 20-item clinical rating scale (the PPP). Subsequently, the validity of the PPP as a pain assessment instrument was evaluated by having parents of 29 children with severe to profound levels of mental retardation provide videotapes of their children in specific pain and non-pain states that were then rated by trained observers using the PPP, and also by ex-amining the relation between PPP ratings and salivary cortisol levels (a marker of stress) during presumed pain states. PPP ratings were found to be stable across raters, to indicate different levels of pain, and to be significantly positively corre-lated with cortisol levels. In a further study, Hunt et al. (2004) replicated the find-ings of significant internal consistency and interrater reliability of the PPP in a new sample of 140 children (mean age = 9 years, 11 months) with mental retardation (median Vineland Adaptive Behavior Composite age equivalent = 7 years; 90% of cases had multiple physical disabilities). Hunt et al. (2004) then demonstrated that mean PPP scores for a subsample of 41 of the children were significantly greater before administration of an analgesic than after, and that the PPP was a practical and sensitive means of assessing postoperative pain in an individualized manner in a subsample of 30 children who received gastrointestinal ($n = 14$) or orthope-dic ($n = 16$) surgeries. In all, this impressive line of clinical studies demonstrated that the PPP is reliable and valid and can be practically used for the clinical as-sessment of pain in children with severe disabilities.

The Pain and Discomfort Scale for Adults with Mental Retardation

To date, neither the NCCPC nor the PPP has been examined in the context of pain assessment or management in adults with mental retardation. Although it is rea-sonable to assume that these scales, developed and validated for children, would also be applicable in the case of adults, this remains to be established. Because of their advanced age and potentially advanced disease state (e.g., neurodegenera-tive disease), it is likely that the assessment of pain in adults with severe neuro-logical impairments is complicated by the presence of chronic pain from various sources. If so, then assessment methods designed to measure acute pain in chil-dren may be relatively less sensitive to pain in adults. Furthermore, standardized assessment of pain in clinical settings is often achieved through the use of a spe-cific set of physical examination steps designed to both elicit and localize potential pain. This is most important in cases of chronic pain, in which the patient may de-velop specific postures or activities to mitigate pain experience (e.g., diminished arm movement related to shoulder or arm joint pain secondary to osteoarthritis) and in which specific manipulations can help identify pain that is otherwise masked (e.g., flexing and extending the arm at its joints). For these reasons, our group developed an adaptation of the NCCPC for use with adults with severe to profound levels of mental retardation (the Pain and Discomfort Scale [PADS]) and a standardized pain assessment procedure for use with the pain scale (the Pain Examination Procedure [PEP]) (Bodfish et al., 2001).

The PADS was developed using the items from the NCCPC (McGrath et al., 1998). The NCCPC has been shown to have adequate reliability and validity characteristics for a clinical rating scale (Breau et al., 2000). The NCCPC items 1) were specifically selected for the identification of pain in people with developmental disabilities and 2) focused on nonverbal behaviors, and the NCCPC scale 3) had been empirically derived and 4) had adequate psychometric properties. We included the 31 NCCPC items as test pool items on the preliminary version of the PADS. We added a 4-point Likert severity rating scale for use in scoring the severity/intensity of each item. This preliminary version was used to screen a sample of 304 adolescents and adults with moderate, severe, or profound mental retardation. Forty-five cases from this sample were retested 1–2 weeks after initial testing to provide data for test-retest reliability analyses. Our intent with this initial data set was to identify those test items that met or exceeded specific, a priori psychometric criteria. Items were retained if 1) the item was endorsed as present for at least 20% of the sample, 2) reliability for the item was greater than 0.60, and 3) the item-total correlation for the item was greater than 0.60. Based on analyses for this initial sample, 3 items were dropped because they were not directly observable in an examination context (eating less, increased sleep, decreased sleep), and 11 items were dropped because they did not meet one or more of the psychometric criteria. This left a revised item pool of 17 items. Based on consultation with pain researchers who had used the Facial Action Coding System to identify specific nonverbal signs of pain in children and in people with developmental disabilities (Craig, 1992; LaChapelle et al., 1998; Oberlander, Gilbert, et al., 1999), we included one new item that focused on specific facial actions (mouth open/lips separated). This left a final revised pool of 18 items for the PADS.

Following this item selection phase, we revised the PADS in two other ways. First, we changed the Likert scoring scheme for item scoring from a generic 4-point severity rating to a more specific 5-point scale that provides specific anchors based on ease of detection and frequency of occurrence. Second, we developed a standardized examination procedure (the PEP) for use with the PADS that was similar to the standard examination procedures used to elicit and localize pain in people without disabilities.

We examined the reliability of the PADS as administered in routine service settings for adults with severe to profound mental retardation in a sample of 65 adults (mean age = 33.6 years; range, 22–68 years) with severe to profound mental retardation (70% of the sample had multiple physical disabilities and comorbid medical conditions). We found that, across a set of four raters, the PADS had acceptable levels of reliability for a clinical rating scale (mean interrater reliability for PADS total score = 0.82; range of interrater reliability across PADS subdomains = 0.64–0.93). We have also examined the validity of the PADS scale and the PEP standardized assessment procedure in a series of validity studies examining a variety of potential pain sources (everyday pain associated with completing activities of daily living, acute pain associated with routine medical procedures, and chronic pain associated with comorbid medical conditions) in samples of adults with severe to profound levels of mental retardation (Figure 11.3).

For people with mental retardation and multiple severe physical disabilities (e.g., spasticity, cerebral palsy, congenital limb malformations), everyday activities

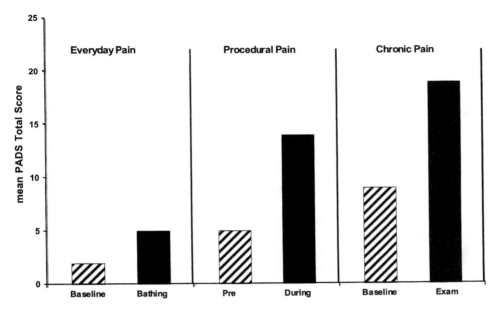

Figure 11.3. Results from PADS assessments for adults with severe to profound mental retardation for a variety of clinical pain sources. *Left,* "Everyday Pain": assessment of patients with multiple severe physical disabilities and chronic painful medical conditions (*n* = 8) both before and during bathing sessions. *Center,* "Procedural Pain": assessment of patients (*n* = 22) both before and during acute medical procedures. *Right,* "Chronic Pain": a comparison of patients with chronic gastrointestinal or musculoskeletal medical conditions or both (*n* = 9) at rest and during the physical examination manipulations of the PEP.

such as bathing and dressing can be sources of significant pain given the amount of movement and exertion involved in even passively assisting with these tasks. In a sample of eight adults with severe to profound mental retardation and multiple physical disabilities, PADS was able to detect significantly increased pain signs during bathing activities compared to a baseline rest condition (see Figure 11.3, left panel).

Individuals with severe to profound mental retardation also frequently undergo a variety of routine medical procedures that can be sources of acute pain (Oberlander, Gilbert, et al., 1999). This includes procedures such as feeding or enteroscopy tube insertions and cleanings, implantation and adjustment of vagal nerve stimulators, frequent blood draws for medical tests, placement of intrathecal baclofen pumps, splinting/casting for contractures, and range-of-motion exercises. We examined acute responses to medical procedures in a sample of 22 adults with severe to profound mental retardation using the PADS assessment both before and during the procedure. The PADS total score was significantly elevated for this group during the medical procedures, suggesting that the PADS was sensitive to acute pain or discomfort reactions in this population (see Figure 11.3, center panel). On average, these procedures produced a 50% increase in observable pain signs. Inspection of individual subject data for this study revealed clear evidence of individual differences in apparent pain reaction, as well as evidence of idiosyncratic modes of pain expression across the participants.

As noted previously, chronic pain conditions may be a particularly important issue for people with severe to profound mental retardation and multiple comorbid physical disabilities, medical conditions, or both. Often the presence of chronic pain can be uncovered in clinical settings through the use of a physical examination with joint manipulations to detect specific pain locations. For this reason, we examined the utility of the PEP in a sample of adults with severe to profound mental retardation and concomitant physical disabilities (e.g., CP, spasticity) and chronic medical conditions (e.g., gastroesophageal reflux, osteoarthritis) (n = 9). During resting baseline conditions, few signs of pain were observable in this group. In contrast, increased pain signs were clearly observed for a majority of the patients (6 of 9) during the brief PEP (see Figure 11.3, right panel). This indicates that the combined PADS + PEP procedure is sensitive to potential signs of chronic pain in individuals with severe to profound mental retardation and also highlights the importance of routine clinical examinations to screen for chronic pain in this group.

In addition to being useful for identifying the presence of pain, standardized pain instruments can also be used to evaluate the efficacy of specific pain management treatments. This is especially critical in the case of people with mental retardation and fragile medical conditions, for whom the addition of potent pain medication treatments is a complex pharmacological issue that must be handled on an empirical basis. For this reason, a sample of 28 adults with profound mental retardation who had medical conditions (e.g., reflux, osteoarthritis) were examined during a baseline (no treatment) condition and then following either medication or nonmedication treatments for pain/discomfort. In all cases, there was evidence of a change in the PADS total score from baseline to treatment, indicating an apparent treatment effect on expressed pain behaviors. Furthermore, the PADS results could be used to optimize treatment selection and scheduling on an individualized basis (e.g., scheduling of daily doses or matching nonmedication treatments to "peak" pain periods during the day).

Together, these studies indicate that the PADS provides a valid measure of nonverbal signs of pain in adults with severe developmental disabilities. We have also found that the PADS and the PEP can be applied by direct health care workers in the course of routine service delivery. On average, a PADS + PEP examination takes trained personnel approximately 10 minutes to administer. Furthermore, our clinical studies suggest that the PADS is sensitive to the variety of sources of pain that are clinically significant for this population, including everyday pain, acute pain responses, and chronic pain. Also, the PADS appears to be sensitive to the effects of treatments directed to alleviate pain. Because patients often manifest idiosyncratic sets of pain signs from within the PADS pain sign pool, the PADS can be adapted to construct an individualized "pain profile" based on repeated observations that confirm a specific pattern for a given individual. Such a clinical adaptation of the PADS often shortens each individual assessment session because only a subset of pain signs are probed, and it also may produce more sensitive assessments of changes in pain state over time or as a result of treatment.

APPLICATIONS OF STANDARDIZED NONVERBAL PAIN SIGNS ASSESSMENT SYSTEMS TO ROUTINE CLINICAL CARE SETTINGS

What do you find when you apply valid methods for measuring pain in people with mental retardation? How often is pain a clinical finding? What are the most likely sources of pain for this group? Does better assessment of pain lead to better treatment? Unfortunately, very little information is available with respect to clinical outcomes of pain management services for adults with mental retardation.

This likely reflects the fact that pain assessment and treatment remains an under-provided service in most clinical settings for this population. However, a few published reports involve the systematic assessment of pain using validated measures of nonverbal pain expression in routine clinical settings for people with mental retardation (Breau, Camfield, McGrath, & Finley, 2003; Hunt et al., 2004; Schwartz, Engel, & Jensen, 1999). Findings from these reports provide information on risk factors for the development of pain, the incidence of pain cases, the prevalence of pain reports in these cases, and common sources of pain in the population. Information from these sources, along with information from the empirical studies of pain sensitivity and pain expression in people with mental retardation, can be used to direct the future development of pain services for these individuals.

Schwartz et al. (1999) examined a series of 93 adults (mean age = 38 years; range = 18–76 years) with CP seen at outpatient medical clinics for CP or served at community group homes for people with developmental disabilities. The majority of the patients had quadriplegia caused by their CP (84%), 54% had spastic CP, and the majority of the patients were fully nonambulatory (94%). Although the majority of the patients studied had only mild levels of mental retardation, the severity of their impairment related to CP compares favorably with that seen in other subgroups of mental retardation with comorbid CP and thus provides a reasonable basis of comparison for individuals with mental retardation and CP as a whole. Furthermore, their mild degree of cognitive impairment made it possible for them to self-report on aspects of their pain experience and thus provide a rich account of the phenomenology of pain in this population that cannot be obtained directly from people with more severe cognitive deficits who cannot self-report. Sixty-seven percent of this group reported one or more areas of chronic pain (minimum of 3 months' duration). Lower extremity pain (66%) and back pain (63%) were the most common complaints, and other frequent pain locations included the neck/shoulder (45%) and hip (39%); the least frequent pain locations were the head and abdomen. Overall, patients reported an average of three distinct pain locations. Pain duration for this group ranged between 8 and 15 years. The majority of the sample reported that their pain occurred on a daily basis. For most, the intensity of pain was rated as mild to moderate, but for a substantial minority (20%), severe daily pain was reported. A variety of pain-exacerbating factors (fatigue, stress, weather changes) and pain-relieving factors (exercise, stretching, resting, massage) were identified.

Breau et al. (2003) examined a series of 94 children and adolescents (mean age = 10 years; range = 3–18 years) with moderate to profound mental retardation who lived either in their natural homes or in group homes. Although the sample consisted of children with disabilities, whose pain experiences may be different from those occurring in adults with disabilities, the range of disabilities studied provides some basis of comparison to adults with severe disabilities. The children were followed prospectively for a period of 1 month. During this time period, 78% of the children experienced pain at least once, and the average pain duration for this time period was 9 hours per week. Common sources of pain were accidental pain (30%), gastrointestinal pain (22%), infections (20%), and musculoskeletal pain (19%). Children with the fewest abilities had significantly more nonaccidental pain, whereas children with more abilities had significantly more accidental pain. These results are very similar to those reported by Hunt et al. (2004), who examined a series of 140 children and adolescents with severe to profound levels of mental retardation and severe physical and medical complications. In this sample, 42% of the children had pain that was rated as severe or very severe that occurred all the time or at least on a daily basis, with the primary pain sources being gastrointestinal (39%) and musculoskeletal (24%).

As a final consideration with respect to the clinical application of pain assessment systems, it is important to discern if systematic assessment efforts can be practically tied to improved treatment outcomes in routine settings. Although no studies to date have addressed this question directly for people with mental retardation, a study of the systematic pain assessment and treatment of adults with late-stage dementia residing in nursing homes provides a reasonable basis of comparison (Kovach et al., 1999). Although people with dementia exhibit normal trajectories of early adaptive development, their late-life neurodegenerative disease renders them functionally similar to adults with mental retardation in terms of cognitive and communication abilities. Like adults with mental retardation, adults with late-stage dementia are at an increased risk for significant pain sources but have limited to no means of expressing pain in a conventional manner.

Kovach et al. (1999) examined the impact of a systematic pain training and pain services program in a sample of 104 adults with end-stage dementia residing in 32 long-term care facilities. This involved a comprehensive four-component training program for nursing staff on the use of a clinical pain service protocol (the Assessment of Discomfort in Dementia [ADD] protocol) developed specifically for use with nonverbal individuals with dementia. The training program covered nonverbal pain assessment, pharmacological and nonpharmacological pain treatments, policy development, staff competencies, and quality improvement. Examination of outcomes revealed that the use of the ADD protocol was associated with 1) a significant decrease in directly observed pain/discomfort signs in patients, and 2) a significant increase in both the use of nonpharmacological pain treatments and the scheduled use of analgesics. Results of questionnaires completed by the nurses involved in the training and program implementation at each facility revealed that the majority found the protocol to be "helpful" (44%) or "very helpful" (44%), although some (12%) believed that it "had no impact." Open-ended responses on these questionnaires indicated that problems nurses had in implementing the protocol were a lack of time, problems getting all staff sufficiently trained on the protocol, and problems related to staff resistance to change. The results provide support for the notion that the pain needs of people with cognitive disabilities associated with dementia can be identified and treated using a standardized nonverbal pain assessment and routine pain treatment approach. However, the results also indicate that a variety of nonpatient and nonpain factors can influence the clinical management of pain in routine settings, including staff attitudes and staff willingness to accept this "new" model of pain awareness and treatment for persons who do not communicate pain in a conventional manner. This is perhaps related to the fact that whereas verbal reports of pain to caregivers are easy to discern, unconventional, nonverbal pain expressions require not only a change in beliefs about how pain is communicated but also a change in response effort to ensure that normally unnoticed nonverbal behaviors are identified.

How can the findings of these studies be translated to guide the routine care of people with mental retardation? First, given research that has shown that detection of pain in this population depends upon the monitoring of nonverbal behaviors, the practicality of this approach needs to be established. Based on the studies of pain assessment outcomes just reviewed, it is clear that nonverbal expressions by people with severe disabilities that signal pain can be monitored in routine settings. These studies involved ongoing pain assessment by typical care providers (parents, nurses, nurses' aides, etc.) (Breau et al., 2003; Hunt et al., 2004) as well as more formal examinations of pain in clinical settings by health care workers (Hunt et al., 2004, Kovach et al., 1999; Schwartz et al., 1999). Second, findings about the prevalence, duration, severity, and sources of pain can be used to determine the parameters of pain monitoring efforts in clinical settings. The findings reviewed indicate that a significant percentage of people with severe to profound mental retardation and concomitant physical and medical conditions experience clinically significant intensities of pain on a daily basis. This indicates that pain monitoring should be a frequent, continuous, and proactive process in clinical settings that serve this population. Furthermore, there is consistent evidence of common risk factors for and sources of pain in this population, including gastrointestinal disorders and musculoskeletal disorders. Thus, individualized routine pain monitoring and management can be designed based on the presence and absence of these conditions. Finally, it is important to recognize that monitoring of nonverbal behaviors that can signal pain, although valid and clinically important, is not the "norm" in routine clinical settings. The original points discussed concerning how care providers come to conceptualize pain experience in people with disabilities are important to consider because care providers' attitudes can determine the fidelity with which pain services are implemented. Even empirically derived and appropriately individualized best practices for pain assessment and management will not achieve optimal patient outcomes in settings where care providers continue to believe that people with mental retardation are insensitive to pain or that pain management is not a priority issue.

CONCLUSIONS

The paradox of pain in individuals with severe to profound levels of mental retardation is that, although there is no evidence that such individuals are insensitive to pain, and in fact they frequently experience pain, common conceptualizations about neurological impairments and cognitive deficits can lead care providers to fail to recognize the significance of pain for this population. A similar paradox existed years ago in the field of pediatrics, and there common misunderstandings about infants' sensitivity to pain were addressed by shifting the focus from pain sensation to pain expression. Following the lead of infant pain research, workers in the field of mental retardation have now firmly established the validity and utility of assessing pain in people with mental retardation using an array of nonverbal pain behaviors. Simply put, nonverbal expressions of pain are now considered to be how people with disabilities self-report their pain. Furthermore, several systems for monitoring nonverbal pain signs in routine service settings have now been developed for this population, and these have been shown to be reliable, valid, and practical as clinical tools. Armed with the knowledge of nonverbal pain expression and the tools to measure it, the task becomes one of applying these tools to teach care providers that people with mental retardation are sensitive to pain and to develop pain management services to ensure that those who are in pain receive adequate pain treatments.

REFERENCES

Anand, K.S., & Craig, K.D. (1996). New perspectives in the definition of pain. *Pain, 67,* 3–6.

Biersdorff, K.K. (1991). Pain insensitivity and indifference: Alternative explanations for some medical catastrophes. *Mental Retardation, 29,* 359–362.

Bodfish, J.W., Harper, V.N., Deacon, J.R., & Symons, F.J. (2001, May). Identifying and measuring pain in persons with developmental disabilities: A manual for the *Pain And Discomfort Scale* (PADS). Available from Western Carolina Center Research Reports, Western Carolina Center, 300 Enola Road, Morganton, NC 28655.

Breau, L.M., Camfield, C.S., McGrath, P.J., & Finley, G.A. (2003). The incidence of pain in children with severe cognitive impairments. *Archives of Pediatrics and Adolescent Medicine, 157,* 1226.

Breau, L.M., Finley, G.A., McGrath, P.J., & Camfield, C.S. (2002). Validation of the Non-communicating Children's Pain Checklist–Postoperative Version. *Anesthesiology, 96,* 528–535.

Breau, L.M., McGrath, P.J., Camfield, C.S., & Finley, G.A. (2002). Psychometric properties of the Non-Communicating Children's Pain Checklist–Revised. *Pain, 99,* 349–357.

Breau, L.M., McGrath, P.J., Camfield, C., Rosmus, C., & Finley, G.A. (2000). Preliminary validation of an observation pain checklist for cognitively-impaired, non-communicating persons. *Developmental Medicine and Child Neurology, 42,* 609–616.

Casamassimo, P.S. (1981). Clinical investigation of relative indifference to pain among adolescent mental retardates. *Journal of Dental Child, 48,* 468–469.

Chambers, C.T., Giesbrecht, K., Craig, D, Bennett, S.M., & Huntsman, E. (1999). A comparison of faces scales for the measurement of pediatric pain: Children's and parents' ratings. *Pain, 83,* 25–35.

Collignon, P., & Giusiano, B. (2001). Validation of a pain evaluation scale for patients with severe cerebral palsy. *European Journal of Pain, 5,* 433–442.

Couston, T.A. (1954) Indifference to pain in low-grade mental defectives. *British Medical Journal, 1,* 1128–1129.

Craig, K.D. (1992). The facial expression of pain. *APS Journal, 1,* 153–162.

Ekman, P., & Friesen, W. (1978). *Investigator's guide to the Facial Action Coding System.* Palo Alto, CA: Consulting Psychologists Press.

Fanurik, D., Koh, J.K., Schmitz, M.L., Harrison, R.D., & Conrad, T.M. (1999). Children with cognitive impairment: Parent report of pain and coping. *Journal of Developmental and Behavioral Pediatrics, 20,* 228–234.

Gadish, H.S., & Gonzalez, J. (1988). Factors affecting nurses' decisions to medicate pediatric postoperative patients in pain [Abstract]. In *Proceedings of the First International Symposium on Pediatric Pain.* Seattle: IASP Press.

Giusiano, B., Jimeno, M.T., Collignon, P., & Chau, Y. (1995). Utilization of a neural network in the elaboration of an evaluation scale for pain in cerebral palsy. *Methods of Information in Medicine, 34,* 498–502.

Grunau, R.E., Oberlander, T., Holsti, L., & Whitfield, M.F. (1998). Bedside application of the bedside Neonatal Facial Coding System in pain assessment of premature neonates. *Pain, 76,* 277–286.

Hadjistavropoulos, T., LaChapelle, D.L., MacLeod, F.K., Hale, C., O'Rourke, N., & Craig, K.D. (1998). Cognitive functioning and pain reaction in hospitalized elders. *Pain and Research Management, 3,* 145–151.

Hadjistavropoulos, T., LaChapelle, D.L., MacLeod, F.K., Snider, B., & Craig, K.D. (2000). Measuring movement-exacerbated pain in cognitively impaired frail elders. *Clinical Journal of Pain, 16,* 54–63.

Hunt, A., Goldman, A., Seers, K., Crichton, N., Mastroyannopoulou, K., Moffat, V., et al. (2004). Clinical validation of the Paediatric Pain Profile. *Developmental Medicine and Child Neurology, 46*, 9–18.

Jancar, J., & Speller, C.J. (1994). Fatal intestinal obstruction in the mentally handicapped. *Journal of Intellectual Disability Research, 38*, 413–422.

Johnston, C.C., & Strada, M.E. (1986). Acute pain response in infants: A multidimensional description. *Pain, 24*, 373–382.

Kovach, C.R., Weissman, D.E., Griffie, J., Matson, S., & Muchka, S. (1999). Assessment and treatment of discomfort for people with later-stage dementia. *Journal of Pain Symptom Management, 18*, 412–419.

LaChapelle, D.L., Hadjistavropoulos, T., & Craig, K.D. (1998). Pain measurement in persons with intellectual disabilities. *Clinical Journal of Pain, 15*, 13–23.

Madonic, M.J. (1954). Congenital insensitiveness to pain. *Journal of Nervous and Mental Disease, 120*, 87–88.

Maurer, H., & Newbrough, J.R. (1987). Facial expression of mentally retarded and nonretarded children: II. Recognition by nonretarded adults with varying experience with mental retardation. *American Journal of Mental Deficiency, 91*, 511–515.

McGrath, P.J., Rosmus, C., Camfield, C., Campbell, M.A., & Hennigar, A. (1998). Behaviours caregivers use to determine pain in non-verbal, cognitively impaired individuals. *Developmental Medicine and Child Neurology, 40*, 340–343.

Merskey, H., & Bogduk, N. (1994). *Classification of chronic pain: Descriptions of chronic pain syndromes and definitions of pain terms* (2nd ed.). Seattle: IASP Press.

Oberlander, T.F., Gilbert, C.A., Chambers, C.T., O'Donnell, M.E., & Craig, K.D. (1999). Biobehavioral responses to acute pain in adolescents with a significant neurologic impairment. *Clinical Journal of Pain, 15*, 201–209.

Oberlander, T.F., & O'Donnell, M.E. (2001). Beliefs about pain among professionals working with children with significant neurologic impairment. *Developmental Medicine and Child Neurology, 43*, 136–140.

Oberlander, T.F., O'Donnell, M.E., & Montgomery, C.J. (1999). Pain in children with significant neurological impairment. *Developmental and Behavioral Pediatrics, 20*, 235–243.

Peine, H.A., Darvish, R., Adams, K., Blakesock, H., Jenson, W., & Osborne, J.G. (1995). Medical problems, maladaptive behaviors, and the developmentally disabled. *Behavioral Interventions, 10*, 149–159.

Prkachin, K.M. (1992). The consistency of facial expressions of pain: A comparison across modalities. *Pain, 51*, 297–306.

Roy, A., & Simon, G.B. (1987). Intestinal obstruction a cause of death in the mentally handicapped. *Journal on Mental Deficiency Research, 31*, 193–197.

Schechter, N.L. (1989). The undertreatment of pain in children: An overview. *Pediatric Clinics of North America, 36*, 781–794.

Schechter, N.L., & Allen, D.A. (1986). Physician's attitudes towards pain in children. *Journal of Developmental and Behavioral Pediatrics, 7*, 350–354.

Schwartz, L., Engel, J.M., & Jensen, M.P. (1999). Pain in persons with cerebral palsy. *Archives of Physical Medicine and Rehabilitation, 80*, 1243–1246.

Stallard, P., Williams, L., Velleman, R., Lenton, S., & McGrath, P.J. (2002). Brief report: Behaviors identified by caregivers to detect pain in noncommunicating children. *Journal of Paediatric Psychology, 27*, 209–214.

Stallard, P., Williams, L., Velleman, R., Lenton, S., McGrath, P.J., & Taylor, G. (2002). The development and evaluation of the Pain Indicator for Communicatively Impaired Children (PICIC). *Pain, 98*, 145–149.

Symons, F.J., Hinze, C., Sutton, K.A., & Bodfish, J.W. (1999, October). Pain management in developmental disabilities. Poster presented at the annual St. Amant Center Conference on Research & Applications Related to Developmental Disabilities, Winnipeg, Ontario, Canada.

Turnquist, K.M., & Engel, J.M. (1995). Occupational therapists' experiences and knowledge of pain in children. *Physical and Occupational Therapy in Pediatrics, 14*, 35–51.

Vortherms, R., Ryan, P., & Ward, S. (1992). Knowledge of, attitudes toward, and barriers to pharmacologic management of cancer pain in a statewide random sample of nurses. *Research in Nursing and Health, 15*, 459–466.

Watt-Watson, J.H. (1987). Nurses' knowledge of pain issues: A survey. *Journal of Pain and Symptom Management, 2*, 207–211.

12

PHARMACOLOGICAL MANAGEMENT OF PAIN IN CHILDREN AND YOUTH WITH SIGNIFICANT NEUROLOGICAL IMPAIRMENTS

Anna Taddio and Tim F. Oberlander

Pharmacological management of pain in children with disabilities is often complicated by the multiple medications used to manage accompanying conditions such as neurological impairment and its sequelae. Medications may be needed to manage seizures, gastrointestinal reflux, or infections, for example; and the combination of medications can have important and potentially adverse implications for effective pain management. Frequently pain management may just require an accurate diagnosis to determine the nature of pain (i.e., neuropathic, inflammatory) leading to selection of the appropriate medication. However, the combination of multiple unexpected pharmacological, enzymatic, genetic, and contextual variables (drug interactions) inherent to this setting may interfere with analgesic efficacy leading to analgesic failure. Knowledge of key pharmacological factors is required to reduce adverse outcomes and optimize pain management. This chapter reviews basic pharmacological approaches to pain management and the impact of analgesics in combination with typical medications used to manage neurological and gastrointestinal conditions, with a view toward illustrating the consequences of polypharmacy and implications this may have for successful pain management.

SETTING THE SCENE: A CLINICAL VIGNETTE

Richard is a 12-year-old with choreoathetoid cerebral palsy who also has gastroesophageal reflux, spasticity, dislocated hips, and a seizure and mood disorder. His cognitive ability is in the low average range, and he communicates effectively through a variety of monosyllabic words, facial expressions, and body movements. He experiences chronic bilateral hip and knee pain. He is fed both orally and via a gastrostomy tube. His medications include phenytoin, omeprazole, chlorpromazine, clonazepam, paroxetine, and salbutamol. In the 3 months preceding this clinic visit, his hip pain has worsened. He was treated with "as needed" ibuprofen and acetaminophen with codeine compound (Tylenol #2). Meperidine was recently added; however, his pain was not relieved. Richard's pain reduced his participation in activities of daily living (dressing, school, visits with friends) and his appetite; disrupted his sleep, mood, and mobility; and increased his rigidity and muscle tone.

In the year prior to his referral for multidisciplinary pain management, Richard's medications were being prescribed by a family physician, a psychiatrist, a pediatrician, and an orthopaedic surgeon across three cities and with no common venue for communication or case coordination. In fact, many of the members of his health care team were not aware of what the others were prescribing. Both his parents and his health care team were increasingly concerned about impact of the pain on his life and were frustrated with the apparent pharmacotherapeutic failure.

This vignette illustrates a number of key features frequently encountered when managing pain in children and youth with complex neurological impairments. First, as discussed elsewhere in this volume (see Chapter 5), pain is a component of daily life with a significant neurological impairment (SNI). Second, daily life with a SNI requires multiple and potentially conflicting medications; and third, despite a thoughtful and systematic approach to Richard's pain using medications that should have adequately managed the pain, the pain still persisted. What had gone wrong? What underlies such pharmacological failure, and what can be done? Analgesic failure may be secondary to pharmacological factors, such as inappropriate drug or dose selection for the type of pain, genetic factors inherent to the individual's capacity to metabolize medications, or the impact of use of multiple drugs that compete for metabolic and excretory pathways, as well as the neurological substrate underlying the SNI itself. Understanding and managing this analgesic failure is the focus of this chapter.

GENERAL APPROACH TO PHARMACOLOGICAL PAIN MANAGEMENT

The pharmacological management of pain requires an understanding of the origin of pain, how the child communicates pain, any previous experiences with pain and pain therapies, and any concerns that the child or family have about it (Rivard, 2001). There is no single agent that is appropriate for all clinical pain situations. In every case, the child's preferences, past experiences, underlying conditions, and concomitant drug therapy should be considered in the management of pain, just as they are commonly appreciated in other child health care settings (see Chapter 10). However, children with a SNI have increased opportunity for pain caused by underlying conditions that are associated with pain as well as painful medical interventions needed to treat them (Oberlander & Craig, 2003). At the outset, the pain management plan requires prestated objectives and outcomes that are specific to the individual and the current clinical condition. Identification of the cause of the pain involves careful and empirical evaluation that includes determination of exacerbating and mediating factors, and an understanding of the pathology or mechanisms contributing to the pain (e.g., neuropathic, inflammatory). It must be recognized, however, that even with all diagnostic avenues explored, the identification of the source of pain is not always possible. In this situation, pharmacological interventions may be used, carefully documenting beneficial or adverse effects. A key objective should be to reduce pain symptoms and improve everyday functioning.

   In an individual with a SNI, a reduction in pain does not always imply an improvement in functioning, as is typically expected for the general population. For example, in using an antispasticity agent to improve neuromuscular tone in a child with spastic quadriplegia, the drug may reduce pain but may also lead to reduced tone. Reduced tone may lead to diminished fine motor skills, reduced ability to stand and transfer, and apparent loss of muscle strength (M. O'Donnell, personal communication, 2005). This leads to even broader effects of increased distress and decreased independence. Continued evaluation of both the symptom and functional outcomes are therefore absolutely essential to any pain or symptom management intervention. Therefore, it is important to recognize that analgesics are chosen after consideration of not only the type and magnitude of pain but concurrent medications and desired outcomes as well. Overall, the success of pain management requires a clearly identified plan and coordinated communication and decision making among the affected individual, caregivers, and clinicians, as well as ongoing reevaluation of pain and of medication side effects.

Acute Pain Management

Acute pain, such as that caused by cutaneous medical procedures, is a common occurrence in children with SNIs. Examples of cutaneous procedures are venipuncture, intravenous cannulation, and intramuscular injection. Pain from procedures can be treated with topical local anesthetics, such as lidocaine-prilocaine (EMLA) cream, amethocaine gel, or liposomal lidocaine cream. For deeper cutaneous pain, such as that caused by lumbar puncture or biopsies, infiltration of local anesthesia via skin that has been previously anesthetized by topical local anesthesia can be performed.

In many situations, local anesthesia alone is insufficient for the management of procedural pain because of the presence of anxiety in the child, which leads to excessive movements and noncooperation. In these cases, additional sedative or analgesic drugs, or a combination, facilitate successful completion of procedures (Fanurik, 1999; Sacchetti et al., 2003). In some circumstances, sedation can be achieved by administering an agent already being used in the child (Sacchetti et al., 2003). This avoids concerns about how the drug will be tolerated. For example, in children taking benzodiazepines or phenothiazines, adequate sedation for procedures may be accomplished by giving the regular benzodiazepine or phenothiazine dose before the scheduled dose time, by administering a small supplemental dose, or by giving a slightly increased dose. Sedation with benzodiazepines causes amnesia, which is particularly useful for children who undergo repeated procedures. For patients with psychotic symptoms, droperidol is particularly useful (Sacchetti et al., 2003). Ketamine, a systemic analgesic, should be avoided in patients with psychiatric symptoms because it may cause emergence reactions (i.e., vivid dreams) that are frightening (Sacchetti et al., 2003). Nonpharmacologic methods of pain relief, such as positioning, distraction, cold or heat application, parental presence, and behavioral interventions, are also useful (Rivard, 2001; Oberlander & O'Donnell, 2001).

Subacute and Chronic Pain Management

The analgesic ladder developed by the World Health Organization (http://www .who.int/cancer/palliative/painladder/en/) as a strategy for the management of cancer pain has been extrapolated to non–cancer-related chronic pain (Gardner-Nix, 2003). This stepwise approach treats mild to severe pain using oral analgesics in the following order until analgesia is achieved: non-opioids (nonsteroidal anti-inflammatory drugs [NSAIDs], acetaminophen); mild opioids (codeine, oxycodone);

and strong opioids (morphine). Adjuvant medications such as topical capsaicin, tricyclic antidepressants, and anticonvulsants are added, as necessary, to improve analgesia. This three-step approach recommends that drugs be given "by the clock" rather than "on demand" and is reported to be effective in more than 80% of patients. Surgical intervention is recommended to provide further pain relief on appropriate nerves if drugs do not achieve the desired effects.

Systemic opioids are the mainstay of analgesia for severe pain. Opioids may be administered by intermittent doses, continuous subcutaneous or intravenous infusion, patient-controlled analgesia, or nurse/parent-controlled analgesia. Nurse/parent-controlled analgesia may be a preferred method over patient-controlled analgesia in children with SNIs because of their physical or cognitive disabilities, or both, which limit effective and safe self-administered analgesia (Lehr, 2003). Respiratory depression is a risk with these methods because self-administration of the dose may occur too frequently. Dosing limits can be programmed into the devices to minimize the risk of overdosing (Lehr, 2003). If patients are experiencing suboptimal analgesia using intravenous opioids, the accuracy of the delivery device and patency of the cannula should be closely examined before increasing the dose. In addition to opioid analgesia, moderate to severe pain can also be treated with local anesthetic blocks either peripherally, regionally, or centrally. Opioids can be added to centrally administered local anesthetic solutions in order to minimize sympathetic or motor blockade caused by local anesthetics.

Coanalgesic medications such as NSAIDs or local/regional analgesia may be coadministered with opioids to improve efficacy and decrease opioid requirements (Morton, 1999). NSAIDs are commonplace for postoperative analgesia management. They have a long duration of action, allow lower opioid doses (thus, fewer opioid-induced adverse effects) and more rapid weaning from opioids, and lack sedative and respiratory depression (Hamunen & Maunuksela, 1996; Morton, 1999). They are contraindicated, however, in patients with asthma, preexisting renal or gastrointestinal diseases, hypovolemia, and concomitant use of interacting drugs such as corticosteroids (Mercadante, 2005). In addition, the use of NSAIDs following orthopedic surgery is controversial because of animal data suggesting that they impair bone healing (Lehr, 2003). It is not clear if this occurs in humans, and additional research is required. Other than these well-known adverse effects, NSAIDs may be associated with drug-induced hepatic injury (Velayudham & Farrell, 2003) and cutaneous reactions, including psoriasis (Tsankov, Angelova, & Kazandjieva, 2000). Acetaminophen also has opioid-sparing effects and is safe when used for postoperative analgesia (Morton, 1999). It should not, however, be used for chronic pain in severe hepatic disease, in the presence of malnutrition, or alongside drugs that promote oxidative metabolism (e.g., phenytoin) or impair conjugation (e.g., fasting), in order to avoid hepatotoxicity (Farrell, 1997).

Routes of Drug Administration

Clinicians should be aware of the various formulations available for many analgesic drugs used in clinical practice. Opioids, for example, are available in different formulations for parenteral administration as well as oral (suspensions, capsules, tablets) and rectal administration. Daily dosing regimens range from single daily administration to multiple doses (reviewed in Gourlay, 1998). Despite differences in pharmacokinetics among the various formulations, the pharmacodynamic effects have been reported to be similar, and the formulation is chosen based on specific patient factors.

Oral administration is preferred for analgesic drugs, whenever feasible and appropriate. However, oral administration of drugs is associated with a long onset of action and a time-consuming titration process. Alternative routes of administration associated with faster onset of action include intranasal and parenteral administration. Intranasal administration involves administration of liquid drugs in the nostril. Intranasal administration and intramuscular injections, however, can be painful and the latter should be avoided. Intravenous administration of drugs leads to a quick onset of action and flexibility with titration of dose. The main limitation, however, is that a form of venous access must be present. Rectal administration is a useful route for opioids, NSAIDs, and acetaminophen, although it must be recognized that, as with the oral route, rectal administration can be associated with a relatively long onset of action (reviewed in Sacchetti et al., 2003). Topical administration of NSAIDs is a new option that may offer an alternative approach.

Monitoring Analgesic Outcomes

Careful evaluation of the outcomes of analgesia should be undertaken with a frequency that is linked to type of pain and interventions. It is particularly important to use validated pain assessment measures. There have been considerable efforts to develop assessment instruments that are useful in home, clinical, and research settings. Self-report tools have been shown to be useful for some children with cognitive impairments (Fanurik, Koh, Harrison, Conrad, & Tomerlin, 1998). More commonly, however, pain has been evaluated using global proxy judgments of pain. Overall, global judgments of pain have been shown to underestimate pain, and, in response, a number of observational studies have been performed that have documented inventories of behaviors considered by observers to be pain-related among children with SNIs (Stallard, Williams, Velleman, Lenton, & McGrath, 2002). These multidimensional instruments are designed to assess pain in children and adults with communication and cognitive impairments and have demonstrated adequate psychometric features during initial reliability and validity testing (Breau et al., 2002, 2004; Collignon & Giusiano, 2001; Hadden & von Baeyer, 2005; McGrath et al., 1998). Additional research is needed to determine the clinical utility of these tools over the broad range of cognitive functioning in children with SNIs. Irrespective of the instruments used, it is clear that pain assessment should be routinely undertaken, regardless of the extent of the disability, particularly when a possible pain source is suspected or extraordinary behavior or context dictates the possibility that pain is present. Caregivers familiar with the child's baseline behavior should always be included in pain assessments because they are sensitive to specific and idiosyncratic changes in the child's behavior (Stallard et al., 2002).

Finally, frequent reexamination of a child with a SNI is needed to determine if there are any emerging alternate or comorbid diagnoses. This is particularly important when pain assessment and treatment may be uncertain or if there is persistent arousal behavior in the presence of appropriate pain management. Pneumonia, pressure sores, occult fractures, and compartment syndrome are examples of conditions that may develop in children with SNIs, particularly in pain-provoking settings (i.e., postoperatively).

Monitoring Adverse Effects

Regular monitoring of potential adverse effects of analgesic drugs should be an integral part of any analgesic regimen. The duration of monitoring depends on the pharmacological characteristics of the specific analgesic being used (i.e., pharmacokinetic and pharmacodynamic profile and length of therapy) and the nature of the underlying pain stimulus. For children receiving opioids, this includes regular assessments of the level of sedation, pulse oximetry, and ventilatory frequency. If opioids are used for acute pain, monitoring should continue beyond the completion of the procedure because adverse effects often occur after the pain stimulus is removed (Sacchetti et al., 2003). If any parameters fall outside of acceptable ranges, appropriate rescue interventions should commence (including administration of oxygen and naloxone) (Morton, 1999).

The potential for significant undesired side effects of many analgesics may be higher in children with developmental disabilities because of their underlying conditions. For example, altered airway reflexes and decreased respiratory reserve resulting from coexisting neuromuscular weakness or scoliosis may put the child at higher risk for respiratory depression when systemic opioids are used. In addition, excessive sedation and respiratory compromise may result from concomitant use of systemic opioids and drugs used to treat nausea, pruritus, or spasticity (i.e., antiemetics, antihistamines, or benzodiazepines, respectively). Oversedation may interfere with communication, and thus appropriate titration of analgesia and reporting of side effects. In addition, oversedation may prevent early opportunities for seating and mobility, possibly contributing to positioning complications such as pressure sores. Pulmonary aspiration may be the consequence of postoperative delayed gastric emptying, ileus, and vomiting, aggravated by opioids and already impaired bulbar reflexes and gastrointestinal motility. Opioid-induced constipation may also complicate preexisting gastrointestinal problems and add a further source of pain.

It should be noted that serious adverse effects of opioids, such as respiratory compromise, are infrequent compared to "nuisance" adverse effects, which can occur in as many as 50% of patients. For frequent adverse reactions, treatment paradigms should be developed to treat these effects (Monitto et al., 2000) rather than stopping the analgesia. Opioid-induced vomiting, itching, urinary retention, and constipation are all relatively frequent adverse reactions and are preventable or at least usually manageable with appropriate interventions. Antiemetics (e.g., metoclopramide, ondansetron) may be used to reduce nausea and vomiting. Antihistamines or small does of naloxone or ondansetron can be used to reduce itching. Urinary retention and constipation are reduced by naloxone. Alternatively, urinary catheterization may relieve retention. Laxatives or suppositories and adequate hydration may be helpful for constipation (Morton, 1999). In addition, opioid-sparing strategies (e.g., NSAIDs and acetaminophen) may be employed in order to reduce these effects (Morton, 1999). Muscle spasms may occur, often seen as chest wall rigidity or adductor muscle spasms (in orthopedic patients), and can be treated with benzodiazepines, but patients should be closely observed for oversedation (Morton, 1999). In general, patients with characteristics that increase the likelihood of adverse effects include those with decreased cardiorespiratory reserve, those with gastrointestinal motility disorders, and those who are unable to communicate (Oberlander & Craig, 2003).

Potential Sources of Variability in Analgesic Responses

Despite the use of appropriate analgesics, administration protocols, and monitoring, unexpected responses may occur in individual patients as a result of drug-drug interactions and underlying genetic factors inherent to the patient.

Drug-drug interactions are defined as "the possibility that one drug may alter the intensity of pharmacological effects of another drug given concurrently"(Nies & Spielberg, 1996). The underlying mechanisms of drug interactions include changes in 1) drug disposition (pharmacokinetics), 2) drug responses (pharmacodynamics), or 3) physical compatibilities (pharmaceutics).

An extensive body of research has focused on drug interactions that alter drug disposition (i.e., drug metabolism). Drug metabolism is the process used by the body to increase the polarity of lipophilic drugs in order to enhance their excretion via the bile or kidney. This is in contrast to relatively polar compounds that are excreted directly via the kidney (Morselli, 1989). Metabolism of drugs occurs mostly in the liver and involves a variety of reactions categorized as phase I (nonsynthetic) and phase II (synthetic) reactions. The cytochrome P-450 (CYP) enzyme system is a major site of drug metabolism and the source of many drug interactions. The P-450 enzyme consists of more than 20 families of related isozymes. The isozymes involved in the metabolism of most drugs are CYP 1A2, CYP 2D6, CYP 2C9, CYP 2C19, and CYP 3A3/3A4 (Bernard & Bruera, 2000). With the exception of CYP 2D6, many isozymes are inducible by drugs and environmental factors (e.g., cigarette smoking, barbecued food), which means that their metabolic capacity may be enhanced. Induction of specific isozymes leads to increased drug elimination for drugs eliminated by those specific isozyme pathways. Conversely, isozymes may be inhibited, leading to decreased capacity and reduced drug elimination. Examples of pharmacokinetic interactions involving analgesics include 1) increased metabolism of methadone by phenytoin, leading to subtherapeutic effects of methadone; 2) inhibition of metabolism of fentanyl by erythromycin and resulting fentanyl toxicity; and 3) inhibition of metabolism of tricyclic antidepressants (TCAs) and selective serotonin reuptake inhibitors (SSRIs) by fluoroquinolones, predisposing to antidepressant-induced side effects.

Pharmacodynamic interactions arise when there is an interaction at the site of action—a receptor or physiological system (Bernard & Bruera, 2000). Examples of pharmacodynamic interactions involving analgesics include 1) opioid toxicity in the presence of NSAID-induced renal impairment, 2) increased analgesia in the presence of opioids and antidepressants or dextromethorphan, and 3) *serotonin syndrome,* which occurs when SSRIs are used with meperidine (see section titled Mental Health: Mood Disturbances and Neuroleptic Medications).

Genetic polymorphism accounts for significant variability in enzyme activity among individuals as well. The implication of this variability in enzyme activity is that the use of a standard analgesic dose may result in dramatically different pharmacological effects. For example, a standard dose of analgesic in an individual who is an extensive metabolizer will lead to subtherapeutic effects. Conversely, the same dose will lead to toxicity in a poor metabolizer. Moreover, if a drug requires metabolism for activation, it would be ineffective in a poor metabolizer but potentially toxic in an extensive metabolizer.

Opioid metabolism is known to be affected in individuals with genetic polymorphisms in hepatic CYP 2D6 isozymes. Codeine, for example, is ineffective in approximately 10% of Caucasians because of the lack of a functional CYP 2D6, the enzyme that is responsible for conversion of codeine to its active metabolite, morphine (Eckhardt et al., 1998). Individuals with poor or limited capacity to metabolize codeine will be at risk for the side effects of the drug without experiencing the analgesic benefits (Eckhardt et al., 1998). In contrast, the clearance of lorazepam is reduced in patients with Gilbert syndrome (Sacchetti et al., 2003). The need to change drug regimens because they are either ineffective or associated with adverse effects may suggest an underlying genetic cause for apparent analgesic failure.

MEDICATIONS USED IN CHILDREN WITH SNIs

Chronic Conditions

Children with SNIs are a heterogeneous group of individuals with a wide variety of underlying medical conditions that include cerebral palsy, traumatic brain injury, congenital central nervous system (CNS) anomalies, seizures, developmental delays, chromosomal syndromes, and metabolic disorders. Many of these conditions require multiple medications that may further complicate the assessment and management of pain. The classes of drugs frequently encountered and their implications for analgesic therapy are reviewed in this section.

CNS Conditions

Spasticity   Children with cerebral palsy experience increased motor tone that leads to frequent spasms, reflexes, and clonus throughout the day and night. Continuous spasms can be a source of ongoing discomfort or pain. Treatment of children with spasticity involves physical therapy, orthopedic surgery, neurosurgery, and pharmacotherapy. Examples of drugs commonly used to manage spasticity are diazepam, baclofen, dantrolene, and botulinum toxin. Visceral spasmodic pain may be managed with anticholinergics and antispasmodics (Oberlander, O'Donnell, & Montgomery, 1999). By decreasing muscular tone, such interventions may indirectly act as analgesics.

Seizures   Many children with SNIs require antiepileptic drugs for seizure disorders. However, both traditional (e.g., phenobarbital, carbamazepine, phenytoin, valproic acid) and newer generation (e.g., vigabatrin, lamotrigine) antiepileptic drugs are a common source of drug–drug interactions (Eriksson, Hoppu, Nergardh, & Boreus, 1996; Sanchez-Alcaraz, Quintana, Lopez, Rodriguez, & Llopis, 2002). For instance, carbamazepine, phenytoin, and phenobarbital all increase levels of CYP 3A4. In the case of carbamazepine, the drug induces its own metabolism as well. The net result is subtherapeutic responses to concomitantly used analgesics metabolized by this isozyme (e.g., methadone and midazolam). Barbiturates induce phase II liver enzymes such as glucuronyltransferase and increase the metabolism of selected analgesic medications (e.g., morphine). This does not affect the initial dosing of an analgesic but may lead to an increase in the amount of subsequent doses (Sacchetti et al., 2003).

Mental Health: Mood Disturbances and Neuroleptic Medications   Depressed mood may also be encountered in individuals with SNIs. SSRIs, TCAs, and monoamine oxidase inhibitors (MAOIs), or a combination of these, are frequently used as antidepressants to counteract CNS symptoms. There is an increasing recognition of potential interactions between analgesics, coanalgesics, and SSRIs (von Moltke, Greenblatt, Schmider, Harmatz, & Shader, 1995). Among the SSRIs, paroxetine, fluoxetine, fluvoxamine, and venlafaxine have been demonstrated to inhibit several cytochrome P-450 isozyme families; however, clinically significant drug interactions are uncommon (Bernard & Bruera, 2000).

Many of the antiepileptic and antidepressant drugs have been demonstrated to have analgesic properties, which can be beneficial in patients with concurrent pain syndromes. However, because these drugs adversely affect psychological functioning as well, they may cause side effects ranging from sedation and confusion to drug-induced depression and mania (Peet & Peters, 1995). These effects potentially complicate pain management in children with SNIs by producing sedation or disruptive behavior that masks pain assessment (Stallard et al., 2002) or by adding to CNS depression caused by concurrent opioid treatment. Conversely, concurrent use of CNS drugs that increase serotonin concentrations in the brain may lead to *serotonin syndrome* (Sporer, 1995). Serotonin syndrome is most frequently reported in patients taking two or more medications from drug classes that increase serotonin concentrations, such as MAOIs, SSRIs, and TCAs. However, meperidine can precipitate serotonin syndrome as well, via inhibition of serotonin uptake (Table 12.1). Features of the serotonin syndrome include altered mental status, autonomic dysfunction, and neuromuscular abnormalities.

Neuroleptic medications, such as thioridazine or haloperidol, are used to treat CNS symptoms. They are cleared by the CYP 2D6 system and may be sources of drug interactions with antidepressants that are metabolized via the CYP 2D6 isozymes (e.g., desipramine) (Ereshefsky, 1996; Gram & Overo, 1972; von Bahr et al., 1991). Neuroleptics may also interact with opioids. For instance, when haloperidol is combined with codeine, the conversion to morphine (CYP 2D6 dependent) may not occur, and analgesic failure may occur, even at higher doses of codeine. If this effect is not recognized, switching to another opioid based on an increased dose of codeine to achieve equianalgesic conversion may result in opioid toxicity (Caraco, Sheller, & Wood, 1996).

Pyresis Individuals with SNIs may have sustained brain injury or stroke and resulting central hyperthermia. Antipyretics such as acetaminophen and ibuprofen are commonly used in these individuals to decrease body temperature, and because they are inherently analgesic as well, they will decrease ongoing pain. Ibuprofen is preferred by some clinicians because it has a longer duration of action compared to acetaminophen and is well tolerated in children (Lesko & Mitchell, 1999). However, both acetaminophen and ibuprofen can lead to serious adverse effects in susceptible populations (see Table 12.1).

Gastrointestinal Disorders

Aspiration or choking may occur in children with SNIs as a result of disorders of swallowing and reflux, or through behaviors that predispose to such disorders (Ruschena et al., 2003). Drugs used to manage these conditions include proton pump inhibitors (e.g., omeprazole), histamine$_2$ receptor antagonists (e.g., ranitidine), anticholinergics, and sucralfate. Omeprazole, which also inhibits the CYP 1A2 isozyme and thus metabolism of diazepam and phenytoin, increasing the potential for oversedation, gait disturbances, and other toxicities from these agents

Table 12.1.   Pharmacologic considerations in children with SNI receiving analgesics

Analgesic	Contraindications	Potential drug interactions*
Opioids	Hypersensitivity Upper airway obstruction, sleep apnea Acute asthma Anemia	Increased opioid effects in patients taking • CNS depressants (benzodiazepines, barbiturates, other CNS depressants) • Cimetidine, diltiazem, verapamil • Anticholinergics Decreased opioid effects in patients taking • Anticonvulsants (carbamazepine, phenobarbital, phenytoin, primidone) • Rifampin • SSRIs (paroxetine, fluoxetine, sertraline), other CYP 2D6 inhibitors Serotonin-like syndrome in patients taking SSRIs
NSAIDs	Hypersensitivity ASA-NSAID–induced asthma Bleeding disorder Renal impairment Peptic ulcer, gastroesophageal reflux disease Concurrent steroids Hypertension Hypovolemia	Increased bleeding in patients taking ASA, anticoagulants Increased blood pressure in patients taking beta-blockers, ACE inhibitors, loop diuretics, thiazide diuretics Increased pharmacologic effects of phenytoin, lithium
Acetaminophen	Hypersensitivity	Decreased pharmacologic effect in patients taking anticholinergics, oral contraceptives Increased pharmacologic effect in patients taking beta-blockers Increased blood pressure in patients taking loop diuretics Decreased pharmacologic effects of lamotrigine
Local anesthetics	Hypersensitivity Myasthenia gravis Epidural or spinal anesthesia contraindicated in CNS/spinal cord disease such as hemorrhage, infection Regional anesthesia contraindicated in infection, hemorrhage, +/–altered anatomy, inability to communicate	Increased pharmacologic effects for epidural administration in patients taking opioids, anticholinergics

Adapted from http://www.oqp.med.va.gov/cpg/PAIN/pain_cpg/algo1frameset.htm.

*Interaction may be specific to only one analgesic in the class or generalizable to entire class, depending on the nature of the interaction.

when used concomitantly (Middle et al., 1995). Reduced consciousness associated with opioid analgesia may predispose to aspiration in children with gastrointestinal disorders (Ruschena et al., 2003). For effective treatment of painful GI conditions (e.g., esophagitis, gastritis) with proton pump inhibitors, it is important to note that any amount of acid will degrade omeprazole (Cornish, 2005). Use of an antacid or ranitidine for the duration of therapy with omeprazole (when broken or crushed) is recommended. Lansoprazole capsules may be opened and the contents administered with food, but G-tube administration should be avoided as it blocks smaller tubes.

Infections

Antimicrobial therapy is frequently required for recurrent respiratory, urinary, and skin infections in children with SNIs. Antimicrobials have substantial potential to interact with analgesics commonly used in this population as well as causing or exacerbating painful conditions. Erythromycin inhibits the CYP 3A4 isozyme and reduces clearance of drugs metabolized by this pathway, such as midazolam and fentanyl (Olkkola et al., 1993). Fluoroquinolones can inhibit CYP P450 3A4 and 1A isozyme activities, leading to toxicity from drugs that utilize these metabolic pathways (e.g., midazolam, TCAs, SSRIs) (Bernard & Bruera, 2000). Antibiotics may be associated with side effects that aggravate underlying conditions in children with SNIs as well. Fluoroquinolones can cause peripheral sensory disturbances, leading to numbness, pain, and muscle weakness (Hedenmalm & Spigset, 1996). Conversely, opioid analgesics can increase the risk of vancomycin-associated *red-man syndrome*, a constellation of symptoms including flushing and pruritus (Wong, Ripple, MacLean, Marks, & Bloch, 1994).

Specific Considerations for Analgesia

Children with SNIs often undergo additional surgeries secondary to their underlying medical condition(s), such as dental and orthopedic procedures. Theoretically, the armamentarium for pain management in these children includes the same drugs as for children without SNIs. Practically speaking, however, analgesic practices in children with SNIs have differed somewhat. In one retrospective report of 42 children, anesthetic administration intraoperatively did not differ between groups (Malviya et al., 2001); however, in another larger prospective study of 290 children, those with SNIs received less opioids in the operating room (Koh, Fanurik, Harrison, Schmitz, & Norvell, 2004). Investigators of the latter study suggested that decreased utilization of opioids was due to concerns that children with SNIs may be more sensitive to the depressive effects of opioids. Postoperatively, similar amounts and types of analgesics were used in the prospective study (Koh et al., 2004), and less were used in the retrospective study (Malviya et al., 2001). The clinical significance of these data are unclear because it is not known if the amount of pain relief achieved for children with SNIs is equivalent to that in children without SNIs because of the inability to assess pain accurately in this population (Koh et al., 2004). In the former study, there was a difference in the intensity of monitoring also; children with SNIs were monitored with pulse oximetry and received supplemental oxygen for longer than other children. However, severe respiratory compromise that required reintubation only occurred in two children with SNIs and did not appear to be related to benzodiazepine use (Malviya et al., 2001).

A more aggressive and closely monitored approach to pain management following surgery has been proposed for patients with chronic disabilities compared to other patients to account for the chronic nature of their disabilities (Rivard, 2001). Children with SNIs undergo repeated complex procedures (e.g., spinal surgery for scoliosis correction, selective dorsal rhizotomy to reduce spasticity) (Chicoine, Park, & Kaufman, 1997). In addition, children with SNIs often have underlying conditions that increase postoperative pain, such as increased muscle tone, anxiety, or fear, further exacerbating pain itself (Malviya et al., 2001; Rivard, 2001). Analgesic regimens should take these factors into account, and determine the medications that will best suit the patient's needs. For instance, antispasmodics should be used if there is spasticity, and midazolam if there is anxiety or distress (Rivard, 2001). Moreover, in the absence of typical means of communication, children with SNIs may be at risk for additional pain resulting from activities of daily living that go unnoticed. Moreover, pain from skin breakdown caused by friction injuries (treated with emollients or dressings) (Association of Women's Health, Obstetric and Neonatal Nurses, 2001) or by irritation at a gastrostomy tube site (treated with protectants such as zinc oxide) is common. In addition, children with SNIs may experience pain from chronic and recurrent conditions that affect the general pediatric population, such as recurrent headaches, abdominal pain, limb pain, musculoskeletal pain, back pain, and fibromyalgia (Palermo, 2000). Thus, children with disabilities can have a background level of pain, and superimposed additional pain from specific stimuli (e.g., transfers, feeding, movement, weight bearing) and their neurological conditions themselves.

The route of administration of analgesics also warrants special consideration in children with SNIs because the choice of formulation to use depends on specific patient factors, such as the presence of a feeding tube. Many children with SNIs have feeding tubes because of underlying swallowing disorders. In children with feeding tubes, liquid formulations of drugs rather than tablets or capsules should be prescribed. When this is not possible, tablets or capsules are usually crushed and mixed with food prior to administration through feeding tubes. Occasionally, the injectable form of the drug can be used. This is done, however, at the risk of changing the pharmacokinetics of the formulation (Mitchell, 2000). Whatever the formulation that is ordered, it is imperative to determine if is suitable for administration through such devices. Different formulations of drugs are designed with the intention of providing specific pharmacological activity, and altering the formulation may lead to either excessive or diminished pharmacological activity.

Many analgesic drugs should not be crushed for ease of administration through a gastric or nasogastric tube. Sustained-release oxycodone should not be crushed, because this formulation is designed to deliver the drug gradually over 12 hours, and crushing the tablet will result in immediate absorption of the entire dose, with potential adverse effects (Cornish, 2005). The acid-suppression agent omeprazole, in contrast, is inactivated by gastric acid, and crushing of the enteric-coated tablet may lead to inactivation by the gastric acid milieu and loss of efficacy (Cornish, 2005). Moreover, some drugs may cause irritation to the gastric mucosa (e.g., NSAIDs) (Marshall, Pai, & Reddy, 1985), may interact with food or the feeding tube (Doak et al., 1998), or because of increased viscosity may obstruct the tube (e.g., clarithromycin, bulk laxatives). The pharmaceutical formulation of some analgesics may therefore limit the use of sustained-release medications such as oxycodone, leading to use of alternative opioids in children with feeding tubes. In contrast, the enteric-coated formulation may still be appropriate for omeprazole with concurrent administration of a histamine$_2$ receptor antagonist or antacid to neutralize stomach pH and protect the omeprazole from acid breakdown while it begins to take effect (usually after 4 days or so). This is supplemented with monitoring of gastric pH to ensure an adequate pharmacological effect. Similarly, phenytoin interacts with nutrients in feeding tubes (Chan, 2002) leading to decreased serum phenytoin concentrations and, thus, increased risk of seizures. In the clinical situation, this is handled with upward adjustment of the dose until the desired effects are achieved. It should be noted, however, that if feedings are discontinued and the drug is switched to an equivalent intravenous administration, the large dosage may lead to serious toxicity (Doak et al., 1998). A list of oral dosage forms that should not be crushed is available (Mitchell, 2000). A list or database of recommended and prohibited medications should be maintained in centers caring for children with feeding tubes, with specific instructions for their administration in order to minimize any potential untoward effects (Cornish, 2005). Referral to this database should be an integral part of prescribing any medication for a child with a SNI.

IMPLICATIONS FOR POLYPHARMACY IN THE MANAGEMENT OF PAIN

Children with SNIs frequently require medications to manage multiple conditions, which directly and indirectly arise from complex neurological conditions, in addition to pain (Table 12.2). In isolation, many of these medications are effective and safe; however, in combination with analgesics, they may lead to decreased efficacy or even pose a health risk. With increasing number of drugs being consumed, there is an increased probability of experiencing an adverse drug reaction (Holdsworth et al., 2003; Impicciatore et al., 2001). In addition, drug interactions may occur, manifesting themselves as exaggerated but otherwise normal pharmacological responses to a drug, or as aberrant, unexpected responses. An interacting drug may alter the pharmacokinetic parameters of another drug, or the pharmacological activity of another drug. Vigilant monitoring is required to avoid serious adverse effects and to optimize clinical effectiveness. For all medications concurrently administered to children with SNIs, a list of specific reactions and interactions that can occur should be identified for clinical staff and parents, with the aim of improving detection and avoiding serious adverse outcomes.

THE CLINICAL VIGNETTE: FOLLOW-UP

A review of Richard's polypharmacy "cocktail" was performed to determine potential sources of the pharmacotherapeutic analgesic failure leading to increased chronic pain and suffering. Initially the combination of medications appeared appropriate for each of his conditions. Upon closer evaluation, however, several factors emerged that may have contributed to his worsening condition. His gastric pain associated with gastroesophageal reflux and esophageal erosion may have worsened because the method for administrating the omeprazole via his gastric tube (i.e., crushing the tablet) was rendered ineffective as a result of breakdown of the drug by the acid milieu. Ibuprofen may have exacerbated his asthma, resulting in frequent night awakenings. Richard may be a poor metabolizer of codeine because of diminished CYP 2D6 activity, which renders it ineffective as an analgesic. Finally, the combination of paroxetine and meperidine may have led to symptoms of the serotonin syndrome as a result of excessively high central nervous system serotonin concentrations.

Once this situation was recognized, the following medications were ordered: chlorpromazine, clonazepam, paroxetine, omeprazole, salbutamol, fluticasone, ran-

Table 12.2. Typical analgesics and adjuvant medications for pain management in children with multiple disabilities

Class	Medication	Indications	Dose	Disadvantages	Advantages
Weak NSAIDs	Acetaminophen	Non-opiod to co-analgesic	10–15 mg/kg/dose PO q4–6h PRN POST OP: 20 mg/kg/dose PO q6h or 35 mg/kg/dose PR q8h × 48 h, then reassess (max 90 mg/kg/day)	Risk of hepatorenal toxicity Mild analgesic effect	Opioid sparing
NSAIDs	Naproxen	Non-opioid co-analgesic Antiinflammatory Bony pain	5–7 mg/kg/dose PO/PR q8–12 h	GI upset, GI bleeding, platelet dysfunction, risk of hepatorenal toxicity	Oral and rectal formulation, BID dosing Extensive pediatric experience
NSAIDs	Ketorolac	Non-opioid co-analgesic Antiinflammatory Bony pain	0.3–0.5 mg/kg/dose q6h IV for 48 h (for short term use only)	GI bleeding, platelet dysfunction, risk of hepatorenal toxicity	Parenteral, may be used IV
NSAIDs (COX2 selective)	Rofecoxib	Non-opioid co-analgesic Antiinflammatory Bony pain	0.5 mg/kg/dose PO (max 50 mg/ 24 h)	Possible less analgesic efficacy than non-selective NSAIDs	Liquid formulation Decreased risk of platelet dysfunction, GI and renal toxicity
Alpha2 Agonists	Clonidine	Non-opioid co-analgesic	2–4 mcg/kg/dose PO q4–6h	Sedation, hypotension	Opioid sparing, sedation

Class	Drug	Indication	Dose	Side effects	Comments
Benzodiazepines	Diazepam		0.1–0.8 mg/kg/24 h PO div q6–8h	Sedation, respiratory depression, paradoxical agitation	Improved tone, non-opioid adjuvant
GABA agonists	Baclofen	Spasticity of spinal or central origin	5 mg PO TID (increased to 80–120 mg/day)* Increase slowly to desired clinical effect	Drowsiness, dizziness, nausea, hypotonia, hypotension	Improved tone, non-opioid adjuvant; intrathecal route available
Anticonvulsants	Gabapentin	Neuropathic pain	5 mg/kg/24 hr PO qhs initially, then increase to BID and then increase to TID and titrate to effect; Maintenance: 8–35 mg/kg/24 hr PO div TID*	Somnolence, dizziness, fatigue, nystagmus	Sedation, neuropathic pain
Calcium flux agents	Dantrolene	Spasticity of spinal or central origin	0.5 mg/kg/dose PO BID, then increase to max 3 mg/kg/dose PO BID–QID (max 400 mg/24 hr)*	Monitor transaminases to detect hepatic injury	Reduces tone by reducing muscle strength

From Oberlander, T.F., & Craig, K.D. (2003). Pain and children with developmental disabilities. In N.L. Schechter, C.B. Berde, & M. Yaster (Eds.), *Pain in infants, children, and adolescents* (2nd ed., p. 599). Philadelphia: Lippincott Williams & Wilkins; reprinted by permission.

*Dose titrated to effects.

itidine, methadone, and morphine. Ranitidine was added for the short term only, and daily pH monitoring was commenced. The NSAIDs administered by gastrostomy tube were stopped, his codeine was switched to methadone (maintenance) and morphine (breakthrough pain) (not dependent on CYP 2D6), and lamotrigine was started (phenytoin increases methadone metabolism). These changes were based on a comprehensive and ongoing multidisciplinary pain management plan that included a case manager and regular communication with Richard, his family, and health care professionals. Within 2 weeks, Richard reported substantially reduced pain and increased appetite, improved sleep patterns and returned to his typical activities of daily living. His family and caregivers were also satisfied with the subsequent substantial reduction of Richard's pain.

In summary, this case illustrates a number of factors that should be considered when managing pain. First, even though appropriate medications (SSRIs, NSAIDs, and opioids) were chosen for his condition (bone pain, depressed mood), his medications were interacting, leading to unwanted side effects (serotonin syndrome, increased rigidity and tone, asthma exacerbation) and increased suffering and pain. The route of administration for his medications (via his gastrostomy tube) may have rendered them ineffective (i.e., omeprazole in an acidic environment), thereby compounding his gastroesophageal reflux/esophageal-related pain. He may also have been genetically predisposed to be a poor CYP 2D6 metabolizer, thereby further reducing the analgesic efficacy. Furthermore, it was clear that comprehensive ongoing communication among his health care team was required to prevent adverse drug reactions and effective treatment.

CONCLUSION

Pain management in children and youth with SNIs requires pharmaceutical approaches that challenge us to think about management strategies that go far beyond choosing appropriate medications. Effective pain control requires knowledge of the underlying conditions and how they influence analgesic efficacy, as well as the pharmacology of analgesics, drug interactions, and specific genetic factors. Regardless of the selection of analgesics, a thorough consideration of possible drug–drug interactions, and monitoring of effects, successful pain management will often also depend on effective communication among all of the members of the health care team and family.

REFERENCES

Association of Women's Health, Obstetric and Neonatal Nurses. (2001). *Evidence-based clinical practice guideline: Neonatal skin care*. Washington, DC: Author.

Bernard, S.A., & Bruera, E. (2000). Drug interactions in palliative care. *Journal of Clinical Oncology, 18,* 1780–1799.

Breau, L.M., Finley, G.A., McGrath, P.J., & Camfield, C.S. 2002. Validation of the Noncommunicating Children's Pain Checklist-Postoperative Version. *Anesthesiology*, 96(3), 528–535.

Breau, L.M., McGrath, P.J., Camfield, C.S., & Finley, G.A. (2002). Psychometric properties of the non-communicating children's pain checklist-revised. *Pain*, 99(1-2), 349–357.

Breau, L.M., McGrath, P.J., Stevens, B., Beyene, J., Camfield, C.S., Finley, G.A., Franck, L., Howlett, A., O'Brien, K., & Ohlsson, A. (2004). Healthcare professionals' perceptions of pain in infants at risk for neurological impairment. *BMC Pediatrics*, 4(1), 23.

Caraco, J., Sheller, J., & Wood, A.J.J. (1996). Pharmacogenetic determination of the effects of codeine and prediction of drug interactions. *Journal of Pharmacology and Experimental Therapeutics, 278,* 1165–1174.

Chan, L.N. (2002). Drug-nutrient interaction in clinical nutrition. *Current Opinion in Clinical Nutrition and Metabolic Care, 5,* 327–332.

Chicoine, M.R., Park, T.S., & Kaufman, B.A. (1997). Selective dorsal rhizotomy and rates of orthopedic surgery in children with spastic cerebral palsy. *Journal of Neurosurgery, 86*(1), 34–39.

Clarkson, A., Ingleby, E., Choonara, I., Bryan, P., & Arlett, P. (2001). A novel scheme for the reporting of adverse drug reactions. *Archives of Disease in Childhood, 84,* 337–339.

Clinical Practice Guidelines. (2005). *Pharmacologic management* (Table OP1—Mechanisms, Contradictions).

Collignon, P., & Giusiano, B. (2001). Validation of a pain evaluation scale for patients with severe cerebral palsy. *European Journal of Pain, 5,* 433–442.

Cornish, P. (2005). "Avoid the crush": Hazards of medication administration in patients with dysphagia or a feeding tube. *CMAJ, 172,* 871–872.

Doak, K.K., Haas, C.E., Dunnigan, K.J., Reiss, R.A., Reiser, J.R., Huntress, J., et al. (1998). Bioavailability of phenytoin acid and phenytoin sodium with enteral feedings. *Pharmacotherapy, 18,* 637–645.

Eckhardt, K., Li, S., Ammon, S., Schanzle, G., Mikus, G., & Eichelbaum, M. (1998). Same incidence of adverse drug events after codeine administration irrespective of the genetically determined differences in morphine formation. *Pain, 76,* 27–33.

Ereshefsky, L. (1996). Drug-drug interactions involving antidepressants: Focus on venlafaxine. *Journal of Clinical Psychopharmacology, 16,* 37S–49S.

Eriksson, A.S., Hoppu, K., Nergardh, A., & Boreus, L. (1996). Pharmacokinetic interactions between lamotrigine and other antiepileptic drugs in children with intractable epilepsy. *Epilepsia, 37,* 769–773.

Fanurik, D., Koh, J.L., Schmitz, M.L., Harrison, R.D., & Conrad, T.M. (1999). Children with cognitive impairment: parent report of pain and coping. *Journal of Developmental and Behavioral Pediatrics, 20*(4), 228–234.

Fanurik, D., Koh, J.L., Harrison, R.D., Conrad, T.M., & Tomerlin, C. (1998). Pain assessment in children with cognitive impairment: An exploration of self-report skills. *Clinical Nursing Research, 7,* 103–119.

Farrell, G.C. (1997). Drug-induced hepatic injury. *Journal of Gastroenterology and Hepatology, 12,* S242–S250.

Gardner-Nix, J. (2003). Principles of opioid use in chronic noncancer pain. *CMAJ, 169,* 38–43.

Gourlay, G.K. (1998). Sustained relief of chronic pain: Pharmacokinetics of sustained release morphine. *Clinical Pharmacokinetics, 35,* 173–190.

Gram, L., & Overo, K.F. (1972). Drug interaction: Inhibitory effect of neuroleptics on metabolism of tricyclic antidepressants in man. *British Medical Journal, 1,* 463–465.

Hadden, K.L., & von Baeyer, C.L. (2005). Global and specific behavioral measures of pain in children with cerebral palsy. *Clinical Journal of Pain, 21*(2), 140-146.

Hamunen, K., & Maunuksela, E.L. (1996). Ketorolac does not depress ventilation in children. *Paediatric Anaesthesia, 6,* 79.

Hedenmalm, K., & Spigset, O. (1996). Peripheral sensory disturbances related to treatment with fluoroquinolones. *Journal of Antimicrobial Chemotherapy, 37,* 831–837.

Herman, R.J., Chaudhary, A., & Szakacs, C.B. (1994). Disposition of lorazepam in Gilbert's syndrome: Effects of fasting, feeding, and enterohepatic circulation. *Journal of Clinical Pharmacology, 10,* 978–984.

Holdsworth, M.T., Fichtl, R.E., Behta, M., Raisch, D.W., Mendez-Rico, E., Adams, A., et al. (2003). Incidence and impact of adverse drug events in pediatric inpatients. *Archives of Pediatrics and Adolescent Medicine, 157,* 60–65.

Impicciatore, P., Choonara, I., Clarkson, A., Provasi, D., Pandolfini, C., & Bonati, M. (2001). Incidence of adverse drug reactions in paediatric in/out-patients: A systematic review and meta-analysis of prospective studies. *British Journal of Clinical Pharmacology, 52,* 77–83.

Koh, J.L., Fanurik, D., Harrison, R.D., Schmitz, M.L., & Norvell, D. (2004). Analgesia following surgery in children with and without cognitive impairment. *Pain, 111,* 239–244.

Lehr, V.T., & BeVier, P. (2003). Patient-controlled analgesia for the pediatric patient. *Orthopaedic Nursing, 22,* 298–304.

Lesko, S.M., & Mitchell, A.A. (1999). The safety of acetaminophen and ibuprofen among children younger than two years old. *Pediatrics* 104(4), e39.

Leuppi, J.D., Schnyder, P., Hartmann, K., Reinhart, W.H., & Kuhn, M. (2001). Drug-induced bronchospasm: Analysis of 187 spontaneously reported cases. *Respiration, 68,* 345–351.

Malviya, S., Voepel-Lewis, T., Tait, A.R., Merkel, S., Lauer, A., Munro, H., et al. (2001). Pain management in children with and without cognitive impairment following spine fusion surgery. *Paediatric Anaesthesia, 11,* 453–458.

Marshall, T.A., Pai, S., & Reddy, P.P. (1985). Intestinal perforation following enteral administration of indomethacin. *Journal of Pediatrics, 107,* 484–485.

Matsui, D., Kwan, C., Steer, E., & Rieder, M.J. (2003). The trials and tribulations of doing drug research in children. *CMAJ, 169,* 1033–1034.

McGrath, P.J., Rosmus, C., Canfield, C., Campbell, M.A., & Hennigar, A. (1998). Behaviours caregivers use to determine pain in non-verbal, cognitively impaired individuals. *Developmental Medicine and Child Neurology,* 40(5), 340–343.

Mercadante, S. (2005). *Special report. World Health Organization guidelines: Problem areas in cancer pain management.* Geneva: World Health Organization.

Middle, M.V., Muller, F.O., Schall, R., Groenewoud, G., Hundt, H.K., Huber, R., et al. (1995). No influence of pantoprazole on the pharmacokinetics of phenytoin. *International Journal of Clinical Pharmacology and Therapeutics, 33,* 304–307.

Mitchell, J.F. (2000). Oral dosage forms that should not be crushed or chewed: 2000 update. *Hospital Pharmacy, 35,* 553–567.

Monitto, C.L., Greenberg, R.S., Kost-Byerly, S., Wetzel, R., Billett, C., Lebet, R.M., et al. (2000). The safety and efficacy of parent-/nurse-controlled analgesia in patients less than six years of age. *Anesthesia and Analgesia, 91,* 573–579.

Morselli, P. L. 1989. Clinical pharmacology of the perinatal period and early infancy. *Clinical Pharmacokinetics, 17*(Suppl. 1), 13–28.

Morton, N.S. (1999). Prevention and control of pain in children. *British Journal of Anaesthesia, 83,* 118–129.

Nies, A., & Spielberg, S.P. (1996). Principles of therapeutics. In J. Hardman, L.E. Limbird, & P.B. Molinoff (Eds.), *Goodman and Gilman's the pharmacological basis of therapeutics* (9th ed., pp. 43–52). New York: McGraw-Hill.

Oberlander T.F., & O'Donnell, M.E. (2001). Beliefs about pain among professionals working with children with significant neurologic impairment. *Developmental Medicine and Child Neurology, 43*(2), 138–140.

Oberlander, T.F., & Craig, K.D. (2003). Pain and children with developmental disabilities. In N.L. Schechter, C.B. Berde, & M. Yaster (Eds.), *Pain in infants, children, and adolescents* (2nd ed., p. 599). Philadelphia: Lippincott Williams & Wilkins.

Oberlander, T.F., & O'Donnell, M.E. (2001). Beliefs about pain among professionals working with children with significant neurologic impairment. *Developmental Medicine and Child Neurology, 43,* 138–140.

Oberlander, T.F., O'Donnell, M.E., & Montgomery, C.J. (1999). Pain in children with significant neurological impairment. *Journal of Developmental and Behavioral Pediatrics, 20,* 235–243.

O'Donnell, M.E., & Armstrong, R. (1997). Pharmacologic interventions for management of spasticity in cerebral palsy. *MRDD Research Reviews, 3,* 204–211.

Olkkola, K.T., Aranko, K., Luurila, H., Hiller, A., Saarnivaara, L., Himberg, J.J., et al. (1993). A potentially hazardous interaction between erythromycin and midazolam. *Clinical Pharmacology and Therapeutics, 53,* 298–305.

Palermo, T.M. (2000). Impact of recurrent and chronic pain on child and family daily functioning: A critical review of the literature. *Journal of Developmental and Behavioral Pediatrics, 21,* 58–69.

Peet, M., & Peters, S. (1995). Drug-induced mania. *Drug Safety, 12,* 146–153.

Rivard, P. (2001). Acute postoperative pain control for children with chronic disabilities. *Orthopaedic Nursing, 20,* 17–21.

Ruschena, D., Mullen, P.E., Palmer, S., Burgess, P., Cordner, S.M., Drummer, O.H., et al. (2003). Choking deaths: The role of antipsychotic medication. *British Journal of Psychiatry, 183,* 446–450.

Sacchetti, A., Turco, T., Carraccio, C., Hasher, W., Cho, D., & Gerardi, M. (2003). Procedural sedation for children with special health care needs. *Pediatric Emergency Care, 19,* 231–239.

Sanchez-Alcaraz, A., Quintana, M.B., Lopez, E., Rodriguez, I., & Llopis, P. (2002). Effect of vigabatrin on the pharmacokinetics of carbamazepine. *Journal of Clinical Pharmacy and Therapeutics, 27,* 427–430.

Sporer, K.A. (1995). The serotonin syndrome: Implicated drugs, pathophysiology and management. *Drug Safety, 13,* 94–104.

Stallard, P., Williams, L., Velleman, R., Lenton, S., & McGrath, P.J. (2002). Brief report: Behaviors identified by caregivers to detect pain in noncommunicating children. *Journal of Pediatric Psychology, 27,* 209–214.

Tsankov, N., Angelova, I., & Kazandjieva, J. (2000). Drug-induced psoriasis: Recognition and management. *American Journal of Clinical Dermatology, 1,* 159–165.

Ulinski, T., Guigonis, V., Dunan, O., & Bensman, A. (2004). Acute renal failure after treatment with non-steroidal anti-inflammatory drugs. *European Journal of Pediatrics, 163,* 148–150.

Velayudham, L.S., & Farrell, G.C. (2003). Drug-induced cholestasis. *Expert Opinion on Drug Safety, 2,* 287–304.

von Bahr, C., Movin, G., Nordin, C., Liden, A., Hammarlund-Udenaes, M., Hedberg, A., et al. (1991). Plasma levels of thioridazine and metabolites are influenced by the debrisoquin hydroxylation phenotype. *Clinical Pharmacokinetics, 49,* 234–240.

von Moltke, L., Greenblatt, D.J., Schmider, J., Harmatz, J.S., & Shader, R.I. (1995). Metabolism of drugs by cytochrome P450 3A isoforms: Implications for drug interactions in psychopharmacology. *Clinical Pharmacokinetics, 29,* 33–44.

Wong, J.T., Ripple, R.E., MacLean, J.A., Marks, D.R., & Bloch, K.J. (1994). Vancomycin hypersensitivity: Synergism with narcotics and "desensitization" by a rapid continuous intravenous protocol. *Journal of Allergy and Clinical Immunology, 94,* 189–194.

IV

EPILOGUE

13

PAIN IN DEVELOPMENTAL DISABILITIES

Lessons Learned

Neil L. Schechter

As with any new and emerging discipline in medicine, our knowledge about pain management in individuals with developmental disabilities is garnered from multiple sources: new information specifically developed to address the unique aspects of this field, extrapolation of research from related or even unrelated disciplines, and clinical trial and error. This chapter focuses on the latter sources of information. Two cases are presented that exemplify some of the complex issues in the management of pain among those whose biology may be unusual and whose communication skills may be limited. The clinical implications that emerge from these cases are discussed along with insights drawn from other related disciplines that might shed additional light on the care of this highly disenfranchised group.

CASE REPORTS

David Grant

David Grant was identified at birth as having a rare genetic disorder characterized by microcephaly, mental retardation, cardiac defects, and a shortened life span. His development progressed as predicted, significantly behind that of his brother, and his communication skills were minimal. His sleep pattern was always aberrant, and he would awaken repeatedly through the night. Pharmacological approaches to his sleep difficulties were never successful, and his parents developed a system of shared responsibility for his care at night so that at least one of them was able to rest. Despite this, David's disposition was sunny and easygoing.

At the age of 5, David became increasingly irritable, and he was eventually diagnosed with gastroesophageal reflux. Medication and positioning were not helpful, nor was surgery. He could tolerate only nasogastric feedings for nutrition. Shortly thereafter, David's personality began to change. He became essentially inconsolable at times and would scream out and tighten his body throughout the day. He always seemed on edge and uncomfortable. David had repeated hospitalizations to evaluate his discomfort, but no obvious source was ever identified. He was given a trial of opioids empirically to determine if his irritability could be reduced. David's irritability diminished somewhat following analgesia, and, as a result, his care providers felt that he was experiencing pain. Even with this intervention, he was inconsolable much of the time, and there was a fine line between relief and excessive sedation. Mrs. Grant experimented with different combinations of the sedatives and analgesics that were prescribed. She would find combinations that were successful for limited periods of time, but then they seemed to inexplicably stop working.

Nighttimes remained particularly difficult for the Grant family. Mr. and Mrs. Grant became increasingly exhausted, and their relationship with their older son began to deteriorate. Even though they had a large, supportive family, David's medical fragility and extensive nursing care requirements precluded anyone but his parents from staying with him, and they essentially had no respite from the demands of caring for him. Even during hospitalizations, the Grants were always present in the hospital, and often the nurses would ask Mrs. Grant's advice on how best to comfort David. When she left for the cafeteria, she would hear David crying in the background. She felt, legitimately so, that her son always seemed to need her. Mrs. Grant and her husband became increasingly exhausted, and the health care team began looking for respite care for David, a child with significant medical needs and limited communication ability who did not sleep through the night and cried most of the day. The appropriate setting was never identified. David was not sick enough for a long-term stay in an acute care facility but was too medically complex for any of the available medical foster homes. All involved with him felt frustrated and exhausted.

This pattern persisted for approximately 4 months until Mrs. Grant put David to bed one night and he did not awaken at the expected 1–2 hours after being put to sleep. She returned to the room and found that David was dead, secondary to aspiration. At the wake, while being consoled by a huge cadre of friends and family, Mrs. Grant stated that at least now David was sleeping and no longer in pain.

Cynthia Thomas

Cynthia Thomas is a young woman with spastic quadriplegia now in her early twenties. She has some dysarthria and is hard to understand. She uses a wheelchair and requires help with transfers. Cynthia has significant learning disabilities, particularly in nonverbal areas, and has genuine difficulties with visuospatial and sequential memory tasks. Despite her disabilities, Cynthia has a wonderful sense of humor, enjoys being with others, and does not seem to take herself too seriously. She describes with great relish her attempt to travel on spring break in college with a number of other students with disabilities. She is fiercely independent and proud. Cynthia's medical condition has subjected her to much pain, including pain from scoliosis and its treatment, pain from contractures and resultant surgeries, frequent spasms, and incident pain associated with movement and therapies. Essentially all of these pain problems, at least historically, have been undertreated.

Cynthia's postoperative pain management has often been markedly inadequate. The general tendency of surgeons to minimize postoperative pain has been even more pronounced in her care. Her care providers often underestimate her intellectual abilities and therefore discount her ability to legitimately report her discomfort. Cynthia, herself, often forgets that she can request pain medication and, because of her problems with time, does not realize when she is able to request her next dose. Therefore, even when she was offered the ability to participate in her own care, such as with the use of patient-controlled analgesia for postoperative pain relief during her scoliosis or release surgeries, she rarely used bolus doses, which led her nurses to assume that she was not having pain. The facial distortions that she demonstrates in association with her cerebral palsy make it harder for care providers to read her facial expression for clues to evaluate her level of discomfort. As a result of these factors, Cynthia was often reluctant to undergo medical procedures and felt helpless even when attempts were made to involve her in her care.

Her pain treatment out of the hospital was similarly compromised. Cynthia's desire for independence often led her to assume responsibility for tasks that she could not, in reality, physically accomplish. For example, when she went to college, she wanted to administer her own pain medication, which she had previously done at home with the help of her parents. A sliding scale of benzodiazepines and opioids were available to her based on her own assessment of her needs. A detailed schedule was developed by Cynthia and her doctors. Despite this, Cynthia's learning problems and disorganization often caused her confusion about her regimen. She would forget which medicine she required, when she was supposed to take it, and whether she actually did take it. This caused havoc in her medical care because the data with which to make judgments were often inaccurate or unavailable. However, her doctors were reluctant to remove this responsibility that she so treasured and took as a sign of increasing and hard-earned independence.

Cynthia also encountered a general lack of expertise in the medical community concerning the management of her pain. She required the assistance of orthopedic surgeons, physiatrists, physical and occupational therapists, as well as clinicians to address her general medical care. Members of her medical team were far-flung (in her home town, at specialized hospitals, in her college town) and did not communicate with each other. Because of limited information, even the experts could not agree on how best to help her. Her pharmacological regimen was also complicated. She had drugs for spasticity and for pain and other drugs to counter the side effects of those drugs.

At this time, Cynthia has graduated from college and is living in an apartment complex designed for individuals with severe physical disabilities. Her care has been consolidated and her pain is adequately managed. It has been a long and tortuous journey, but she is optimistic about her future.

CASE DISCUSSION

These cases are offered to point out some of the genuine complexity and variability in dealing with pain in a population with disabilities. Although a unique literature is emerging for defining and treating these issues, there is much to be learned from clinical anecdotes and from extrapolation from other literatures. An attempt is made to address some of these issues, which have been divided arbitrarily into assessment and clinical care.

Assessment

A number of complex issues emerge regarding the assessment of pain in individuals with developmental disabilities. Many of these have been covered in other chapters in this volume, but, because of the importance of adequate assessment, they are reviewed in this section.

Recognition of Pain

The clinician who is even considering developing a specific pain treatment plan for a patient has already made two important assumptions: 1) that an individual is actually capable of experiencing pain, and 2) that pain is itself worthy of treatment, that is, that the treatment is not worse than the symptom and that its successful management will make a difference in the life of the treated individual. Although these assumptions seem on the surface to be self-evident and to represent universal truths for all patients, this is not always as clear.

Clinicians have historically tended to discount the possibility of pain in certain populations. Until relatively recently, for example, pain in infants and young children tended to be ignored (Eland, 1977; Mather & Mackie, 1983; Schechter, Allen, & Hanson, 1986). Surgeries were performed on infants without anesthesia; postoperative analgesia in children was minimal or nonexistent; and painful procedures were performed without sedation. These clinical practices reflected the underlying attitudes of the practicing community—that children because of the immaturity of their nervous systems did not experience pain the way adults did (Schechter & Allen, 1986). The fact that children did not display behaviors thought to represent pain and often did not request pain relief further bolstered these practices. When a body of research began to emerge that contradicted these attitudes, indicating that infants as early as the second trimester have the neuroanatomical and neurochemical capability to experience pain (Anand & Hickey, 1987) and that alternative ways of assessment demonstrated far more pain than had been assumed (Finely & McGrath, 1997), attitudes and practice behaviors began to change. Newer surveys suggest that essentially all providers who care for children believe that children experience pain (Broome, Richtsmeier, Maikler, & Alexander, 1996; McLauglin, Hull, Edwards, Cramer, & Dewey, 1993).

Although this issue is well resolved for typically developing children, the situation is far from resolved for individuals like David and Cynthia. Some medical care providers have historically believed that the nervous systems of individuals with developmental disabilities are sufficiently different from the norm that their pain perception may be diminished or nonexistent. Cynthia would often say that few believed that she was experiencing pain because the source of her pain was not obvious and because her outward response to pain was nontraditional.

The research supporting the notion that individuals with disabilities may experience pain differently or not at all is both confusing and controversial. Investigators have explored this phenomenon at both the biochemical and clinical levels. For example, a series of papers both support and refute the contention that endogenous opioid peptides are increased in children with autism. The finding of elevated endogenous opioids has been offered to support the reported observation that children with autism are less responsive to painful stimuli than are agematched peers. There is still significant ongoing controversy regarding these theories, and more research is needed before they can be either accepted or rejected (Hunter, O'Hare, Harron, Fisher, & Jones, 2003; Shattock, Hooper, & Waring, 2004). Other investigators have compared the responses of individuals with and without developmental disabilities to similar painful stimuli. Gilbert-MacLeod, Craig, Rocha, and Mathias (2000) observed the response patterns of children with and without disabilities to the normal bumps and bruises that accompany childhood. They found that, compared to children without disabilities, children with disabilities had a moderated response to normal trauma and often did not seek attention from adults for their injuries. Biersdorff (1994) likewise identified an unconventional pain response in adults with disabilities, which he thought might reflect basic biophysical differences such as an elevated pain threshold. Oberlander, Gilbert,

Chambers, O'Donnell, and Craig (1999) identified a difference in response to immunization in children with disabilities as compared to age-matched peers. All of these investigators perceived that the differing response patterns were at least in part explained by poorer social communication of pain rather than less pain and emphasized the need to recognize and anticipate pain in this population regardless.

As for the second assumption that there is value in pain treatment, research has identified negative long-term consequences, both biological and psychological, if pain is inadequately addressed (Goldschneider & Anand, 2003; Weisman, Bernstein, & Schechter, 1998). As a result of this research as well as our deepening understanding of the nature of pain and how to treat it more effectively, there has been a significant change in practice behavior. Now, pain that is predictable and for which treatment algorithms can be developed and easily implemented, such as postoperative pain, is more effectively treated (Johnston, Abbott, Gray-Donald, & Jeans, 1992). Unfortunately, pains that are less predictable, more chronic, and without obvious source are still poorly addressed because they require not only the assumption that the individual could be experiencing pain but also more rigorous monitoring and assessment. Although their postoperative and procedure pain would probably be better treated today, the chronic, persistent pains that David and Cynthia experienced would still probably not be well recognized because they could not be predicted or anticipated. In this way, except for the additional complexity of their pain assessment, their care would probably be similar to that of age-matched peers.

Issues of Intellectual Capacity and Learning Disabilities

Self-report is well recognized as the "gold standard" of pain assessment (Finley & McGrath, 1997). Traditionally, typically developing children older than the age of 7 or 8 use adult visual analogue scales because it is assumed that they possess the underlying psychological processes necessary to quantify their discomfort. Children between 3 and 7, who typically have some ability to internally survey their pain and quantify it, can often use less abstract versions of the visual analogue scales such as cartoon faces, color scales, and the like. For children younger than 3 years, composite measures have been developed using physiological and behavioral markers to assess pain.

The applicability of these measures to individuals with developmental disabilities is complicated by a host of factors. First, physicians tend to overestimate a child's intellectual ability if the child is not dysmorphic and is well dressed (Korsch, Cobb, & Ashe, 1961). Therefore, it is imperative to actually know the child's cognitive status before assigning a specific type of self-report measure. Even that knowledge, however, is often not adequate. These scales are based on the notion that the child's development, whatever its level, is uniform. Individuals with disabilities, however, are often not merely delayed (i.e., acting as would a younger child). They may also have significant unevenness in their learning profiles, which may further complicate assessment. For example, Cynthia's severe learning disabilities in areas of sequential memory made it difficult for her to provide information regarding her pain even though she was able to seriate and appeared to have the cognitive ability to quantify her discomfort.

Besides issues of intellectual capacity and learning style, other disabilities may impact on our ability to interpret discomfort in individuals with disabilities. For example, Cynthia's dysarthria limits the ability of her providers to understand her speech. Clinicians would nod as though they understood her, when in fact they did not, so as not to offend or patronize her. In retrospect, she might have been better served by use of a communication board. The frequent facial movements that she demonstrates are additional impediments to using traditional assessment methods for her, and well-meaning clinicians may misinterpret facial tics as pain grimaces.

Use of Functional Measures

For Cynthia, therefore, using assessment techniques that focus on her functioning and not solely on her report are an essential aspect of adequately monitoring her pain, both its intensity and its qualities. These techniques emerged from the chronic pain literature (Bursch, Walco, & Zeltzer, 1998), where it was recognized that children and adults with persistent pain would often rate their pain intensity as unchanging (e.g., always 10 of 10), despite demonstrating changes in mood and function. As a result, clinicians began to informally incorporate questions about overall functioning into their analyses. Sleep, appetite, social involvement, hardiness and endurance, and mood were all considered when attempting to evaluate the degree of discomfort an individual was experiencing and assess the impact of an intervention. Such measures should be considered as part of an overall assessment strategy, and an emerging literature supports their value (Eccleston, Malleson, Clinch, Connell, & Sourbut, 2003; Walker & Greene, 1991). The difficulty is, of course, having adequate knowledge of the individual's baseline functioning so that changes from baseline can be appreciated. Parents are invaluable in providing that information.

Proxy Reporters

A seminal clinical and ethical issue in individuals whose pain cannot be adequately assessed by the treating team is the use of proxy reporters to assess pain. Parents are often the proxy reporters, and, although their evaluation is essential and perhaps the most important variable in appreciating pain in individuals with developmental disabilities, the subjectivity of their report needs to be taken into account. Parents may feel guilty, stressed, or anxious, and this may impact on their interpretation of their child's symptom. David's parents, for example, were completely exhausted. They never slept, and the burden of providing his care never left them, even in the hospital. Given the essential subjectivity of pain assessment, wherein subtle clues may be all that we have on which to base treatment decisions, relying on fatigued and demoralized individuals to be the sole arbiters of pain and suffering in their children is problematic at best. The extensive literature on parenting children with disabilities demonstrates the enormous resiliency of families, but the impact of guilt and chronic sorrow should not be underestimated (Olshansky, 1962). Parents may react in any number of ways. Conflicting feelings of guilt about what their child must endure, embarrassment about calling the doctor yet again, total exhaustion, and feelings of helplessness and loss of control may cause families to under- or oversurvey their child's behavior for evidence of discomfort. It is important, therefore, to recognize that pain assessment in individuals with disabilities should not be reduced to a single instrument, even if modified for this population, or to the reports of a single individual. If pain can be anticipated (i.e., from a surgery or a procedure), it should be prevented in the same way that the pain of all individuals should be addressed. If it is unpredictable, multiple sources of information should be used to assess it, including parental and provider reports as well as functional measures.

Clinical Care

Experience and extrapolation from other literatures offers some practical insights into the issues encountered in the clinical care of children and adults with developmental disabilities.

Coordination of Care

Children and adults with developmental disabilities often require the services of multiple physicians to address their complex needs. David's care team included geneticists, general pediatricians, gastroenterologists, neurologists, pain specialists, and home care nurses. Each had an important role to play, would make suggestions to his parents, and prescribed medications, but unfortunately each often would not talk to the others involved in David's care. As a result, David's mother felt that she was "a general contractor" who was somehow responsible to coordinate the input of all of the "subcontractors." To change metaphors, there was no obvious captain of the ship, and, as a result, David's mother was somehow responsible for navigating it. Cynthia and her family faced similar issues.

Such a situation is typical for children with developmental disabilities as well as children with life-threatening diseases. The Institute of Medicine report on palliative care for children identified lack of coordination of care as one of the most difficult problems that parents encountered:

> In parents' stories of their experiences with a child's life threatening illness and death, two frequent themes are the burden of coordination of the many elements of their child's care and sustaining trusted relationships. Parents find themselves spending hours on the phone trying to identify, schedule, and coordinate providers and services and also to struggle with health plan requirements and procedures. They may have to ensure that essential medical information and care plans accompany their child from one provider to another and still repeatedly explain the child's history and their experiences and preferences regarding the child's care. (Field & Berman, 2003, pp. 187–188)

Communication and coordination are therefore important in all aspects of the care of children with developmental disabilities. The treatment of pain and related symptoms is particularly vulnerable to mismanagement if multiple providers are involved. Oversedation is possible if many subspecialists are prescribing variations of the same drugs for different pain problems. Serotonin syndrome is another distinct possibility (Gillman, 1999). Therefore, the pain management of children with developmental disabilities should be centralized if possible. Even though pain may stem from different biological systems, it is advantageous if only one individual is prescribing analgesics, sedatives, antidepressants, and hypnotics.

Psychosocial Variables

A host of psychosocial variables may influence the care that children with developmental disabilities receive by affecting the families in which they live. It is intuitive that caring for a child with any chronic disorder increases stress and the likelihood of parental depression. This hypothesis is supported by research on the families of children with chronic pain (Hunfield et al., 2001), biochemical genetic disorders (Waisbren, Rones, Read, Marsden, & Levy, 2004), muscular dystrophy (Nereo, Fee, & Hinton, 2003), and cerebral palsy (Manuel, Naughton, Balkrishnan, Patterson Smith, & Koman, 2003). In most studies, parental stress is increased, quality of life deteriorates, social life becomes restricted, and depression increases dramatically. Obviously, these factors that impact so dramatically on families alter their ability to shoulder the burdens of care that these children require, not the least of which is assessment and management of pain. As the mother of a child with cerebral palsy put it:

> Sometimes I feel like a doctor, therapist, nurse, chauffeur, inventor, builder, computer expert, communication expert . . . so many things; I sometimes forget I am still a mom. (Tuna, Unalan, Tuna, & Kokino, 2004, p. 647)

Because the nature of pain is so multifactorial and its assessment so inherently subjective, parental depression, exhaustion, anger, guilt, embarrassment, and sadness may influence their interpretation of their child's pain ratings and behaviors. Siblings also shoulder additional burdens. Meta-analyses from the chronic illness literature speak to the importance of not only addressing sibling concerns that are causing family upheaval but also anticipating those that may be bubbling quietly below the surface (Sharpe & Rossiter, 2002).

It is imperative, therefore, that the psychosocial functioning of the family be considered when dealing with the medical care of children with developmental disabilities. The medical provider should specifically inquire about depression, exhaustion, and stress directly as well as indirectly through assessing parental functioning. Although caring for these children will still remain challenging, endorsing for the family how difficult it is, that the feelings that they have are normal, and that the care they are providing is essential is often validating and helpful for families who may feel unappreciated and as though they are shouldering burdens that are unique. Identifying counselors who are familiar with the issues involved in caring for a child with a disability and are not patronizing or overly solicitous is often helpful for parents, as are referrals to support groups. Finally, helping the family identify respite care opportunities is enormously helpful. Respite care will allow the family to replenish its psychological resources, decrease resentment, and enhance its functioning. David's family would have benefited dramatically from a short period of respite care wherein the needs of his brother could be addressed and the stress of being continuously "on call" could be eliminated at least for a short while.

Procedure Pain

Children and adults with developmental disabilities are subjected to frequent medical procedures. These range from nonpainful procedures that require cooperation, such as imaging studies, to procedures that are associated with minor discomfort, such as phlebotomy or venous cannulation, to procedures that are quite painful, such as bone marrow aspirations, pin removals, and the like.

A few factors that are unique to children with developmental disabilities may impact on their experience during these procedures. Preparation prior to medical procedures is now standard care for most children and adults. Discussion in a developmentally appropriate manner prior to the procedure about what will happen and how it will feel has been shown in multiple studies to reduce anxiety and pain during the subsequent procedure (Peterson, 1989; Zeltzer, Jay, & Fisher, 1989). Advanced preparation may not be feasible in some children with developmental disabilities, however, if they have extreme limitations in their cognitive abilities. Preparation may also be inadequate if the clinician either under- or overestimates the child's intellectual capabilities. Regardless, it is important for the medical team to understand not only the child's physical problems but his or her level of development. This also speaks to the potential for increased impact of procedures on children with disabilities, who may be subjected to procedures without the often calming knowledge of what is happening to them, why it is occurring, and when it will end.

Additional research from the cancer literature may provide further insight into the experience of children with developmental disabilities/neurological impairments who are undergoing painful procedures. Studies now suggest that in individuals subjected to sequential painful procedures, the adequacy of pain control during the initial procedure may impact on the pain associated with subsequent procedures. In one study (Weisman et al., 1998), individuals who received adequate sedation initially during a bone marrow aspiration reported less pain on subsequent bone marrow aspirations than did a group who had a placebo analgesic initially, even though both groups had similar sedation/analgesia in the subsequent marrow aspirations. This finding was statistically significant only in the group of children younger than age 8. In the group of children older than 8, additional discussion and preparation could allay fears and concerns about the upcoming procedure. This knowledge changed the subsequent experience. In the younger group, however, preparation was unable to undo their initial negative experience because of normal age-related cognitive limitations, and, as a result, they experienced more pain. This finding may have relevance to a group with developmental disabilities whose intellectual understanding of the procedure may be less mature; their understanding may resemble that of the younger group in the study.

Pharmacological Interventions

Pharmacological therapy in children with developmental disabilities is often complicated. Factors that might explain this complexity are biological differences in these individuals, lack of ability to adequately monitor the efficacy of the drug secondary to communication gaps between the patient and the provider, pain problems that are unique to this population, limitations in the ability to assess nonpain symptoms in noncommunicating patients (nausea, fatigue), and the general limitation of research on pharmacological agents in children.

Individuals with developmental disabilities may have altered or idiosyncratic responses to medications. This is certainly the clinical experience of many who work in this field. There is no uniform explanation for this phenomenon given the wide variation of individuals who are categorized as having developmental disabilities. This variability in drug response seen in a subset of patients may merely be a reflection of their biological variability and may reflect differences in the way drugs are metabolized or their impact at the end organ. Regardless, differences in the metabolism of certain drugs and in their side effect profiles have been reported in individuals with developmental disabilities. The subset of individuals in whom this is so needs to be rigorously studied to understand the underlying biological variability.

It may be, however, that some of the observed differences may also stem from our inadequacy to recognize and assess pain in this population, a recurrent theme throughout this book. As a result, we are often left with only crude approximations of relief (decrease in crying time, less fidgetiness, decreased irritability), which may in fact miss subtle improvements that have occurred secondary to our interventions. For example, if pain improves the equivalent of 3 units on a traditional visual analogue 10-point scale (from 8 to 5), it would be hard to detect this change on the relatively unsophisticated instruments we have available to use with noncommunicating patients. We are even less sophisticated when it comes to measuring nonpain symptoms and medication side effects. For example, unless there is vomiting associated with it, nausea is difficult to recognize. Individuals who experience persistent nausea often report that it is as disabling, disheartening, and unpleasant as pain, yet this symptom eludes our measurement capabilities despite the availability of potential treatments.

There are also pains that are somewhat unique to individuals with developmental disabilities. For example, spasms associated with cerebral palsy can be almost incapacitating. There are some pharmacological approaches available to us, but the research literature is limited, and most practitioners are not comfortable with these medications.

Finally, there are the general limitations that exist on all medications for smaller specialized populations. The enormous expense necessary to bring a new drug to market creates a significant disincentive for the pharmaceutical industry to develop new medications for narrow populations. Children in particular are therapeutic orphans because they represent a smaller market and because research on them is often ethically and methodologically complex. Individuals with developmental disabilities present similar challenges—they are a small market, assessment is complicated, and issues of consent are challenging.

SUMMARY

This book addresses for the first time in a comprehensive way the pain problems that individuals with developmental disabilities encounter. Although a body of information is now emerging on this long-ignored population that can help us address their pain, a wealth of clinical experience and extrapolation from other literatures can provide additional insight.

The cases of David Grant and Cynthia Thomas are instructive in their demonstration of the wide range and variability of issues that these individuals can encounter. David had severe mental retardation and a limited life expectancy. His short life was marred by inadequately treated pain. Cynthia, who is more able to advocate for herself, struggled not only with communicating the details of her pain but also with the complex issues of autonomy and dependence.

In this chapter, some of the relevant issues regarding the management of pain in this population were reviewed. Most of these issues have been thoroughly discussed throughout this volume, but their clinical relevance calls for reemphasis.

Assessment is the cornerstone of adequate treatment, and the issues of assessment in individuals with developmental disabilities are manifold. Self-report is often impossible or unreliable, and proxy reporters, although well meaning, have inherent bias. Use of functional measures requires detailed baseline information and must be individualized for each person. Although these issues complicate assessment, they do not abrogate its importance in pain treatment.

Clinically, individuals with complex medical problems often have pain problems in many realms. Coordination of care is essential to assure that someone is responsible for pain management. Without a coordinated approach, pain is often easily ignored by assuming another provider will handle it or addressed by multiple clinicians with the attendant risk of overmedication. Compliance with any medical regimen in this population involves the whole family. The needs of family members are often suppressed and ignored because each individual perceives that he or she must first address the seemingly endless needs of the dependent charge. Feelings inevitably bubble to the surface that can undermine the family unit and the subsequent care of the individual with disabilities. Procedures, which are a fact of life in many medically complex individuals, need to be planned for adequately. Medications need to be carefully monitored because most lack supportive controlled research to determine their safety and efficacy.

These caveats are offered only as a cautionary note, not to imply futility or to undermine the critical importance of addressing pain in this population. Approaches to pain management in individuals with developmental disabilities need to be crafted from the combination of available information and the creation of new information. This volume, by calling attention to the needs of this underserved population and cataloging what we already know, is an important first step.

REFERENCES

Anand, K.J.S., & Hickey, P.R. (1987). Pain and its effects in the human neonate and fetus. *New England Journal of Medicine, 317,* 1321–1329.

Biersdorff, K.K. (1994). Incidence of significantly altered pain experience among individuals with developmental disabilities. *American Journal on Mental Retardation, 98,* 619–631.

Broome, M.E., Richtsmeier, A., Maikler, V., & Alexander, M. (1996). Pediatric pain practices: A national survey of health professionals. *Journal of Pain and Symptom Management, 11,* 312–320.

Bursch, B., Walco, G.A., & Zeltzer, L. (1998). Clinical assessment and management of chronic pain and pain-associated disability syndrome. *Journal of Developmental and Behavioral Pediatrics, 19,* 45–53.

Eccleston, C., Malleson, P.N., Clinch, J., Connell, H., & Sourbut, C. (2003). Chronic pain in adolescents: Evaluation of a programme of interdisciplinary cognitive behaviour therapy. *Archives of Disease in Childhood, 88,* 881–885.

Eland, J.M. (1977). The experience of pain in children. In A. Jacob (Ed.), *Pain: A source book for nurses and other health professionals* (pp. 453–471). Boston: Little, Brown.

Field, M.J., & Behrman, R.E. (Eds.). (2003). *When children die: Improving palliative and end-of-life care for children and their families* (pp. 187–188). Washington, DC: National Academies Press.

Finley, G.A., & McGrath, P.J. (Eds.). (1997). *Measurement of pain in infants and children* (Problems in Pain Research and Management, Vol. 10). Seattle: IASP Press.

Gilbert-MacLeod, C.A., Craig, K.D., Rocha, E.M., & Mathias, M.D. (2000). Everyday pain responses in children with and without developmental delays. *Journal of Pediatric Psychology, 25,* 301–308.

Gillman, P.K. (1999). The serotonin syndrome and its treatment. *Journal of Psychopharmacology, 13,* 100–109.

Goldschneider, K.R., & Anand, K.J.S. (2003). The long term consequences of pain in neonates. In N.L. Schechter, C.B. Berde, & M. Yaster (Eds.), *Pain in infants, children, and adolescents* (2nd ed., pp. 58–70). Philadelphia: Lippincott, Williams & Wilkins.

Hunfeld, J.A., Perquin, C.W., Duivenvoorden, H.J., Hazebroek-Kampschreur, A.A., Passchier, J., van Suijlekom-Smit, L.W., et al. (2001). Chronic pain and its impact on quality of life in adolescents and their families. *Journal of Pediatric Psychology, 26,* 145–153.

Hunter, L.C., O'Hare, A., Herron, W.J., Fisher, L.A., & Jones, G.E. (2003). Opioid peptides and dipeptyl peptidase in autism. *Developmental Medicine and Child Neurology, 45,* 121–128.

Johnston, C.C., Abbott, F.V., Gray-Donald, K., & Jeans, M.E. (1992). A survey of pain in hospitalized patients aged 4–14 years. *Clinical Journal of Pain, 8,* 154–163.

Korsch, B., Cobb, K., & Ashe, B. (1961). Pediatricians' appraisals of patients' intelligence. *Pediatrics, 27,* 990–1003.

Manuel, J., Naughton, M.J., Balkrishnan, R., Patterson Smith, B., & Koman, L.A. (2003). Stress and adaptation in mothers of children with cerebral palsy. *Journal of Pediatric Psychology, 28,* 197–201.

Mather, L., & Mackie, J. (1983). The incidence of postoperative pain in children. *Pain, 15,* 271–282.

McLaughlin, C.R., Hull, J.G., Edwards, W.H., Cramer, C.P., & Dewey, W.L. (1993). Neonatal pain: A comprehensive survey of attitudes and practices. *Journal of Pain and Symptom Management, 8,* 7–16.

Nereo, N.E., Fee, R.J., & Hinton, V.J. (2003). Parental stress in mothers of boys with Duchenne muscular dystrophy. *Journal of Pediatric Psychology, 28,* 473–484.

Oberlander, T.F., Gilbert, C.A., Chambers, C.T., O'Donnell, M.E., & Craig, K.D. (1999). Biobehavioral responses to acute pain in adolescents with a significant neurological impairment. *Clinical Journal of Pain, 15,* 201–209.

Olshansky, S. (1962). Chronic sorrow: A response to having a mentally defective child. *Social Casework, 43,* 190–193.

Peterson, L. (1989). Coping by children undergoing stressful medical procedures: Some conceptual, methodological and therapeutic issues. *Journal of Consulting and Clinical Psychology, 57,* 380–387.

Schechter, N.L., & Allen, D. (1986). Physicians' attitudes toward pain in children. *Journal of Developmental and Behavioral Pediatrics, 7,* 350–354.

Schechter, N.L., Allen, D.A., & Hanson, K. (1986). Status of pediatric pain control: A comparison of hospital based analgesic usage in children and adults. *Pediatrics, 77,* 11–15.

Sharpe, D., & Rossiter, L. (2002). Siblings of children with a chronic illness: A meta-analysis. *Journal of Pediatric Psychology, 27,* 699–710.

Shattock, P., Hooper, M., & Waring, R. (2004). Opioid peptides and dipeptidyl peptidase in autism [Letter]. *Developmental Medicine and Child Neurology, 46,* 357–358.

Tuna, K., Unalan, H., Tuna, F., & Kokino, S. (2004). Quality of life of primary caregivers of children with cerebral palsy: A controlled study with Short Form-36 questionnaire. *Developmental Medicine and Child Neurology, 46,* 647–648.

Waisbren, S.E., Rones, M., Read, C.Y., Marsden, D., & Levy, H.L. (2004). Brief report: Predictors of parenting stress among parents of children with biochemical genetic disorders. *Journal of Pediatric Psychology, 29,* 565–570.

Walker, L.S., & Greene, J.W. (1991). The Functional Disability Inventory: Measuring a neglected dimension of child health status. *Journal of Pediatric Psychology, 16,* 39–58.

Weisman, S.J., Bernstein, B., & Schechter, N.L. (1998). Consequences of inadequate analgesia during painful procedures in children. *Archives of Pediatrics and Adolescent Medicine, 152,* 147–149.

Zeltzer, L.K., Jay, S.M., & Fisher, D.M. (1989). The management of pain associated with pediatric procedures. *Pediatric Clinics of North America, 36,* 941–964.

14

TRANSLATIONAL RESEARCH PERSPECTIVES AND PRIORITIES

Frank J. Symons and Tim F. Oberlander

The work represented by this volume highlights the complex and challenging nature of pain in individuals with developmental disabilities and the inherently interdisciplinary nature of this field. An interdisciplinary intersection can be uncertain territory, filled with multiple converging but often divergent assumptions, perspectives, and research traditions. This dynamic space is filled with the promise of generating novel solutions for long-standing problems. Although within-discipline inquiry in pharmacology, physiology, molecular biology, genetics, anthropology, and psychology has led to remarkable advances in understanding pain, it is likely that the next advances will come from the intersections of these fields.

In addressing pain in individuals with developmental disabilities, the field requires us to build interdisciplinary networks investigating multiple interrelated components of the brain, behavior, and clinical sciences that ultimately lead to transforming new knowledge into novel therapeutic approaches. Beyond the obvious need for new basic knowledge, there are contextual barriers that need to be crossed. These range from disciplinary jargon and cultural differences among scientists and clinicians, with their specific disciplinary backgrounds, to structural problems within academia. Further, a drive to achieve first-authored publications and the perception that interdisciplinary research reduces chances for tenure and promotion also complicates this situation (National Academy Press, 2000). These barriers need to be overcome, and, indeed, there is emerging recognition of a significant commitment to *translational research* cutting across funding agencies that has been aptly described in the National Institutes of Health "Roadmap" (http://nih roadmap.nih.gov/initiatives.asp).

In this chapter, we explore a number of related translational research perspectives and priorities central to addressing the urgent clinical and research challenges facing our understanding of pain among individuals with developmental disabilities. As a starting point, it is worth recapping several major issues raised by the contributors. In terms of the current status of pain assessment and treatment among programs for individuals with intellectual and communication disabilities, severe neuromotor impairments, and related developmental disabilities, pain management is not routinely considered a part of care. Although everyday pain and discomfort appear to be substantial among individuals with a range of developmental disorders and related disabilities; until recently this has been overlooked by the scientific and health care community. Moreover, postoperative pain appears to be undertreated, and, more generally, conditions associated with chronic pain are often not considered for pain management in this population. Many questions underlie these clinical observations for which we simply do not have answers based on reliable, credible empirical evidence. Are individuals with developmental disabilities less sensitive or reactive to painful events? Notably, what are the common beliefs about pain in people with developmental disabilities across health care and related care providers? What is the best or the most efficient way to identify pain if a person cannot self-report? What are the mechanisms that underlie pain most commonly associated with different developmental disabilities? What is considered best practice in the management of pain in individuals with cognitive, communicative, and motor impairments associated with developmental disabilities?

The contributors to this volume provide a foundation from which to address such pressing questions. There can be little doubt that attitudes and beliefs about pain in individuals with developmental disability affect clinical practice. Craig's discussion concerning the definition of pain forces a broader appreciation for the nuances of the construct itself, whereas Sobsey provides an important ethical framework to consider issues inherent in pain in specialized and vulnerable populations. Kehl and Goldetsky's overview of the neurobiological mechanisms underlying pain emphasizes the remarkable advances made from the basic sciences and reminds us of the work required to link these basic findings with clinical practice. The review by Bottos and Chambers point out the scope of the problem, and the contributions of Breau, Stevens, and Grunau, as well as Engels and Kartin, Kennedy and O'Reilly, and Taddio and Oberlander, suggest the myriad developmental, functional, pharmacological, and behavioral consequences associated with pain and its impact on daily life. O'Donnell proposes use of a conceptual framework that helps account for the multiple functional impairments in the context of everyday pain compounding the inherent impairments of a developmental disability. The reviews by Breau, McGrath, and Zabalia and by Bodfish and colleagues indicate that pain can be measured reliably among individuals with developmental disabilities using observable, nonverbal behaviors. Finally, Schechter effectively ends at the beginning by providing two penetrating case histories illustrating the clinical complexities and scientific uncertainties posed by pain in developmental disability.

TRANSLATIONAL BARRIERS AND FRAMEWORKS

With this discussion as a starting point, what, then, are the translational issues facing the study of pain in developmental disabilities? What barriers may interfere with moving knowledge from research to practice? In all areas of science, advances in methodology and measurement go hand in hand with advances in substantive knowledge. New technologies in studying the human brain make it possible to engage in systematic study of the neural circuitry and mechanisms underlying the complexities of the human pain experience. Despite substantial advances in the neuroscience of pain, we still have much work to do to translate this knowledge into reliable and valid interventions with measurable real-world effects. As mentioned previously, there can be numerous barriers to interdisciplinary research. In addition to substantive issues specific to disciplinary inquiry, there are at least two "meta-level" challenges that can limit the realization of a translational research agenda predicated on interdisciplinary research. The first may be referred to as a "linkage" problem: How do we build sustainable and productive links among disciplines? The second may be referred to as "levels of analysis" problem: How do we integrate findings based on different scales (metrics), time frames (slow versus fast reactivity), account for reactivity system discordances (i.e., biological and behavioral discordances or typical developmental processes that are inherently discordant), and categories of measurement specific to any given discipline? The former requires a sound understanding of the mechanisms that constitute the pain system. The latter involves moving back and forth between the basic neurological substrate of pain and pain behavior in social contexts. As Salzinger (1992) observed, writing from a different position on translational research issues, there can be serious interpretive problems when we seek to correlate the blood levels of metabolites of some single neurotransmitter, measured correct to the nearest nanogram, with behavioral ratings measured correct to the nearest rater. In short, the precision of measurement has to be balanced against the ambiguity of interpretation when all relevant pieces of the phenomenon under investigation remain unknown.

Current advances in the two primary spheres of research in pain—brain and behavior—provide an opportunity to make new connections between data that can inform assessment, treatment and practice. The relationship among basic and clinical nodes need to be organized in a conceptual framework designed to begin to define the process of successful interdisciplinary and translational research that addresses the problem of pain in developmental disability. The framework should include

- A statement of the specific problem framed at the behavioral level (e.g., procedural pain associated with intramuscular botulinum toxin injection for the treatment of spasticity)

- The incidence and prevalence of the problem (e.g., for what percentage of individuals with cerebral palsy is procedural pain associated with Botox injection?)

- The outcomes associated with the problem (e.g., what specific consequences are associated with procedural pain of this type?)

- The mechanisms (neural and behavioral) underlying the problem (e.g., what underlying circuitry is mediating the pain signal associated with deep intramuscular injection/needling? what are the effects of different caregiver behavior on the expression of pain/discomfort during such procedures?)

- Identified interactions with other risk factors (e.g., is the procedural pain different for individuals with different forms of cerebral palsy associated with different conditions?)

- Preclinical models of the problem (e.g., is there a relevant preclinical model that could be developed or that already exists for this type of clinical pain problem?)

- Interventions and their relative efficacy and effectiveness for the problem (e.g., what evidence-based approaches could be used in a randomized trial for the treatment of this type of pain?)

In addition, there should be a justification of why the proposed interdisciplinary approach is an improvement over past approaches at solving the problem, together with a specific interdisciplinary plan and proposed time line to bring to scale and test the feasibility of theoretically derived interventions.

At this point, the standard model of progress tends to rely on a unidirectional flow of information from the basic sciences to the clinical disciplines, with the former often proceeding relatively independently from the latter's needs (Stokes, 1997). An alternative model of progress might be characterized as bidirectional, in which basic and clinical needs inform each other. In a bidirectional model, translational research may develop and advance in more sustainable ways because the agenda is driven (and constrained) by a broader array of contextual factors, including disciplinary culture, local capacity, and specific group processes, all with reference to the nature of the problem (i.e., its significance, history, models, designs, and tools). Although not always discussed as such, much of the problem of extending findings from bench to bedside has to do with understanding the conditions of knowledge production and the way that the scientific method produces reliable and generalizable knowledge (Latour, 1999). Mao (2002) commented on exactly this notion in a topical review addressing the gap between basic and clinical research in pain. In this context, it is emphasized that the clinical value of any given basic research paradigm will be determined, in part, by the goodness of fit between critical features of the preclinical model and the critical features of clinical pain.

TRANSLATIONAL FRONTIERS

This volume reflects the substantial work that has been accomplished over the past few decades to understand pain in individuals with a disability. Much work still needs to be done. Despite work to study pain behaviors and to quantify, assess, and manage pain in a variety of populations of individuals with disabilities across the age spectrum, numerous questions remain. At a very basic level, our understanding of relations between altered neurological function and the pain system remains incomplete. Specifically, we need to address how a neurological injury, particularly one that occurs at critical times in neural development, alters the structure and function of the pain system. Similarly, we need to improve our understanding of how social and cognitive impairments influence the expression of pain, and the implications this might have for intervention strategies that reduce suffering in situations in which individuals experience repetitive painful events. Furthermore, work needs to be directed toward understanding the impact that family and social influences, mental illness, and culture have on the pain experience in this population. Finally, we need to seek ways to translate research into meaningful clinical and public health policies specific to individuals with developmental disabilities. This latter task requires us to confront the need to integrate new knowledge into everyday individual and organizational behavior that leads to substantive changes in the ways we think about and practice pain management in all settings.

Basic Science Frontiers

Despite the progress of preclinical experimentation, the findings from basic studies often reflect only a very small part of clinical pain problems (Mao, 2002). Even with changes to the definition of pain (see Chapter 2), the inherent heterogeneity associated with developmental disabilities requires considerable skill on the part of clinical researchers to accommodate the ambiguity associated with pain assessment and its measurement. Among the most compelling conceptual shifts in the understanding of pain regulatory mechanisms has been the notion of an active rather than passive nervous system (Melzack, 1999). A steadily growing body of empirical findings from multiple levels of inquiry (molecular, genomic, proteomic, cellular) has followed in tandem, providing convincing evidence of remarkable plasticity in pain regulatory networks. As one example, basic findings from research examining neuropathic pain suggest that peripheral or central neural tissue injury can set up long-lasting spinal and supraspinal reorganization partly through a process referred to as central sensitization (Woolf & Salter, 2000). Evidence suggests that this reorganization can extend to higher cortical areas, including the forebrain. What is not entirely clear are the circumstances under which such plasticity (e.g., forebrain changes) may be adaptive and promote functional recovery, or may be maladaptive and prevent or prolong functional recovery and thus undermine treatment. Work by Casey, Lorenz, and Minoshima (2003) suggested that the forebrain of individuals with chronic neuropathic pain can undergo pathologically induced changes that may impair clinical response to treatment because of reductions in the functional connectivity of subcortical pathways. A key challenge here is to determine how a neurological injury, leading to a developmental disability, disrupts the neural substrate that becomes the pain system. Similarly, how does injury or disruption to the development of one system lead to altered function of other systems (i.e., hypothalamic-pituitary-adrenal axis regulation, autonomic stress reactivity) that goes on to be expressed as altered pain behaviors? A clue to understanding how neurological injury influences the growth and development of the pain system may come from an emerging literature examining the long-term sequelae of early repetitive pain in term and preterm infants (Grunau, 2005). Of particular relevance is that some individuals with a developmental disability may, *by virtue of the (often unknown) underlying neurological impairment,* have altered functional connectivity in areas of the brain responsible for nociceptive processing. In this sense, they may be at risk for specific components of the pain experiences. The question is not simple and is translational by its very nature.

At a very basic level, we need to learn more about how genetic and metabolic defects that lead to developmental disability directly contribute to altered pain system function. Opportunities to examine this question may come from detailed studies of biobehavioral pain responses in individuals with Down syndrome, fragile X syndrome, or Lesch-Nyhan syndrome. To date, very limited work has examined basic sensory mechanisms related to nociception and pain in animal models of such developmental disorders. Similarly, examination of pharmacological factors associated with known genetic disorders need to be included in these pain paradigms to help understand differences in neural, autonomic, and neuroendocrine responses.

Clinical Frontiers

A major challenge facing clinical pain research is our ability to assess and quantify painful experiences in ways that are meaningful to individuals and caregivers alike. Of what use is an expression of pain without a meaningful response? Understanding the afferent and efferent arms of the pain experience is key to effective pain management. To move in the direction of understanding both mechanism (e.g., changed sensory threshold) and outcome (i.e., improved functioning), our ability to quantify sensory and pain parameters in individuals with cognitive and communicative skills that are compromised because of congenital or acquired neurological impairment must be improved. Defrin and colleagues (2004) reported on an unbiased (i.e., reaction time–free) method of testing pain thresholds in individuals with specific cognitive impairments. Similar work needs to be extended to larger trials with individuals with a range of cognitive and related neurological impairments. In studies of individuals with severe neurological impairment associated with developmental disabilities, including cognitive impairment and social-emotional disorders such as autism, a body of work is emerging that is explicitly designed to identify non–language-based pain-related behaviors associated with acute and chronic pain episodes (see Chapters 2, 10, and 11). More work is needed to understand relationships between pain and differing levels of consciousness (e.g., coma, brain injury) and mental illness, both of which may compound life with a developmental disability. In particular, research is needed to examine how the presence of mood, affective, and psychotic disorders alters the expression (i.e., relationships between anxiety disorder and expression of pain) and management (i.e., polypharmacy issues; see Chapter 12) of pain. Results consistently show that pain behavior among nonverbal individuals with developmental disabilities and related disorders corresponds to the timing of the noxious or painful event. The studies demonstrate that the magnitude of pain expression in nonverbal individuals with a range of severe neurological impairments can be reliably quantified. Objective measurement of pain expression in highly vulnerable specialized populations shows that painful events reliably lead to the same kinds of nonverbal pain expression seen in people without severe neurological impairments. This suggests that there is little reason to preclude such individuals from pain research designed to improve clinical practice.

Studies need to be undertaken that include individuals with developmental disabilities. In the past, such individuals were excluded explicitly from pain research. To understand the specific nature of pain, research designs should be directed at studying differences between individuals with and without disabilities, but should also include between and within subject designs (i.e., each subject used as his or her own control). The recent advances in behavioral pain assessment through rating scales and the application of facial coding and related technologies should be capitalized on in larger scale studies designed to address issues of treatment efficacy, predictors of treatment response, and individual differences in outcomes for the treatment and management of pain. Developmental disability should not be an exclusion criterion. Large-scale pain assessment and treatment studies should include populations representative of those who actually present to health services for treatment. In parallel, additional clinical work is necessary to examine more closely the specific signs and symptoms of pain and discomfort within and among individuals with a range of developmental disability. For example, the relation between sleep, pain, and developmental disability is not well understood despite the fact that sleep problems are pervasive among many individuals with developmental disabilities, and there are many beliefs and anecdotes about how sleep regulation could improve health and well-being, including pain and discomfort. Investigating such a complex relationship could, in turn, improve our basic understanding of the neurobiology of pain. Finally, we must use this new clinical knowledge to develop a focus that leads to interventions that improve pain management that are specific to varying levels of cognitive, social, and motor abilities.

Organizational and Service Delivery Frontiers

Regardless of advances in basic and clinical knowledge, without the infrastructure and organizational support to translate new knowledge into practice, advances in pain management will be slow and ineffective. Underlying much of the discussion in several chapters of this volume are implicit assumptions about the nature of pain assessment and treatment in the context of a medical model (i.e., pain as a medical problem or disorder). An alternative, which is not necessarily contradictory, is to consider pain and discomfort in the context of a habilitative model, in relation to quality of life and everyday function. From this perspective, numerous features of health care service delivery related to pain and quality of life, *based on what we already know,* could be addressed through an applied interdisciplinary research agenda. General training for all care staff should be provided to increase awareness of pain, pain types, and idiosyncrasies in pain expression. Key staff (direct care staff, nurses, and psychologists) should be trained in state-of-the-art objective pain assessment methods. Pain clinics or consultative teams with expertise in developmental disabilities should be established to advise on individual cases and to consult on hospital inpatient units, on surgery units, and in orthopedic clinics. Pharmacy and medical staff should be trained on current medication treatment guidelines and issues unique to increased risk of drug interactions (e.g., with anticonvulsants, with psychotropics) or preexisting cardiac or respiratory conditions. Training and knowledge transfer need to be consistent with the needs and expertise of these professionals at the moment they need the skills. Applying "just-in-time learning" focused on adult learners will be a key to moving the practice of pain management forward in this field. Teaching curricula specifically related to pain in individuals with developmental disabilities are beginning to emerge (see the International Association for the Study of Pain [IASP] web site: http://www.iasp-pain.org/index.html) and should become an inherent part of health care professionals' educational experience. Consistent with current standards, pain should be made the "fifth vital sign" in ongoing nursing/medical monitoring for individuals with developmental disabilities living in group home or similar aggregate care arrangements. Last, the potential impact of pain on quality-of-life indicators should be considered in person-centered planning.

Basic and Clinical Science Integration

Clinical and basic research scientists need common ground to develop collaborative laboratory and clinical research programs. Venues might range from common work and meeting spaces to shared work on animal models of developmental disorders and pain research that address basic and clinical questions in combined research models. The separation of research activities should be bridged by deliberate pre- and postdoctoral cross-training programs to foster integration between new clinicians and researchers. Additional mechanisms, such as career development awards through the National Institutes of Health and similar awards through the Canadian Institutes of Health Research and the Medical Research Council in the United Kingdom, could provide partial support for mid-career interdisciplinary training. Considering that the research and clinical work in pain in developmental disability are just emerging, the future agenda seems clear.

REFERENCES

Casey, K.L., Lorenz, J., & Minoshima, S. (2003). Insights into the pathophysiology of neuropathic pain through functional brain imaging. *Experimental Neurology, 184,* 80–88.

Grunau, R.E., Holsti, L., Haley, D.W., Oberlander, T., Weinberg, J., Solimano, A., et al. (2005). Neonatal procedural pain exposure predicts lower cortisol and behavioral reactivity in preterm infants in the NICU. *Pain, 113,* 293–300.

Latour, B. (1999). *Pandora's hope.* Cambridge, MA: Harvard University Press.

Mao, J. (2002). Translational pain research: Bridging the gap between basic and clinical practice. *Pain, 97,* 183–187.

Melzack, R. (1999). From the gate to the neuromatrix. *Pain Supplement, 6,* 121–126.

National Academy Press. (2000). *Bridging disciplines in the brain, behavioral, and clinical sciences.* Washington, DC: Author.

Salzinger, K. (1992). Connections: A search for bridges between behavior and the nervous system. *Annals of the New York Academy of Sciences, 658,* 276–286.

Stokes, D.E. (1997). *Pasteur's quadrant: Basic science and technological innovation.* Washington, DC: Brookings Institution Press.

Woolf, C.J., & Salter, M.W. (2000). Neuronal plasticity: Increasing the gain in pain. *Science, 288,* 1765–1768.

INDEX

Entries with *f* indicate figures; those with *t* indicate tables.